Handbook of Advanced Cancer Care

Patients with advanced cancer increasingly receive end-of-life care from a variety of nonspecialist physicians and nurses. These professionals need to be able to assess the original diagnosis and the appropriateness of patient referral, set a treatment or palliation program, and recognize and plan for the clinical problems associated with specific primary tumors. However, there is no comprehensive source of information available to them at a level between specialist oncology texts and nursing texts. To remedy this, two eminent physicians from one of the world's foremost cancer centers have drawn together a remarkable team to provide a handbook which covers the full range of problems nonspecialists will encounter. This highly accessible text covers general principles in oncology, the primary tumors one by one, and management of specific symptoms and syndromes. It will be invaluable to primary care physicians, surgeons, non-oncology subspecialists, nurses, therapists, and trainees.

Dr Michael J. Fisch is Assistant Professor of Medicine at the University of Texas M.D. Anderson Cancer Center.

Dr Eduardo Bruera is Professor and Chair of the Department of Palliative Care and Rehabilitation Medicine at the University of Texas M.D. Anderson Cancer Center.

Handbook of
Advanced Cancer Care

edited by

Michael J. Fisch

and

Eduardo Bruera

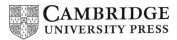

CAMBRIDGE
UNIVERSITY PRESS

PUBLISHED BY THE PRESS SYNDICATE OF THE UNIVERSITY OF CAMBRIDGE
The Pitt Building, Trumpington Street, Cambridge, United Kingdom

CAMBRIDGE UNIVERSITY PRESS
The Edinburgh Building, Cambridge CB2 2RU, UK
40 West 20th Street, New York, NY 10011-4211, USA
477 Williamstown Road, Port Melbourne, VIC 3207, Australia
Ruiz de Alarcón 13, 28014 Madrid, Spain
Dock House, The Waterfront, Cape Town 8001, South Africa

http://www.cambridge.org

First published 2003

Printed in the United Kingdom at the University Press, Cambridge

Typefaces Minion 10.5/14 pt, Formata and Formata BQ   *System* LATEX 2_ε [TB]

A catalogue record for this book is available from the British Library

Library of Congress Cataloging in Publication data
Handbook of advanced cancer care / [edited by] Michael J. Fisch, Eduardo D. Bruera.
    p.   cm.
Includes bibliographical references and index.
ISBN 0 521 01043 8 (pbk.)
1. Cancer – Palliative treatment – Handbooks, manuals, etc.   2. Terminal care – Handbooks, manuals, etc.
3. Cancer – Nursing – Handbooks, manuals, etc.   I. Bruera, Eduardo.   II. Fisch, Michael J., 1964–
RC271.P33 C356   2003
616.99′406 – dc21   2002073305

ISBN 0 521 01043 8 paperback

To our spouses and children whose love and sacrifice allow us the privilege to care for patients and families with advanced cancer

Susan, Amanda, and Ryan Fisch
Maria, Ed, Sophia, and Sabastian Bruera

Contents

Part III   Management of specific symptoms and syndromes

Contributors

James L. Abbruzzese
Department of Medical Oncology,
GI Oncology (Box 426)
U.T. M.D. Anderson Cancer Center
1515 Holcombe Boulevard
Houston, TX 77030, USA

Sam H. Ahmedzai
Section of Palliative Medicine
Department of Surgical and
Anesthetic Sciences
University of Sheffield, Floor K
Royal Hallamshire Hospital
Sheffield, S10 2JF, UK

Heather-Jane Au
Department of Medicine
Cross Cancer Institute
11560 University Avenue
Edmonton, AB, Canada T6G 1Z2

Walter F. Baile
Department of Psychiatry (Box 100)
U.T. M.D. Anderson Cancer Center
1515 Holcombe Boulevard
Houston, TX 77030, USA

Stephen A. Bernard
C.B. #7305
University of North Carolina
3009 Old Clinic Building
Chapel Hill, NC 27599-7305, USA

Charles D. Blanke
OHSU-Hem/Medical Oncology Division
Oregon Health & Science University
3181 SW Sam Jackson Park Rd, MC L-580
Portland, OR 97202-3011, USA

Diane C. Bodurka
Department of Gynecologic Oncology (Box 67)
U.T. M.D. Anderson Cancer Center
1515 Holcombe Boulevard
Houston, TX 77030, USA

J. J. Body
Institut Jules Bordet
Rue Heyer Bordet, 1
1000 Brussels, Belgium

Michael J. Boyer
Department of Medical Oncology
Sydney Cancer Centre
Missenden Road
Camperdown, NSW 2050, Australia

Rae Zyn H. Brana
Department of Surgical Oncology (Box 444)
U.T. M.D. Anderson Cancer Center
1515 Holcombe Boulevard
Houston, TX 77030, USA

Robert Buckman
Department of Medical Oncology
University of Toronto Sunnybrook Cancer
Center
Toronto, Canada

Mabel Caban
Baylor College of Medicine
Houston, TX 77030, USA

Carlos Centeno
Centro Regional de Medicina Paliativa y
Dolor
Hospital Los Montalvos
37192 Los Montalvos
Salamanca, Spain

Nessa Coyle
Memorial Sloan–Kettering Cancer Center
1275 York Avenue
New York, NY 10021, USA

Larry D. Cripe
Division of Hematology/Oncology
Indiana University Medical Center
535 Barnhill Drive, Room 473
Indianapolis, IN 46202-5149, USA

Christopher K. Daugherty
University of Chicago
5841 S. Maryland Avenue, MC 2115
Chicago, IL 60637-1470, USA

Romano T. DeMarco
Indiana University Cancer Pavilion
Urology Department (Rt 420)
425 University Boulevard
Indianapolis, IN 46202-5143, USA

Paul M. DesRosiers
Indiana University Medical Center
535 Barnhill Drive, RT 041
Indianapolis, IN 46202, USA

Larry Driver
Department of Symptom Control and
Palliative Care
U.T. M.D. Anderson Cancer Center
1515 Holcombe Boulevard
Houston, TX 77030, USA

Barry A. Eagel
Beth Israel Medical Center
Department of Pain Medicine and Palliative
Care
Phillips Ambulatory Care Center
10 Union Square East
New York, NY 10011, USA

Tim Eisen
Department of Oncology
University College London, 5th Floor
91 Riding House Street
London, W1P 8BT, UK

Ahmed Elsayem
Department of Palliative Care and
Rehabilitation (Box 8)
U.T. M.D. Anderson Cancer Center
1515 Holcombe Boulevard
Houston, TX 77030, USA

Douglas B. Evans
Department of Surgical Oncology (Box 444)
U.T. M.D. Anderson Cancer Center
1515 Holcombe Boulevard
Houston, TX 77030, USA

Robin L. Fainsinger
Royal Alexandra Hospital
10240 Kingsway Avenue, Room 2108
Edmonton, AB, T5H 3V9 Canada

Barry W. Feig
Department of Surgical Oncology, R10.2205
U.T. M.D. Anderson Cancer Center
1515 Holcombe Boulevard
Houston, TX 77030, USA

Michael Fisch
Division of Cancer Medicine (Box 8, Rm
P12.2911)
U.T. M.D. Anderson Cancer Center
1515 Holcombe Boulevard
Houston, TX 77030, USA

Richard S. Foster
Indiana University Cancer Pavilion
Urology Department (Rt 420)
425 University Boulevard
Indianapolis, IN 46202-5143, USA

Kathryn G. Froiland
Department of Nursing (Box 82)
U.T. M.D. Anderson Cancer Center
1515 Holcombe Boulevard
Houston, TX 77030, USA

Rob Glynne-Jones
Mount Vernon Hospital
Centre for Cancer Treatment
Rickmansworth Road
Northwood, HA6 2RN, UK

Carmen González
Avenida de Burtos 16B
Esc. 2, Bajo B
28036 Madrid, Spain

Neil A. Hagen
Tom Baker Cancer Center
1331 9th Street NW
Calgary, AB, T2N 4N2 Canada

Mark Harries
CRC Department of Medical Oncology
The Royal Marsden Hospital
Downs Road
Sutton, SM2 5PT, UK

Roy S. Herbst
Thoracic/Head and Neck Medical
Oncology (Box 8)
U.T. M.D. Anderson Cancer Center
1515 Holcombe Boulevard
Houston, TX 77030, USA

Vincent Hsieh
Palliative Care Program
Georgetown University Medical Center
3800 Reservoir Road
Washington, DC. 20007, USA

Jane Ingham
Georgetown University Medical Center
3800 Reservoir Road NW
Washington, DC 20007, USA

William Paul Irwin, Jr
Department of Obstetrics and
Gynecology
UVA Health System, Box 387
Charlottesville, VA 22908, USA

Aminah Jatoi
Department of Medical Oncology
Mayo Clinic
Rochester, MN 55905-0001, USA

John J. Kavanagh
Gynecologic Medical Therapeutics
U.T. M.D. Anderson Cancer Center
1515 Holcombe Boulevard
Houston, TX 77030, USA

Maria Kelly
Department of Radiation Oncology
University of Virginia Health Science Center
(Box 383)
Charlottesville, VA 22908, USA

Merrill S. Kies
Thoracic/Head and Neck Medical Oncology
(Box 432)
U.T. M.D. Anderson Cancer Center
1515 Holcombe Boulevard
Houston, TX 77030, USA

Stephen D. King
Seattle Cancer Care Alliance
825 Eastlake, G-6602
PO Box 19023
Seattle, WA 98109, USA

Julia Ladd Smith
Division of Oncology
University of Rochester
224 Alexander Street
Rochester, NY 14607-4002, USA

Peter G. Lawlor
Palliative Care Program
University of Alberta Hospital
Room 3T1.08 Walter Mackenzie Ctr.
8440-112 Street
Edmonton, Alberta, Canada

Renato Lenzi
Department of GI Oncology/Dig Disease
(Box 78)
U.T. M.D. Anderson Cancer Center
1515 Holcombe Boulevard
Houston, TX 77030, USA

Edward H. Lin
Department of Medical Oncology, GI Onc
(Box 426)
U.T. M.D. Anderson Cancer Center
1515 Holcombe Boulevard
Houston, TX 77030, USA

A. Marlene Lockey
U.T. M.D. Anderson Cancer Center (Box
103)
1515 Holcombe Boulevard
Houston, TX 77030-4009, USA

Charles L. Loprinzi
Medical Oncology
Mayo Clinic
Rochester, MN 55905-0001, USA

Isabelle Mancini
Institut Jules Bordet
Rue Heger Bordet, 1
1000 Brussels, Belgium

Laura McClure-Barnes
Vanderbilt University Medical Center
Division of Hematology/Oncology
1956 The Vanderbilt Clinic
Nashville, TN 37232-5536, USA

Kathy D. Miller
Department of Hematology/Oncology
Indiana University Cancer Pavilion

535 Barnhill Drive, IP 473
Indianapolis, IN 46202, USA

Letha E. Mills
Dartmouth Hitchcock Medical Center
1 Medical Center Drive
Lebanon, NH 03756-001, USA

Pamela N. Munster
Lee Moffitt Cancer Center and Research
Institute
MRC 3E, Room 4072B
Tampa, FL 33612, USA

Derek B. Murray
5 Comely Bank Place
Edinburgh EH4 1DT, Scotland

Rudolph M. Navari
Department of Preprofessional Studies
250 Nieuwland Science Hall
University of Notre Dame
Notre Dame, IN 46556-5670, USA

Hans Neuenschwander
FMH Medicina Interna
Specialita Oncologia
Via Trevano 62
6900 Lugano, Switzerland

Craig R. Nichols
Division of Hematology/Oncology
Oregon Health & Science University
3181 SW Sam Jackson Park Rd, OP28
Portland, OR 97201-3011, USA

Scott North
Department of Medicine
Cross Cancer Institute
11560 University Avenue
Edmonton, AB, T6G, 1Z2 Canada

Juan M. Núñez-Olarte
Unidad Cuidados Paliativos
Hospital General Universitario Gregario
Marañon

C/Dr Esquerdo 46
28007 Madrid, Spain

Doreen Oneschuk
Grey Nuns Community Hospital
1100 Youville Drive NW (Room 5211)
Edmonton, Ab, T6L 5X8, Canada

J. Lynn Palmer
Department of Biostatistics (Box 213)
U.T. M.D. Anderson Cancer Center
1515 Holcombe Boulevard
Houston, TX 77030, USA

Silvia Paz
Department of Surgical and Anaesthetic
Sciences
University of Sheffield, Floor K
Royal Hallamshire Hospital
Sheffield S10 2JF, UK

Lukas Radbruch
Pain Clinic
Department of Anaesthesiology
University of Cologne
50924 Cologne, Germany

Paul W. Read
Department of Radiation
Oncology
University of Virginia Health
Sciences Center
Box 383, Charlottesville
VA 22908, USA

Mary Ann Richardson
National Institutes of Health
National Center for Complementary/
Alternative Medicine
6707 Democracy Blvd., #106
Bethesda, MD 20892-2182, USA

Carla Ripamonti
Palliative Care Division
National Cancer Institute
Via Venezian, 1
20133 Milan, Italy

Cheryl Rutledge
Division of Hematology/Oncology
Indiana University Medical Center
535 Barnhill Drive, Room 473
Indianapolis, IN 46202-5149, USA

Alan Sandler
Vanderbilt University Medical Center
Division of Hematology/Oncology
1956 The Vanderbilt Clinic
22nd Avenue South
Nashville, TN 37232-5536, USA

Alvaro Sanz
Centro Regional de Medicina Paliativa y Dolor
Hospital Los Montalvos
37192 Los Montalvos
Salamanca, Spain

David Seitz
Department of Hematology/Oncology
Indiana Cancer Pavilion, RT 473
535 Barnhill Drive
Indianapolis, IN 46202-5289, USA

Ki Y. Shin
Symptom Control and Palliative Care (Box 8)
U.T. M.D. Anderson Cancer Center
1515 Holcombe Boulevard
Houston, TX 77030, USA

Thomas J. Smith
Division of Hematology/Oncology
PO Box 980230
1101 E. Marshall Street
Richmond, VA 23298-0230, USA

David B. Solit
Memorial Sloan–Kettering Cancer Center
1275 York Avenue
New York, NY 10021, USA

Sharon E. Soule
Department of Hematology/Oncology
Indiana Cancer Pavilion, RT 473
535 Barnhill Drive
Indianapolis, IN 46202-5289, USA

Florian Strasser
Department of Internal Medicine
Kantonsspital
9000 St Gallen
Switzerland

Christopher Sweeney
Department of Hematology/Oncology
Indiana University Cancer Pavilion
535 Barnhill Drive, IP 473
Indianapolis, IN 46202, USA

Robert D. Timmerman
Indiana University Cancer Pavilion
535 Barnhill Drive, RT 041
Indianapolis, IN 46202, USA

Paul W. Walker
Department of Symptom Control and
Palliative Care (Box 8)
U.T. M.D. Anderson Cancer Center
1515 Holcombe Boulevard
Houston, TX 77030, USA

Suzie Whelen
Massey Cancer Center
Medical College of Virginia
401 College Street, #980230
Richmond, VA 23298-0230, USA

Lori Wood
Department of Medical Oncology
QE II Health Sciences Center
4th Floor, Bethune Building
1278 Tower Road
Halifax, Nova Scotia, Canada B3H 2Y9

Anna Wreath Taube
Grey Nuns Community Hospital
5211 1100 Youville Drive NW
Edmonton, AB T6L 5X8, Canada

Donna S. Zhukovsky
Department of Symptom Control and
Palliative Care (Box 8)
U.T. M.D. Anderson Cancer Center
1515 Holcombe Boulevard
Houston, TX 77030, USA

Ralph Zinner
Thoracic/Head and Neck Medical Oncology
(Box 80)
U.T. M.D. Anderson Cancer Center
1515 Holcombe Boulevard
Houston, TX 77030, USA

Preface

As medical oncologists specializing in palliative care in a Comprehensive Cancer Center, we face several enormous challenges. First, the care of our patients requires fundamental understanding of basic principles of cancer care – including chemotherapy, radiation therapy, surgery, family dynamics, ethics, etc. Moreover, we must have fundamental knowledge about the natural history, biology, and treatment of the patient's individual cancer. Finally, we need to be able to recognize and manage common syndromes and scenarios that can influence the quality of life and possibly the length of life for the advanced cancer patient. As we peruse our bookshelves and libraries, there are many wonderful references to assist us in this difficult quest. There are major textbooks of oncology, surgery, radiation oncology, nursing, internal medicine, pain, and palliative medicine. There are also smaller handbooks of cancer chemotherapy or palliative care with shorter chapters. Of course, there are drawers full of sentinel articles and our favorite review articles as well.

In the United States alone, there are more than half a million patients living with and subsequently dying from advanced cancer each year. The healthcare workforce caring for these patients is obviously not limited to cancer specialists and palliative care experts. A significant portion of the care provided to advanced cancer patients is delivered by physicians, nurses, allied health professionals, and students who have only limited training and experience in cancer care and/or palliative medicine. This trend is likely to continue in the future because of the increasing number of cancer patients and the relative shortfall of specialized health professionals. For the non-oncology health professional, it is not practical to have a large number of textbooks and references related to cancer care. And if such resources were available, it is rare indeed that a person could spend much time reading through the multiple, complex articles and chapters available. Indeed, in our experience, few of our clinical colleagues in nursing or medicine can honestly report having read a single book chapter in its entirety in the past 3 months, and most have not read an entire review article more than five pages in this time either. This does not reflect professional disinterest or laziness, it reflects the real time constraints of health professionals and the need for new ways to combine and deliver information so that it can be used by these dedicated people to improve patient care.

Since half of all patients diagnosed with invasive malignancy are ultimately unable to be cured of their disease, the spectrum of outpatient care and especially in-patient care is biased towards advanced cancer. At M.D. Anderson Cancer Center, an informal survey of the numerous non-oncology health professionals revealed great enthusiasm for a book on advanced cancer with concise, readable chapters that contains relevant information about principles of cancer care, specific cancers, and specific syndromes. The target audience for this book is the health professional involved in caring for persons with advanced cancer. The book is not intended for specialists in oncology, but rather for primary care physicians, surgeons, non-oncology subspecialists, nurses, physical therapists, pharmacists, speech patholo-gists, social workers, house officers, and undergraduates in medicine – all of whom commonly play a vital role in the multidisciplinary care of advanced cancer patients.

This target audience tends to be less interested in the academic style of writing that is heavily referenced and detailed, and somewhat avoidant of practical statements that cannot be supported by rigorous evidence. Expert clinicians are often excellent educators at the bedside or doing "chalk-talks," but their pearls of wisdom are hard to find in books. In this book, we asked expert clinicians from around the world to explain their topic to our target audience in the most easily digestible form and style they could muster. We did not force any specific format on the chapters – each author could choose a writing format with which he/she could be most effective for the topic at hand. The authors were asked to include sentinel references, best reviews, and relevant web sites at the end of each chapter. They were asked to avoid including references within the text (something that proved to be almost irresistible to academic clinicians).

This handbook is thus the result of a unique writing assignment and unique combination of topics organized around the theme of advanced cancer care. The editors recognize that there is substantial variability in advanced cancer care around the world, and each chapter may reflect the local/regional context experienced by the specific author. We are hopeful that this book will assist our clinical colleagues worldwide in delivering better care to patients and families affected by advanced cancer.

Michael J. Fisch

Eduardo Bruera

Acknowledgements

We are grateful to Richard Barling and Pauline Graham of Cambridge University Press for the opportunity to pursue this unique project. We thank our many contributors who had the courage to adjust their writing style to accommodate this project. We offer special thanks to Martha Sandoval and Katja Sullivan for administrative assistance. We are grateful to our colleagues in Palliative Care at M.D. Anderson for their contributions to the book itself, to our understanding of palliative care, and to our protected time as we prepared the book.

Part I

General concepts in oncology

Principles of diagnosis and staging

John J. Kavanagh

U.T. M.D. Anderson Cancer Center, Houston

Introduction

The development of prognostic data and therapeutic outcomes in cancer is dependent upon meaningful communication among physicians, educators, health administrators, and all parties concerned with improving the care of malignancies. In order to ensure accurate descriptions of cancers, and allow comparisons of data and treatment methodologies, various cancer staging systems were developed. As cancer care became more complex over the years, multidisciplinary methods of treatment became essential. The importance of reproducible and functional staging systems for cancer are the cornerstone in the conduct of trials, introduction of new technologies, and comparisons of treatment. This is a summary of the evolution and current uses of these various staging methodologies.

Principles of cancer staging

The utility of a cancer staging system will depend on its accurate reflection of the natural history of the disease and the functional ability of healthcare givers to utilize these staging descriptions. Malignancies reflect a continuum of varying natural histories and are a dynamic process. Although no staging system can precisely take into account all variables, there must be enough functionality that will reflect this natural history. The staging ideally represents a point in time where the malignancy can be easily defined, utilized by all parties caring for the patient, and results in the accumulation of meaningful information. Therapeutic modalities can be used for comparing outcomes, planning policy, and advising individual patients. The staging system must also be flexible enough that it takes into account the development of new knowledge allowing appropriate modification of the various stages as necessary.

A second principle is the functional utility of the system in the hands of the caregivers. It must be efficient and practical in nature. The staging must interdigitate with the actual care patterns and allow the incorporation of these data for analysis.

The staging should also be detailed enough to allow meaningful conclusions, but not too complex that it can only be used by highly skilled personnel. One of the most important considerations in the collection of data is that it not be perceived as inefficient and/or irrelevant to patient care.

A third and increasingly important principle is the integration of the collection of data into a format that reflects modern information technology. The databases developed must be consistent and allow computer-based analysis on an international basis. As information is distributed to the caregiver the information flow becomes just as important for individual treatment planning. This relatively new concern over information technology integration is being addressed by several groups such as statisticians, computer scientists, and epidemiologists. Yet to be addressed will be issues of confidentiality, proprietary rights, and access to the information.

A fourth principle of staging is cost efficiency. With the increased use of healthcare economic analysis, staging systems must now consider their intrinsic cost. Careful consideration must be given to the necessity of various staging procedures. In addition, there will be increasing use of outcomes analysis concerning the utility of various staging evaluations themselves.

A fifth, and most important aspect of a staging system, is its validity and reproducibility. Succinctly, is the decision making based on staging reflective of reproducible clinical practice? Is there sufficient objectivity in the decisions regarding staging of a patient that it may be translated on an international basis? Are the staging procedures involved too complex or subjective in interpretation that compromise the consistency of data reporting? Can the staging decisions and data be audited for confirmation and validity? These are questions that become more important as our medical statistics and clinical research designs increase in sophistication.

A final concern is the integration of laboratory based or molecular data into a staging definition. This is a new problem that confronts individuals dealing with the reporting of cancer outcomes data. There is no doubt that molecular-based prognostic data will soon enter into our clinical management. It is not clear how this will impact prospectively on staging patients. It is also unclear how such information can be used on a retrospective basis for analysis. The problem is qualitatively different than the introduction of a radiographic or surgical technique. These newer prognostic criteria will be based on either a serologic measurement or some type of pathologic evaluation of specimens. Most of these newer molecular techniques will initially be difficult, but quite quickly available to the routine laboratory.

History

There have been many systems of cancer staging over the years. Gynecologists involving numerous organizations and disciplines used a staging system for cervical cancer that dated back to the League of Nations system for cervical cancer published in 1920.[1] The TNM (Tumor, Node, Metastasis) system was introduced by Denoix approximately 50 years ago. This was published as a formal proposal in 1944 in a bulletin of the National Institute of National Hygiene of Paris.[2] The TNM system has become a cornerstone of an international basis for describing these stages of cancer and comparing end results. The International Union Against Cancer (UICC) and the American Joint Committee on Cancer (AJCC) were constituted to develop a joint system based on the TNM classification. This evolved gradually in the 1950s and there were various publications with differing stages. Eventually, a consensus was reached in the 1980s that resulted in the publication of the *Manual for Staging of Cancer* by the AJCC and the *TNM Classification of Tumors* by the UICC.[3] It is important to note that these institutions represent predominantly American–European consensus. The collaboration between these two organizations has been essential in creating a relatively uniform TNM system that can be internationally applied. It is also endorsed by the American College of Surgeons, American College of Physicians, American Cancer Society, and National Cancer Institute along with the multiple organizations participating in the UICC. Through the years these staging manuals have had several revisions.[4,5]

The utility of cancer staging is dependent upon the histopathologic description of the tumor. At this time the histopathologic classification is largely morphologic based. There is not agreement among pathologists as to which histopathologic classifications of cancer should be used in the TNM staging system. The World Health Organization has provided international criteria for these histologic classifications of malignancy since the 1950s. There is also a numerical coding system know as the ICD–O, i.e., International Classifications of Diseases for Oncology. The numerical coding allows for more accurate reporting of data when integrated into the staging systems. The use of this system has been recommended by multiple organizations in order to make the TNM staging more clinically meaningful.[6,7]

TNM system rules

The staging system is based on the extent of the primary tumor (T), presence of regional lymph node metastasis (N), and the extent of distant metastasis (M). Each major category is then given a numerical component. These data are then summarized and the patient is given a stage according to a diagram. Depending on each disease site there may be a clinical classification based on clinical findings and imaging modalities. This is cTNM or TNM. There may also be a pathologic classification know as pTNM. There can also be a retreatment classification which is used with recurrences requiring further treatment. This is known as rTNM. Finally, there is an autopsy staging depending on postmortem data that is known as aTNM.

Another principle of the staging is that if there is doubt concerning the accuracy of the TNM then the lower stage should be applied. In the case of multiple tumors the highest T category is selected for staging description. The TNM categories may be expanded for the purposes of research, but the original definitions may not be changed. Finally, in the case of an unknown primary, staging will be determined on the most probable primary site of origin.

Certain classifications will require histopathologic grading. The system uses a G classification. GX means grade can not be assessed. G1 is well differentiated and G4 is undifferentiated. The most undifferentiated area of the tumor is used for the purposes of grading.

An added complexity of the TNM system has been multidisciplinary or neo-adjuvant care and longer disease-free intervals. Prefixes are then used. rTNM means a recurrent tumor which has been restaged after a disease-free interval. If there are multiple primary tumors at a single site then the highest T is used and number of tumors noted, i.e., $T_3(4)$. yTNM means that the classification was performed during or following multimodality therapy.

An essential part of the TNM system is to eventually classify the patient within a stage. These stages range from I to IV. The stage will be determined by a table with the various parameters of the TNM components. Another aspect is the cancer staging data form. These are forms that correspond to particular aspects of each malignancy. The TNM and other criteria are filled out and the stage noted. This remains within the medical record and serves as the baseline stage of the patient. It may be modified in the future as previously described.

It is most important to note that the staging classifications do not address the issues of quality of life, psychosocial issues, toxicity, or morbidities of therapy. The primary purpose of the staging data is to determine the extent of the cancer and eventually analyze patterns of care and outcomes along with the conduct of clinical research.

Examples of staging

Lung cancer

The staging of lung cancer follows the TNM system. The primary site is characterized by size and invasive nature. T1 is a tumor 3 cm or less in dimension. T2 size is more than 3 cm or it involves the main bronchus, nearness to the carina, or invasion of the visceral pleura. Regional lymph node disease is usually defined by radiographic and/or surgical staging. NX means they can not be assessed and N0, no metastases. N1–N3 represent various degrees of involved lymph nodes. Distant metastases are M0 with no distant metastases and M1, with distant metastases (Table 1.1). This may be seen in the stage grouping in Table 1.2. Histopathologic

Table 1.1. Definition of TNM

Primary tumor (T)

TX   Primary tumor cannot be assessed, or tumor proven by the presence of malignant cells in sputum or bronchial washings but not visualized by imaging or bronchoscopy.

T0   No evidence of primary tumor.

Tis   Carcinoma in situ.

T1   Tumor 3 cm or less in greatest dimension, surrounded by lung or visceral pleura, without bronchoscopic evidence of invasion more proximal than the lobar bronchus[a] (i.e., not in the main bronchus).

T2   Tumor with any of the following features of size or extent:
        More than 3 cm in greatest dimension
        Involves main bronchus, 2 cm or more distal to the carina
        Invades the visceral pleura
        Associated with atelectasis or obstructive pneumonitis that extends to the hilar region but does not involve the entire lung.

T3   Tumor of any size that directly invades any of the following: chest wall (including superior sulcus tumors), diaphragm, mediastinal pleura, parietal pericardium; or tumor in the main bronchus less than 2 cm distal to the carina, but without involvement of the carina; or associated atelectasis or obstructive pneumonitis of the entire lung.

T4   Tumor of any size that invades any of the following: mediastinum, heart, great vessels, trachea, esophagus, vertebral body, carina; or separate tumor nodules in the same lobe; or tumor with a malignant pleural effusion.[b]

Regional lymph nodes (N)

NX   Regional lymph nodes cannot be assessed

N0   No regional lymph node metastasis

N1   Metastasis to ipsilateral peribronchial and/or ipsilateral hilar lymph nodes, and intrapulmonary nodes including involvement by direct extension of the primary tumor

N2   Metastasis to ipsilateral mediastinal and/or subcarinal lymph node(s)

N3   Metastasis to contralateral mediastinal, contralateral hilar, ipsilateral or contralateral scalene, or supraclavicular lymph node(s)

Distant metastasis (M)

MX   Distant metastasis cannot be assessed

M0   No distant metastasis

M1   Distant metastasis present.[c]

Source: Fleming ID, Cooper JS, Henson DE et al. (ed.) *AJCC Cancer Staging Handbook*, 5th edn, pp. 117–27. Philadelphia, PA: Lippincott–Raven, 1998.

[a] The uncommon superficial tumor of any size with its invasive component limited to the bronchial wall, which may extend proximal to the main bronchus, is also classified T1.

[b] Most pleural effusions associated with lung cancer are due to tumor. However, there are a few patients in whom multiple cytopathologic examinations of pleural fluid are negative for tumor. In these cases, fluid is nonbloody and is not an exudate. When these elements and clinical judgement dictate that the effusion is not related to the tumor, the effusion should be excluded as a staging element and the patient should be staged T1, T2, or T3.

[c] M1 includes separate tumor nodule(s) in a different lobe (ipsilateral or contralateral).

Table 1.2. Stage grouping

Stage grouping of the TNM subsets has been revised as follows:			
Occult Carcinoma	TX	N0	M0
Stage 0	Tis	N0	M0
Stage IA	T1	N0	M0
Stage IB	T2	N0	M0
Stage IIA	T1	N1	M0
Stage IIB	T2	N1	M0
	T3	N0	M0
Stage IIIA	T1	N2	M0
	T2	N2	M0
	T3	N1	M0
	T3	N2	M0
Stage IIIB	Any T	N3	M0
	T4	Any N	M0
Stage IV	Any T	Any N	M1

Source: Fleming ID, Cooper JS, Henson DE et al. (ed.) *AJCC Cancer Staging Handbook*, 5th edn, pp. 117–27. Philadelphia, PA: Lippincott–Raven, 1998.

grade is from GX where no grade can be assessed and from G1–G4 for gradually less differentiation. An example of a lung staging diagram can be seen in Fleming et al., pp. 117–27.[4]

Because of the common nature of the tumor, with a fairly predictable natural history and therapy options, the staging of lung cancer has been quite useful in the conduct of studies and prognosis. Therefore, it represents one of the best models for staging cancer.

Gynecologic cancer

The International Federation of Gynecology and Obstetrics (FIGO) has been active in staging gynecologic cancers for many years. In an attempt to blend the TNM and FIGO systems there is a synthesis of both systems. The end result is essentially the same. However, it is most common that the FIGO system is used in clinical practice and in the conduct of studies. The nature of each staging system can be seen in Table 1.3 (ibid Pecorelli et al., pp. 63–78).[1]

At this time the principles of surgical staging combined with the importance of residual disease remains essential to clinical understanding and the conduct of studies in this disease. It is probable that this system will remain relatively intact pending the discovery of any unusual predictive diagnostic serum marker or radiological technique.

Table 1.3. Carcinoma of the ovary – staging

FIGO stages	TNM categories
Primary tumor cannot be assessed	TX
No evidence of primary tumor	T0
I Tumor limited to the ovaries	T1
IA Tumor limited to one ovary; capsule intact, no tumor on ovarian surface: no malignant cells in ascites or peritoneal washings	T1a
IB Tumor limited to both ovaries; capsule intact, no tumor on ovarian surface: no malignant cells in ascites or peritoneal washings	T1b
IC Tumor limited to one or both ovaries with any of the following: capsule ruptured, tumor on ovarian surface, malignant cells in ascites or peritoneal washings	T1c
II Tumor involves one or both ovaries with pelvic extension	T2
IIA Extension and/or implants on uterus and/or tube(s); no malignant cells in ascites or peritoneal washings	T2a
IIB Extension to other pelvic tissues; no malignant cells in ascites or peritoneal washings	T2b
IIC Pelvic extension (IIA or IIB) with malignant cells in ascites or peritoneal washings	T2c
III Tumor involves one or both ovaries with microscopically confirmed peritoneal metastasis outside the pelvis and/or regional lymph node metastasis	T3 and/or N1
IIIA Microscopic peritoneal metastasis beyond pelvis	T3a
IIIB Macroscopic peritoneal metastasis beyond pelvis 2 cm or less in greatest dimension	T3b
IIIC Peritoneal metastasis beyond pelvis more than 2 cm in greatest dimension and/or regional lymph node metastasis	T3c and/or N1
IV Distant metastasis (excludes peritoneal metastasis)	M1

Source: Pecorelli S, Jones HW, Ngan HYS, Bender HG, Benedet JL. Cancer of the ovary. In *Staging Classifications and Clinical Practice Guidelines of Gynecologic Cancers*, FIGO Committee on Gynecologic Oncology, pp. 1, 63–78. London: Elsevier, 2000.

Leukemia

The acute leukemias represent an extremely diverse group of malignancies. The original understanding was based on morphologic analysis. Now it is based on morphologic, immunologic, and cytogenetic evaluation.[8–10] These are often done in highly specialized laboratories. Therapeutic approaches can differ according to these various characteristics. The particular staging of this malignancy is dynamic in nature because of the rapidly changing nature of the field. An example is seen in Table 1.4. This description applies for acute lymphocytic leukemia. The staging

Table 1.4. Morphologic, immunologic, and cytogenetic classification of acute lymphocytic leukemia (ALL)

Category	Karyotype	Cell markers								FAB morphology
		Tdt	Ia	CD19	CD10	Cylg	Slg	CD7	CD2	
Early T precursor ALL	t or del 9p	+	−	−	−	−	−	+	−	L_1 or L_2
T-cell ALL	t(11;14), 6q−	+	−	−	−	−	−	+	+	L_1 or L_2
Early B precursor ALL	t(4;11), t(9;22) = Ph+	+	+	+	−	−	−	−	−	L_1 or L_2
Common ALL (cALLa)	6q−, near haploid t or del (12p), t(9;22) 9p− hyperdiploid (> 50)	+	+	+	+	−	−	−	−	L_1 or L_2
Pre-B ALL	t(1;9), t(9;22) 6q− hyperdiploid (> 50) t(8;14), t(2;8), t(8;22)	+	+	+	+	+	−	−	−	L_1 or L_2
B-cell ALL	Burkitt's lymphoma translocation, t(8;14), t(8;22), t(2;8), 6q−	−	+	+	±	±	+	−	−	L_3

Source: O'Donnell JR. Acute leukemias. In *Cancer Management: A Multidisciplinary Approach*, 3rd edn, pp. 575–96. Melville, NY: PRR, 1999.

Note: cALLa, common acute lymphocytic leukemia antigen; CD, cluster of differentiation; Cylg, cytoplasmic immunoglobullin; Ia, I antigen; Ph, Philadelphia chromosome; Slg, surface immunoglobulin; Tdt, terminal deoxynucleotide.

systems for the acute leukemias are subject to extensive debate and differing philosophies on therapy. Such staging systems will remain within the realm of fairly specialized hematologists who have an interest in these diseases. Cooperative group studies engaging in the treatment of the disease tend to pick the most essential characteristics for the purposes of stratification and therapy. There is significant debate concerning the "staging" of the hematologic malignancies with the introduction of newer molecular markers.

Summary

The staging of malignancy has evolved over many years. The most commonly used solid tumor staging system is the AJCC/UICC, arrived at through a number of consensus meetings. This has worked very well in a number of solid tumors for the purpose of prognosis, treatment, and the conduct of treatment trials. In the area of gynecology the FIGO and UICC has a synthesized version, which has proved functional in nature. The hematological diseases and lymphomas remain fairly specialized and subject to significant change, based on morphologic, immunologic, and cytogenetic techniques. These diseases require very specialized approaches and consensus before beginning a trial.

Staging systems, however, do not address the quality of life of patients, nor do they address any issues of palliative care. Staging systems are focused on the essential statistical issues of stratification, characterization of patients, and cancer survival analysis including life tables, Kaplan–Meier methods, and multivariate analyses. In the future, one would anticipate that there will be a greater integration of psychosocial instruments into staging, to allow investigators a better sense of the quality of life and palliative care issues of patients with cancer.

REFERENCES

1 Pecorelli S, Jones HW, Ngan HYS, Bender HG, Benedet JL. Cancer of the ovary. In *Staging Classifications and Clinical Practice Guidelines of Gynecologic Cancers*, FIGO Committee on Gynecologic Oncology, pp. 1, 63–78. London: Elsevier, 2000.

2 Denoix PF. TNM classification. *Bull Inst Nat Hyg Paris* 1994;1:1–69 and 1944;5:52–82.

3 Rubin P, McDonald S, Keller JW. Staging and classification of cancer: A unified approach. In *Principles and Practice of Radiation Oncology*. 2nd edn, pp. 162–72. Philadelphia, PA: Lippincott–Raven, 1992.

4 Fleming ID, Cooper JS, Henson DE et al. (ed.) *AJCC Cancer Staging Handbook*, 5th edn, pp. 117–27. Philadelphia, PA: Lippincott Raven, 1998.

5 International Union Against Cancer. *TNM Classification of Malignant Tumors*, 4th edn. Berlin: Springer–Verlag, 1987.

6 World Health Organization. *WHO International Histological Classification of Tumors*, Vol. 1–25. Geneva: WHO, 1967–1981; 2nd edn, Berlin: Springer–Verlag, 1988–1992.

7 World Health Organization. *WHO International Classification of Diseases for Oncology*, 2nd edn. Geneva: WHO, 1990.

8 World Health Organization. *International Classification of Diseases for Oncology*. Geneva: WHO, 1976.

9 O'Donnell JR. Acute leukemias. In *Cancer Management: A Multidisciplinary Approach*, 3rd edn, pp. 575–96. Melville, NY: PRR, 1999.

10 Krueger GR, Medina JR, Nein HO et al. A new working formulation of non-Hodgkin's lymphomas: A retrospective study of the new NCI classification proposal in comparison to the Rappaport and Kiel classification. *Cancer* 1983;52:833.

11 Hoelzer D, Thiel E, Loffler H et al. Prognostic factors in a multicenter study for treatment of acute lymphoblastic leukemia in adults. *Blood* 1988;71:123–31.

2

Principles of palliative chemotherapy

Michael Fisch

U.T. M.D. Anderson Cancer Center, Houston

Introduction

Patients with advanced cancer are heterogenous not only with respect to the underlying histology and biology of their cancer, but also in other important ways. Advanced cancer patients also vary with respect to their overall health status, their preferences, the local extent of their underlying disease, the number of sites of their metastatic spread, the overall bulk of their cancer, and their sources of suffering. One of the most important decisions that must be made in caring for these patients is determining the role of anticancer therapy in the comprehensive plan of care. This important decision has implications regarding the number and type of health providers involved in the care, the proper setting for the delivery of care, the third-party and out-of-pocket costs of care, the level of family support necessary to implement the care properly, and the overall trajectory of care. This chapter will address the use of systemic anticancer therapy for advanced cancer patients with a focus on five major questions: (1) Is there a conceptual framework that can be used to inform this decision? (2) What is the range of possible specific goals for this therapy? (3) What are the most useful predictors of response to therapy? (4) What are the broad categories of therapies that are commonly used? (5) How are patients followed once therapy is started?

A conceptual framework

An investment broker might ask a client what his or her financial goals are and get a generic reply such as "I want the largest possible return on my investment with the least possible risk." What would be the analogous, generic reply for an advanced cancer patient describing his or her personal goal to an oncologist? One might suppose that the reply to an oncologist would be "I want to live as long as possible and as well as possible." One way to demonstrate this goal conceptually is illustrated in Figure 2.1. If one were to plot quality of life versus quantity of life, the area under

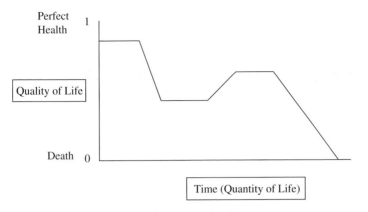

Figure 2.1   The overall goal: to increase the area under the curve.

the curve would be one reliable way to summarize the end results of a portion of life for an individual. For example, a treatment that prolongs survival slightly but diminishes quality of life profoundly would not produce much of an incremental gain in the area under the curve. Likewise, a treatment that improves quality of life greatly without improving survival might be beneficial, unless the duration of improvement was particularly short. Using this conceptual model, each treatment decision must involve some judgement about the possible direction, magnitude, and duration of effects on quality of life as well as the expected effect on quantity of life.

In order to apply this conceptual model, one must also have a specific notion of what is meant by quality of life for the individual. Quality of life is a multidimensional concept that includes health domains (such as physical and psychological function) and nonhealth domains (such as social, economic, family, and spiritual well-being). Each individual puts these various domains into a particular personal and cultural context, and the importance of each domain may be different from person to person and may vary within-person over time.

If the goal in caring for advanced cancer patients is to improve quality of life over time, one might still struggle in understanding individual treatment decisions without some conceptual model related to the relationship between disease management (control of the cancer itself) and suffering management (control of the effects of the illness on the individual). Figure 2.2 illustrates the traditional view about this interaction, in contrast to a revised view and a "realistic" view. The traditional view in cancer care has been that the cancer is treated as long as it is feasible, and when the disease is refractory or the patient is too ill or otherwise unsuitable for cancer treatment, then palliative measures are undertaken. A revised view incorporates some component of palliation in combination with cancer treatment from the outset, and the assumption is that there is a more-or-less linear decline in the relative role of cancer treatment as the patient approaches the end of life. The

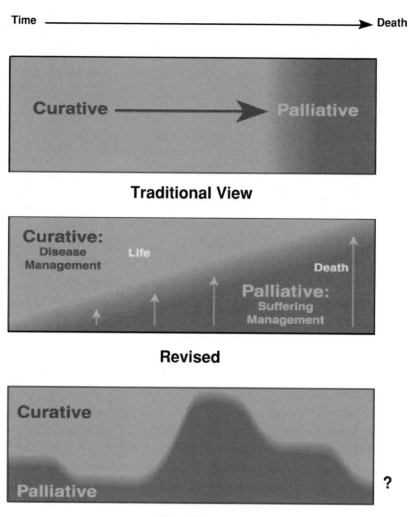

Figure 2.2   Coordinating disease management with symptom management.

third panel in Figure 2.2 describes what seems to be the most realistic viewpoint from the standpoint of trying to maximize quality of life over time – that there ought to be a nonlinear and highly individual set of relationships between cancer therapy and purely palliative therapy over time. It would follow, then, that the ideal treatment plan and setting at the end of life is highly sensitive to the individual and his or her own health preferences and circumstances (as well as nonhealth-related preferences and circumstances).

How can one communicate these conceptual ideas to individual patients? Figure 2.3 provides an example of a visual model that might be useful in explaining to patients the goals of care at any given point in time. The model represents the

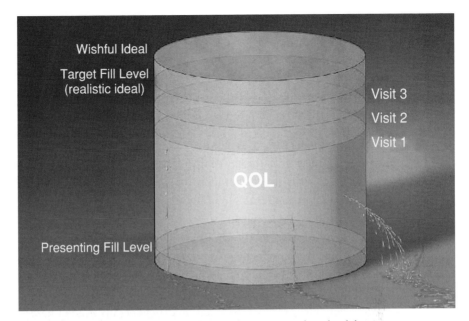

Figure 2.3   The quality of life tank model for explaining the conceptual goals of therapy.

oncologist as the "quality of life tank manager." The goal is to identify the "realistic ideal" level of fill in the quality of life tank, and then to take action to find the sources of leaks in the quality of life tank and correct them in the most feasible, effective, and rapid manner. If uncontrolled systemic disease or locally uncontrolled disease is the cause of major problems, and if the disease might be responsive to therapy, then anticancer therapy is often worth pursuing. In addition, if the patient is struggling with symptoms (i.e., pain, fatigue, nausea, sleep disturbance, etc.), then specific action to assess and manage those problems has the promise of improving the patient's quality of life. The art of filling this tank is not only related to finding and correcting the leaks, but also in making a sound judgement about the realistic ideal that is appropriate for the given patient. For some patients, the realistic ideal may be cure of cancer and eventually winning an Olympic medal. For most patients, the realistic ideal involves more modest achievements, such as eating better and sleeping better with less pain and a more normal mood. It should be noted that it is both common and appropriate for patients to speak about their "wishful ideal." The patient may say "I wish I never had this cancer" or "I wish that I could see my child grow up and go to college." Sometimes, these statements make the nurse or oncologist feel sad or helpless (or both). One appropriate way to handle these wishful statements from patients or family members is to simply acknowledge them in an empathetic manner, and perhaps offer a reflective statement such as "I wish things were different for you. I can see how painful this is for you and your family."

This can help set the stage for a transition where the clinician then identifies the realistic ideal and some specific actions that might help move the patient towards that level of fill in his or her quality of life tank.

What are the possible goals of systemic anticancer therapy?

With the above-mentioned conceptual framework in mind, one might understand palliative chemotherapy as a disease management strategy where the intent is to increase the area-under-the-curve through the effects of chemotherapy on quality of life more so than quantity of life. Sometimes the treating physician is making a judgement that the patient's physical well-being is being diminished by the cancer and that shrinking or stabilizing the cancer on a systemic basis may produce a net benefit. In some instances, the physician may decide that the use of systemic therapy may also directly or indirectly provide relief of psychological distress to the patient. Practice patterns vary widely regarding these judgements.

While there is no way to determine what response might be achieved for individual patients, physician expectations are generally guided by both their own anecdotal experience as well as by evidence in similar groups of patients available through clinical trials. Most physicians incorporate both kinds of information (data and anecdote), but the weight given to each kind of information is highly variable, and the quality and quantity of relevant data that are understood by the physician and applied to each decision are also variable. Table 2.1 lists the most commonly reported clinical trial endpoints in cancer research. For any given study, one or more of these endpoints is likely to be reported in a numerical format. The most relevant endpoints for the purpose of individual treatment decisions depend on the viewpoint of the patient and the judgement of the physician. Overall survival is the least disputable with respect to its importance. Complete response rates are considered highly relevant also, for this refers to complete resolution of the cancer for some period of time. Clinical benefit may refer to a combination of complete and partial response rates plus stable disease for some specific period of time.

Table 2.1. Clinical trial endpoints

Overall survival
Disease-free survival
Progression-free survival
Complete response
Partial response
Stable disease
Clinical benefit
Relief of symptom(s)
Overall quality of life

Table 2.2. Performance status by Eastern Cooperative Oncology Group (ECOG) and Karnofsky criteria

Grade	Description
0	Fully active, able to carry on all predisease performance without restriction (Karnofsky 90–100)
1	Restricted in physically strenuous activity, but ambulatory and able to carry out work of a light or sedentary nature such as light house work or office work (Karnofsky 70–80)
2	Ambulatory and capable of all self-care, but unable to carry out any work activities. Up and about more than 50% of waking hours (Karnofsky 50–60)
3	Capable of only limited self-care, confined to bed or chair more than 50% of waking hours (Karnofsky 30–40)
4	Completely disabled. Cannot carry out any self-care. Totally confined to a bed or chair (Karnofsky 10–20)

Alternatively, "clinical benefit" may refer to a specific formula that includes response, functional status, and symptom status.

What factors help predict response to systemic anticancer therapy?

The single most powerful predictor of response to systemic therapy is the patients' performance status. Performance status refers to the level of activity that the patient is able to perform as judged by the clinician on the basis of the patient's history and physical examination. One could summarize use of this parameter as a prediction of outcome succinctly as "winners win and losers lose." Widely used measures of performance status include the Karnofsky Performance Status (KPS), which is scaled from 100% (perfect) to 0 (dead). The Zubrod scale ranges from 0 (best) to 4 (worst) and has been adapted by the Eastern Cooperative Oncology Group (ECOG) (Table 2.2). Performance status is such an important factor for symptom status, response to therapy, and survival that it is often used as an enrollment criterion and/or a stratification factor for clinical trials. For example, a lung cancer study might specify that only patients with Zubrod performance status 0 or 1 are eligible. This might be based on data suggesting that patients with poor performance status have an unfavorable risk–benefit ratio for similar kinds of therapy. Alternatively, the study might include a wide range of patients with stratification by performance status level in order to ensure that all treatment arms are well balanced with respect to this parameter.

For patients with advanced solid tumors, it is also clear that not all metastatic sites are equal – some respond better than others. Patients with spread of cancer (metastases) to visceral sites such as bone, liver, or brain have a worse prognosis and are less likely to respond to therapy than patients with involvement of other sites such as lung, lymph nodes, and/or soft tissue. In addition to the type of metastatic site, the overall bulk of disease and the number of different metastatic sites is also both prognostic of outcome and predictive of response to therapy.

Another major factor that oncologists consider when evaluating systemic therapy options for advanced cancer patients is the effect of prior therapy. Generally speaking, the best outcomes are obtained with the first attempt at therapy. The expectations for response fall dramatically with each subsequent "line" of therapy. A "round" or "cycle" of therapy refers to the repeated administration of the same drug or drug combination on a given schedule between treatments. In contrast, a second or subsequent "line" of therapy refers to a switch to a new drug or drug combination, where the switch is motivated by lack of response or excess of toxicity to the previously used treatment regime. As a general rule of thumb, second-line therapy is associated with one-third to one-half the response rate (or less) compared with the initial therapy. This reflects the fact that oncologists never save their bullets – they use the most effective treatments up front. It also reflects the fact that the biology of the cancer may change due to treatment exposure. The tumor cells that remain after first-line therapy often have a higher proportion of resistant cells compared with the original situation. In addition, it is important to note both the magnitude and duration of response to first-line therapy. Once again, the dictum "winners win and losers lose" applies. Specifically, those patients with a good response and a durable response to first-line therapy are more likely to respond to second-line therapy at the time of progression.

Other predictors that are often considered before initiating systemic therapy include the patient's chronological age and the level of family and social support available. The basis for taking chronological age into consideration is controversial. There are prospective studies that show that the effect of age is negligible when regression analyses are applied taking other factors into account. However, it is clear that advancing age brings, on average, competing health risks that may serve to reduce the overall benefit of therapy. For those older adults who do receive systemic therapy, full doses of the medications are generally used because of data in several diseases (non-small cell lung cancer, breast cancer, and others) suggesting that low-dose therapies produce inferior outcomes in older patients. With respect to the importance of family and social support, it is clear that most therapy is now given on an outpatient basis and thus the patients' family and/or friends serve an important monitoring role. Without a social network for both monitoring and taking action in the event of treatment toxicities, patients are at greater risk for death and adverse events from treatment.

Table 2.3. Response definitions for solid tumors

Complete response[a]
   Disappearance of all target lesions
Partial response[a]
   30% decrease in the sum of the longest diameters
Stable disease
   Absence of a complete or partial response
Progressive disease
   20% increase in the sum of the longest diameters

[a] Complete and partial responses should be confirmed
by repeat assessments 4 weeks after onset.

How are patients followed for response to therapy?

The specific definitions for complete response, partial response, and stable disease
have been defined by a task force established by the European Organisation for
Research and Treatment of Cancer (EORTC), the National Cancer Institute (NCI),
and the National Cancer Institute of Canada (NCI–C) (Table 2.3). These definitions
are the RECIST criteria (Response Evaluation Criteria in Solid Tumors). In general,
oncologists ascertain response in their patients using the same conventional definitions that are used for clinical trials. Target lesions are identified, where a target
lesion refers to a measurable cancer lesion that is ≥ 2.0 cm in longest diameter. A
maximum of 10 total lesions (no more than five lesions per organ) are identified and
the disease is quantified by taking the sum of these unidimensional measurements.
For hematological malignancies, the specific definitions of response vary by disease.
For example, a hematological remission for acute myelogenous leukemia is defined
differently than it is for multiple myeloma or chronic lymphocytic leukemia.

   Finally, the methods used to ascertain the benefit of using systemic therapy reflect the fact that most of the existing systemic therapies are intended to shrink
tumors and produce clinical benefits because of this tumor shrinkage. Traditionally, oncologists identify active cytolytic agents and combine agents with distinct
mechanisms of action and mechanisms of tumor resistance as well as nonoverlap-
ping toxicity. In this traditional model, higher drug doses are expected to produce
better tumor shrinkage (provided that toxicity is acceptable). More recently, there
has been a trend towards the use of sequential single agents administered in a
weekly or biweekly fashion (so-called "dose-dense" therapy). This newer model
for chemotherapy administration has gained some momentum in the management of breast cancer, and it is being tested in other solid tumors. Fortunately,
progress in cancer treatment is not limited to innovative dosing and scheduling of

Table 2.4. Categories of commonly used systemic cancer therapies

Older	Newer
Cytolytic chemotherapy	Monoclonal antibody targets
Alkylating agents	CD20
Antimetabolites	HER-2 receptor
Platinum compounds	CD52
Taxanes	CD33
Anthracyclines	Anti-angiogenesis targets
Vinca alkaloids	Humanized anti-VEGF
Antitumor antibiotics	Small molecule inhibitors of VEGF
Miscellaneous agents	receptor tyrosine kinases
Biological agents	Other agents
Interferons	Tyrosine kinase inhibitors
Interleukins	Imatinib mesylate
Hormonal therapy	Cancer vaccines
Corticosteroids	Gene therapy
Androgens	Retinoids
Estrogens	Anti-sense oligonucleotides
Anti-androgens	Radiation response modifiers
Anti-estrogens	
Progestins	
Aromatase inhibitors	
LHRH analogues	

existing cytolytic agents. Recent advances in the understanding of the molecular biology of cancer have led to the discovery of new biologic targets and new drugs. Table 2.4 summarizes the categories of newer therapies in contrast to the older therapies. One feature that many of the newer therapies share is that they are expected to have a cytostatic (tumor stabilizing) effect rather than a cytolytic (tumor shrinking) effect. These drugs have been generally better tolerated than traditional cytolytic agents. Less toxicity translates into less complex, less expensive, and less time-consuming supportive care for those patients who continue to receive "active" anticancer systemic therapy. Moreover, these drugs often do not have additional activity against cancer or toxicity against normal cells when given in higher doses. These therapeutic advances have created new challenges in clinical trial design and response evaluation. Physicians may eventually follow specific biological endpoints for some of these new agents, but the standard strategies are still evolving. Due to the rapid progress in cancer therapeutics and the trend towards more tolerable systemic anticancer therapy, it is conceivable that a growing proportion of patients will be offered systemic anticancer therapy of some kind towards the last weeks to days of life. This changing cancer treatment landscape will undoubtedly create new opportunities and challenges in the delivery of end-of-life care.

BIBLIOGRAPHY

Sentinel articles

Burris HA, Moore MJ, Anderson J, Green MR, Rothenberg ML, Modiano MR. Improvements in survival and clinical benefit with gemcitabine as first line therapy for patients with advanced pancreas cancer: a randomized trial. *J Clin Oncol* 1997;15:2403–13.

Cassell EJ. The nature of suffering and the goals of medicine. *N Engl J Med* 1982;306:639–45.

Doyle C, Crump M, Pintilie M, Oza AM. Does palliative chemotherapy palliate? Evaluation of expectations, outcomes, and costs in women receiving chemotherapy for advanced ovarian cancer. *J Clin Oncol* 2001;19:1266–74.

Geels P, Eisenhauer E, Bezjak A, Zee B, Day A. Palliative effect of chemotherapy: Objective tumor response is associated with symptom improvement in patients with metastatic breast cancer. *J Clin Oncol* 2000;18:2395–405.

Karnofsky DA, Abelmann WH, Craver LF, Burchenal JH. The use of nitrogen mustards in the palliative treatment of carcinoma. *Cancer* 1948;1:634–56.

Korn EL, Arbuck SG, Pluda JM, Simon R, Kaplan RS, Christian MC. Clinical trial designs for cytostatic agents: are new approaches needed? *J Clin Oncol* 2001;19:265–272.

Motzer RJ, Mazumdar M, Bacik J, Berg W, Amsterdam A, Ferrara J. Survival and prognostic stratification of 670 patients with advanced renal cell carcinoma. *J Clin Oncol* 1999;17:2530–40.

Quill TE, Arnold RM, Platt F. "I wish things were different": expressing wishes in response to loss, futility, and unrealistic hopes. *Ann Intern Med* 2001;135:551–5.

Saxman SB, Propert KJ, Einhorn LH et al. Long-term follow-up of a phase III intergroup study of cisplatin alone or in combination with methotrexate, vinblastine, and doxorubicin in patients with metastatic urothelial carcinoma: a cooperative group study. *J Clin Oncol* 1997;15:2564–9.

Tannock IF, Osoba D, Stockler MR, et al. Chemotherapy with mitoxantrone plus prednisone or prednisone alone for symptomatic hormone-resistant prostate cancer: a Canadian randomized trial with palliative end points [see comments]. *J Clin Oncol* 1996;14:1756–64.

Therasse P, Arbuck SG, Eisenhauer EA et al. New guidelines to evaluate the response to treatment in solid tumors. *J Natl Cancer Inst* 2000;92:205–16.

Zubrod CG, Schneiderman M, Frei E et al. Appraisal of methods for study of chemotherapy of cancer in man. Comparative therapeutic trial of nitrogen mustard and triethylene thiophosphoramide. *J Chron Dis* 1960;11:7–33.

Review articles/book chapters

Ellison NM. Palliative chemotherapy. *Am J Hospice Palliat Care* 1998;15:93–103.

Ellison NM. Palliative chemotherapy. In *Principles and Practice of Supportive Oncology*, ed. A Berger, RK Portenoy, DE Weissman, pp. 667–79. Philadelphia, PA: Lippincott–Raven, 1998.

3

Principles of palliative surgery

Barry W. Feig

U.T. M.D. Anderson Cancer Center, Houston

Introduction

Surgical oncology is a diverse and challenging subspecialty. Despite the obvious intricacies of surgery in complex oncologic cases, the role of palliative surgery is perhaps one of the most complex aspects of surgical oncology. The decision to perform palliative surgery requires an understanding of the potential morbidities and mortalities associated with surgical procedures. This must be balanced against the natural history of the underlying malignancy along with possible benefits, such as the patient's quality of life and potential life expectancy. Most often there is not a single correct approach when evaluating palliative surgical options. A treatment approach can only be determined through evaluation of all potential risks and benefits in conjunction with extensive discussion with the patient and family.

The decision to perform a palliative operation is usually based on a number of factors including the life expectancy of the patient, the quality of the patient's life, the expected benefit of the operation, and the availability of less invasive palliative approaches. In general, performing a palliative operation will not extend the life expectancy of the patient. Although this may be intuitively obvious, it is often difficult for patients and families to understand and accept this hypothesis. Before commencing with a palliative operation, it is important that both the patient and their family understand this concept. This fact has to be established before the issue of attempting to improve quality of life can be addressed. To this end, it is important that the patient and family understand what are realistic expectations of a proposed surgical intervention. The five essential roles of the surgeon in the palliation of an advanced cancer are: (1) the initial evaluation of the disease; (2) local control of the disease; (3) the control of discharge or hemorrhage; (4) the control of pain; and (5) reconstruction and rehabilitation. Table 3.1 provides an example of a relevant surgery in each category. A more general definition that we have found to be applicable and clinically useful is that a palliative operation is an

Table 3.1. Common palliative surgical procedures

Initial evaluation of disease
   e.g., staging laparotomy for advanced ovarian carcinoma
Local control of disease
   e.g., salvage cystectomy or pelvic exteneration
Control of discharge, hemorrhage, or fungating tumor
   e.g., mastectomy to remove a foul-smelling breast mass
Control of pain
   e.g., decompressive laminectomy for a refractory vertebral tumor
Reconstruction and/or rehabilitation
   e.g., intramedullary fixation of a femur involved with tumor

attempt to relieve a symptom or improve the quality of life in a patient with an otherwise untreatable/incurable malignancy. At the M.D. Anderson Cancer Center, we strongly believe that there is no role for the expectant palliation of symptoms in this patient population. Unfortunately, in the oncologic patient, palliative operations often are addressing acute exacerbations of chronic ongoing conditions (i.e., chronic partial small bowel obstruction which has now become complete). It can therefore be difficult to quantify for patients the amount and length of benefit that a surgical intervention could provide. In general, if the surgical intervention can alleviate the symptomatology caused by an acute exacerbation then this may provide a palliative benefit to the patient. Unfortunately, there are few studies that address the issue of the benefits of palliative surgery. These studies are extremely difficult to perform, as the endpoints are vague and difficult to define. Therefore, the majority of decisions as to when to perform palliative surgery are based on subjective criteria and anecdotal data.

There are clearly instances where surgical intervention can achieve at least a temporary palliative effect. For example, drainage of a malignant fluid collection in the chest, pericardial cavity or abdominal cavity (malignant ascites) can achieve a rapid, dramatic improvement in symptoms in many cases. Although these symptoms can often be relieved with a relatively minor invasive procedure (i.e., thoracentesis, chest tube, paracentesis), the methods frequently result in reaccumulation of fluid and resultant symptoms. Often, to provide a longer period of relief of these symptoms, a more invasive surgical procedure is required (i.e., pericardial window, peritoneovenous shunt, pleurodesis).

Another common area where surgery can play a role in palliation is in patients with obstruction of a hollow viscous secondary to their tumors. This occurs most commonly in the bowel and the biliary tract. Palliation of biliary tract obstructions can frequently be achieved with endoscopic stenting. Similarly, near-obstructing lesions of the stomach, esophagus, and large bowel can be palliated with endoscopic

Table 3.2. Common palliative interventional procedures

Ablations of unresectable tumors
    Endoluminal laser ablation
    Radiofrequency ablation
    Embolization/chemoembolization
Shunting of uncontrolled fluids
    Peritoneovenous shunting of ascites
    Pleuroperitoneal shunting of malignant pleural effusion
    Pericardial window for pericardial effusion
Stenting of obstructed viscera
    Ureteral
    Tracheobronchial
    Esophageal
    Biliary

stenting in a significant number of cases. Unfortunately, obstruction of the small bowel usually requires surgical intervention via laparotomy to provide relief of obstruction. Endoluminal laser ablation can also be used for tumors in the esophagus and large bowel to relieve obstructive symptoms. Similarly, this approach can be used via a bronchoscope to relieve obstructions of the bronchial tree. Common palliative interventional procedures are summarized in Table 3.2.

Although less common, tumor resections are occasionally performed for palliation. The most common reasons to resect a tumor in the palliative setting is when there are complications which interfere with the quality of life of the patient such as extensive bleeding or a fungating necrotic tumor. In the former case, repeated hospitalizations for bleeding requiring blood transfusion not only raises ethical concerns regarding extensive use of blood products in a palliative setting, but also raises questions regarding the quality of life, when patients repeatedly have to come to the hospital to receive blood transfusions. In the latter case, removal of a fungating necrotic tumor can often relieve a patient of a burdensome wound care problem as well as that of the socially difficult problem of being able to keep clean and free of odor. Other common palliative scenarios include ureteral stenting for ureteral obstruction, decompressive laminectomy for spinal cord compression, and intramedullary fixation of a pathological fracture of a long bone. Many of these situations present as acute changes and are considered emergencies, as the consequences of not intervening can be significant. Unfortunately, in the acute setting it is extremely difficult to discuss with the patient and family the potential benefits as well as the risks and consequences of a major invasive procedure. In general, discussions concerning the expected outcome and course of disease in patients in the palliative setting should be discussed with the patient and family prior to an acute medical crisis. Obviously, not every scenario can be discussed ahead of time, however, if patients and families are informed about their overall course and prognosis prior to an acute event, they can be better prepared to make a decision regarding their desire for a major intervention. Unfortunately, in order to achieve some of the objectives as outlined above, these surgical interventions can result in a significant alteration of lifestyle. This includes the possibility of a permanent colostomy in patients with bowel obstruction or amputation to remove a fungating necrotic extremity tumor, or a mastectomy to provide local control of a fungating breast cancer. In addition, these procedures may require extensive surgery which could result in an extended period of time as an inpatient. Obviously, a postoperative complication can result in an extended hospitalization and even death.

Conclusion

The decision to undertake a palliative operation usually requires extensive discussion regarding potential risks and benefits. Unfortunately, these parameters are often vague and subjective, making an informed decision difficult for patients. Obviously, a small operation with a short hospitalization that would provide palliation of a symptom as well as a reasonable quality of life for a year would be a straightforward scenario with an easy answer for both the patient and physician. In contrast, an operation that does not improve the quality of life and only allows the patient to suffer further deterioration also allows for a relatively straightforward decision on the part of physician and patient. Unfortunately, most palliative scenarios are somewhere between these two extremes. In these cases, extensive discussion and education is necessary so that patients and families can be guided in making an informed decision. In order to achieve a successful outcome surgical intervention must improve the patient's quality of life without introducing significant additional burden to the patient and the family.

BIBLIOGRAPHY

Sentinel articles

Krouse RS, Nelson RA, Farrell BR et al. Surgical palliation at a cancer center. *Arch Surg* 2001;136:773–8.

Markman M. Surgery for support and palliation in patients with malignant disease. *Semin Oncol* 1995;22(Suppl. 3):91–4.

Miner TJ, Jaques DP, Tavar-motamen H et al. Decision making on surgical palliation based on patient outcome data. *Am J Surg* 1999:177:150–4.

Reviews

Ball AB, Baum M, Breach NM et al. Surgical palliation. In *Oxford Textbook of Palliative Medicine*, ed. D Derek, GWC Hanks, N MacDonald, pp. 282–97. Oxford: Oxford University Press.

Baron, TH. Expandable metal stents for the treatment of cancerous obstruction of the gastro-intestinal tract. *N Engl J Med* 2001;344:1681–7.

Schmidt RG, Winkler GA. Palliative orthopedic surgery. In *Principles and Practice of Supportive Oncology*, ed. Berger et al., pp. 639–50. Philadelphia, PA: Lippincott–Raven, 1998.

4

Radiotherapy for palliation of symptoms

Carlos Centeno[1] and Carmen González[2]

[1] Hospital Los Montalvos, Salamanca, Spain
[2] Hospital Universitario Gregorio Marañón, Madrid, Spain

Principles of palliative radiation therapy

Between 30 and 50% of the patients who reach the service of radiotherapy are treated with radiotherapy with palliative intention. Palliative radiotherapy aims at an improvement or elimination of symptoms that are due to an incurable cancer, and it is effective in 75% of the cases. A treatment of palliative radiotherapy must relieve rapidly and for a long time, must interfere as little as possible with the general state of the patient and his or her way of living, and must lack, as much as possible, important secondary effects.

In some cases, besides aiming at relieving the symptoms, radiotherapy (RT) aspires to increase survival, even though there may not exist a clear increment in the usual cure rates. Such is the case, for instance, in glioblastoma multiforme, lung cancer in stage IIIB, and cervical cancer in stage IVA. In these cases, radiation is carried out as if the objective were curative (high doses, standard fractionation) even if the possibilities for a cure are remote. Thus, the difference between a radical approach and a palliative one is difficult to determine. Even in patients whose disease is disseminated, palliative radiotherapy must be conditioned to the concrete characteristics of each case, avoiding quick or easy treatments that do not consider the benefits of other approaches more suitable for the patient and his/her life expectations. This is the case, for example, of a young patient with breast cancer with only one bone metastasis or another one with the same metastasis but from lung cancer and general deterioration.

Palliative radiotherapy for symptom relief should be given as soon as possible when it is indicated. But emergency treatments with radiation are not always are palliative ones. In some cases, such as in superior vena cava syndrome in lymphoma or in spinal cord compression in Ewing sarcoma, radiotherapy must both control the symptoms and seek the antineoplasic effect characteristic of high doses, without interfering with later treatments that will be necessary for the cure.

Table 4.1. Indications for palliative radiation therapy

Metastatic disease
Bone metastases
Hepatic metastases
Brain metastases
Pathological fractures
Spinal cord compression
Choroidal metastases
Suprarenal metastases
Painful or compressive masses or nodes

Incurable or locally advanced diseases
Pancreas adenocarcinoma
Splenomegaly
Endobronchial relapse
Hemorrhages
Glioblastoma multiforme
Advanced pelvic disease in rectal cancer
Recurrent and advanced locoregional disease from breast cancer
Dyspnea
Tumoral ulcers

From the technical point of view, palliative radiotherapy must fulfill the following general principles:

- The type of palliative radiation and its complexity (external radiotherapy, intraoperative, hemibody irradiation, stereotaxic radiosurgical, etc.) must be adapted to each case.
- The radiation field must be wide, but always protecting the critical areas.
- Short fractions and high doses per fraction are preferred.
- While being treated, the patient must be in the most comfortable position.
- Delays should be avoided by using the unit or the treatment available and which takes the shortest time, especially if the patient cannot keep the treatment position due to pain or dyspnea.

The indication for palliative radiotherapy can be symptomatic treatment of metastases, treatment of tumors locally advanced or incurable, and treatment of recurrences in previously radiated areas (see Table 4.1). Radiotherapy can be applied in order to relieve any type of symptoms due to any kind of tumors and localizations, as long as the exact goal is clearly defined as well as the doses for delivery and the volume to be radiated. It is crucial that the general state of the patient allows for a precise administration of the treatment.

Radiotherapy in bone pain

Bone metastases represent 50% of the total amount of palliative treatment administered in a radiotherapy service. External radiotherapy with an analgesic purpose is the treatment for localized bone pain from metastases, since besides relieving the pain, it improves the mechanical conditions of the patient, it prevents the appearance of fractures or compression, it slows local tumor growth and it reduces the need for analgesics. Asymptomatic localizations must be treated only if there exists a risk for fracture or in order to prevent neurological deficits. There are no guidelines as to doses and schedules. There have been tests with several fractions (5 or 10 fractions) as well as with single-dose therapy (8–9 Gy). Prospective studies confirm that the safety and efficiency of both patterns are similar, both relieving the pain within 2 or 3 weeks after the treatment in more than 70% of cases (Table 4.2). The only noticeable difference is that patients with single doses need reirradiation more frequently. In general, patients with long life expectancy (only one metastasis, good general performance status, controlled primary tumor, or patients with a good response to a systemic therapy) can be candidates for multiple fractions, high doses, and bigger volumes, while patients with short life expectancy may be more suitable for one-dose radiations and a smaller volume. Half of the patients with life expectancy longer than 1 year will remain free of pain in the area treated. Overall, the average duration of the effect lasts longer than 3 months and signs of relief become noticeable between 3 and 14 days after starting the treatment. If pain is recurrent (3–30% of cases), reirradiation can be considered as long as it does not exceed the highest dose bearable by the spinal cord or the nearby critical organs. This way, effective relief can be achieved in most of the cases.

Hemibody external radiation can also attain good bone pain control in patients with multiple bone metastases. It is carried out by administering only one fraction onto a hemibody, superior (6 Gy) or inferior (8 Gy). Unlike localized radiotherapy, most of the patients experience pain relief within the first 48 hours, independently of the radiosensitivity of the tumor. Analgesia is obtained in 70% of patients (complete response in more than 50%) and it is maintained until death. In hemibody irradiation, toxicity, especially digestive and hematological, is more important, which implies that the selection criteria must be more strict and it needs a bigger support treatment. The most serious, but uncommon (1%), complication may be pneumonitis. In the inferior half body, gastrointestinal toxicity appears sometimes (25%). Hemibody irradiation is not recommended for patients with low white blood cell counts, very poor condition or short life expectancy of a few weeks.

Intravenous single doses of radioactive isotopes that give out beta radiations such as strontium (Sr89) have been administered in order to relieve bone pain. This treatment is useful in 40–90% of the cases. The effect is manifested in the first 2 weeks and

Table 4.2. Prospective studies of localized external radiotherapy in the treatment of osseous metastases (MTS)

Author	No. of patients	Fractionation	Pain response (%)	Statistical significance
Tong	1016	Single MTS:		NS
		20 Gy/5 fr	53	
		40.5 Gy/15 fr	61	
		Multiple MTS:		
		15 Gy/5 fr	49	
		20 Gy/5 fr	56	
		25 Gy/5 fr	49	
		30 Gy/10 fr	57	
Madsen	57	20 Gy/2 fr	48	NS
		24 Gy/6 fr	48	
Blitzer	759	Single MTS:		$P = 0.0003$
		20 Gy/5 fr	37	
		40.5 Gy/15 fr	55	
		Multiple MTS:		$P = 0.0003$
		15 Gy/5 fr	36	
		20 Gy/5 fr	40	
		25 Gy/5 fr	28	
		30 Gy/10 fr	46	
Okawa	80	30 Gy/15 fr	76	NS
		22.5 Gy/5 fr	75	
		20 Gy/10 fr bid	78	
Rasmusson	217	15 Gy/3 fr	75	NS
		30 Gy/10 fr	80	
Niewald	100	20 Gy/5 fr	68	NS
		30 Gy/15 fr	83	
Price	288	8 Gy/1 fr	45	NS
		30 Gy/10 fr	28	
Cole	29	8 Gy/1 fr	90	NS
		24 Gy/6 fr	86	
Hoskin	270	8 Gy/1 fr	69	$P < 0.001$
		4 Gy/1 fr	44	
Steenland	1171	8 Gy/1 fr	72	NS
		24 Gy/6 fr	69	
Bone Pain Trial Working Party	761	8 Gy/1 fr	78	NS
		20 Gy/5 fr	78	
		30 Gy/10 fr		
RTOG 97-14	open	8 Gy/1 fr		
		30 Gy/10 fr		

it can increase in the following months. Radioisotopes can be administered only in centers where there is a Nuclear Medicine Service. Treatment with Sr89 is indicated in patients with refractory pain, especially multifocal, secondary to osteoblastic lesions. The candidates for this kind of treatment are patients with a life expectancy longer than 3 months, enough medullary reserve, and without plans for future chemotherapy. Nonetheless, it is not appropriate as the only treatment for patients with severe pain because its analgesic effect is revealed slowly. Other isotopes that are less toxic and act faster are currently being studied, such as Samarium or Renium.

Radiotherapy in visceral pain

A tumor can produce pain when it grows and invades or compresses an organ. Even though radiotherapy is used less than for bone pain, it is also useful for the symptomatic treatment of hepatic metastases, tumoral splenomegaly, and other cases of visceral pain.

Hepatic pain can be effectively treated with low doses of radiation since the liver is relatively sensitive to it. There is a certain resistance to palliative RT in cases of hepatic metastases for fear of radiation-induced hepatitis, but in fact, analgesia is achieved with quite low doses. Lymphomas and other more radiosensitive tumors show a better response than gastric or pancreatic adenocarcinomas. Radiotherapy is advisable in cases of painful hepatomegaly, especially when it is massive or quickly established, and when there is no good response to analgesics or corticosteroids. Randomized studies show that radiation of the whole liver, or if possible and in order to reduce toxicity, of smaller volumes, achieves improvement of the pain in every two out of three patients. Hepatomegaly, nausea, vomiting, ascites and even tests of hepatic function also improve. Radiotherapy is administered in 7–8 fractions for 2–3 weeks, with total doses of 25–30 Gy. Toxicity is moderate, and it shows in the way of tiredness and nausea due to sensitiveness of the hepatic cell, and it might be higher if the patient has previously received chemotherapy.

Symptomatic splenomegaly generally appears in chronic leukemia, myelo-dysplastic syndromes and non-Hodgkin's lymphomas. The treatment normally chosen is splenectomy, but radiation can also be an option when the disease is very advanced or the patient has deteriorated and surgery is not advisable. Since the splenic tissue is extremely sensitive to radiation, it is necessary to administer very low total doses (10 Gy) in fractions smaller than the usual (1 fraction of 0.8 Gy per day), with daily reductions of the field of treatment. This way, pancytopenia is moderated and tolerance is improved.

Radiotherapy can also be an option in cases of persistent visceral pain, such as pain due to renal or pancreatic tumors that cannot be operated upon. It can treat pain or bile obstruction produced by tumoral lymph nodes of the portal area, suprarenal metastases, etc.

Pain due to infiltration of plexus or peripheral nerves

Any tumor can grow compressing or invading a peripheral nerve. The pain is of radicular type and it precedes the appearance of neurological symptoms. As will be explained later, corticosteroids, together with radiotherapy, are the elected treatment. The brachial and lumbosacral plexuses are frequent places for metastasic deposits or tumoral relapses. In these cases, a neuropathic pain appears, which has a bad prognosis for its symptomatic control.

The most frequent cause of pain by affecting the brachial plexus is the recurrence of breast cancer after mastectomy in the axilla or in the supraclavicular fossa. A differential diagnosis must be carried out with radioinduced plexopathy. Tumors of the superior sulcus (Pancoast syndrome), neck tumoral nodes, and thyroid tumors can also affect the brachial plexus. When a previous radiation has not been carried out, the treatment chosen for controlling the pain in the area is radiotherapy. Doses of 40–50 Gy in 4–5 weeks are normally enough for the relief of the symptoms. As a rule, the improvement is short-lasting. As for the involvement of the presacral plexus, the most frequent cause is the relapse of rectal cancer after surgery. Presacral involvement is rare in patients who have not undergone surgery. This syndrome has been related to the surgical destruction of the presacral fascia and with the delay of pelvic radiation after surgery. With radiotherapy, relief is achieved in 80% of the cases, even when the tumoral growth is reduced only slightly. Ten fractions of 3 Gy in 2 weeks is a suitable guideline.

Tumors in the head and neck, as well as pelvic ones, can produce pain by compression or invasion of peripherial nerves. Treatment with radiotherapy reduces pain as it reduces tumoral pressure, inflammatory reaction over the nerves, and local liberation of the nociception mediators. The palliative dose is normally lower than the one needed for tumor control, and it depends on the tumor radiosensitivity and the localization and extension of the tumor. Doses of 25–30 Gy, over 2 or 3 weeks, can be enough to control the pain. If the initial response is good, an additional radiation dose can be considered in order to extend the interval free of symptoms.

Pathological fractures

A pathological fracture does not necessarily define the patient as a terminal patient. In patients with a generally bad performance status and limited functional or vital prognosis, it is possible to attain good palliation through nonsurgical ways: limb immobilization, traction, and/or administration of a single dose of radiotherapy (8–10 Gy).

Aside from these situations, in the oncological patient, the treatment of a pathological fracture is based on orthopedic stabilization, radiotherapy, and the use of an analgesic treatment. Radiotherapy must always follow orthopedic stabilization because it diminishes the risk of new bone fractures given that the initial lesion favors the expansion of the tumor through the hematoma. There is no contraindication for its use over metallic fixings. In the case of long bones, radiation of the whole bone is recommended as opposed to only the area of the fracture, using either short fractionations (5 fractions of 4 Gy) or a single fraction (6–10 Gy).

Brain metastases

Whole brain irradiation is the standard palliative treatment for patients with brain metastases (see Chapter 35). Around 80% of patients obtain an important relief of the symptoms of intracranial pressure, convulsions, or headaches. Other symptoms that also improve, although not as much (60–70%) are paresis, dysarthria, aphasia, cognitive impairment, and alterations in the cerebellum and the cranial nerves. The improvement allows for a lowering or even removing of corticoids within a month after radiotherapy. Treatments of 1 or 2 weeks (of 20 or 30 Gy) are as effective as longer ones. In the case of patients with a prognosis of survival of only 1 or 2 months, shorter cycles of only one or two fractions can also be considered. Accelerated fractionations or the use of radiosensitizers have not revealed benefits in randomized trials.

Patients with single brain metastases and with absent, minimal, or stable extracerebral disease can benefit from surgical resection and posterior whole brain radiotherapy. In the case of a single metastasis (or two or three located in the same hemisphere) smaller than 3.5 cm, stereotactic radiotherapy is indicated as overtreatment after whole brain irradiation, as an alternative to surgery in areas that cannot be well accessed and as a rescue for patients with single recurrent metastasis after previous radiotherapy. Local control is achieved in 73–98% of the cases with an average of survival of 11 months and only 8% of local relapse per year. It must be accompanied by cranial radiotherapy and doses between 12 and 20 Gy.

The beginning of the whole brain treatment may produce an increase of the edema in the brain. Therefore, at the start an increase of corticotherapy is recommended. It must be drawn to the attention of the patients that they may have headaches or nausea during the first few days of the treatment. Another side effect that may affect the patients in the last months of their life is temporal alopecia.

Palliative radiotherapy does not prevent more than half of the patients with brain metastases from dying with recurrence of symptoms as a consequence of progression in the brain. The average duration of the response is 10 weeks. Even though reirradiation is possible, it is not usual to carry it out due to a general wearing out of the patient. Instead, corticosteroids and analgesics are used as palliative measures.

Tumoral ulcers

Ulceration of tumoral growth may cause great discomfort in a patient with cancer in an advanced stage. It is more frequent in cases of local recurrences in the thoracic wall in breast cancer, in recurrent nodes in the neck and inguinal area, and in the local progression of epitheliomas, which are normally located in the face. Administering a radiotherapy treatment while the skin is still intact can effectively prevent ulceration of the tumor. When ulceration has already occurred, the treatment becomes more complicated. However, radiotherapy with single doses (8–10 Gy) or fast fractionations (five fractions of 4 Gy), together with local cures and topic treatments, can have a palliative role, as it reduces tumoral growth, inhibits superficial hemorrhages, and avoids later complications.

Tumoral bleeding

Hemoptysis secondary to a bronchial tumor, hematuria, rectal and vaginal bleeding secondary to a pelvic tumor improve with radiation in 70% of cases. Multiple fractionations have been used, ranging from a single dose of 10 Gy to doses of 50 Gy with standard fractionation. In general, in the case of locally advanced tumors (stage IIIB in lung, rectal cancer, prostate with vesicle affected, etc.) that have not been previously treated with radiotherapy, it is advised to use fields confined to the tumor, with high doses in longer fractionations. Relief takes place in 80% of the cases, it lasts longer, and the percentage of complications and toxicity is drastically lower.

In patients who have been previously irradiated and/or have metastases, the volume of the irradiation may be more limited, and the doses per fraction may be higher (3–4 Gy) with hypofractionation. In cases of vaginal bleeding from relapse of a gynecological tumor previously radiated, local brachytherapy achieves, with little added toxicity, a quick and long-lasting control of the hemorrhages, since a higher dose is administered over the whole bleeding surface.

Dyspnea

The obstruction of the airway may be produced by tracheal or endobronchial tumors or by the extrinsic compression of tumors or lymphatic nodes that spread through the mediastinum. It is clinically presented as dyspnea, stridor, hemoptysis, and sometimes as pneumonia, atelectasia, etc. Radiotherapy, whether external or endobronchial, attains a good control of the symptoms independently of the origin of the obstruction.

Endobronchial brachytherapy consists of the placement of a radioactive isotope, usually Ir-192, through a rigid bronchoscopy, in the tumor area. Sources of high dose rate are used, administering a high dose in each session (6–10 Gy) in less than 30 minutes. Its main indication is small endobronchial recurrences in patients previously irradiated. The length of the lesion must not exceed 5 cm and tracheo-esophageal fistulae must be avoided. Two-thirds of the patients experience an improvement of the tumor and the symptoms. Its most frequent complications are hemorrhages, perforation, pneumothorax, and bronchospasm.

External beam radiation is useful in cases of obstruction by extrinsic compression of the airway. External radiotherapy together with expandable prostheses is the best option for the treatment. External radiotherapy is indicated as an emergency in cases of existence of tumors that close the airways. There are no contraindications according to the type of tumor or the general state of the patient, as long as he or she can remain still during the 5–10 minutes that irradiation lasts. Fractionations will depend on the state of the patient and the volume of the tumor. Excellent results are achieved both with single doses and with longer fractionations. If the patient had already received radiotherapy as part of the initial treatment, reirradiation can be considered. In these cases, life expectancy of the patient, time passed since the last irradiation, and truthful information about the risks of irradiation as well as about therapeutic abstention determine the way to proceed.

Superior cava vein syndrome (SCVS)

The treatment of superior cava vein syndrome (SCVS) has two goals: symptom relief and improvement of the primary malignant process (see Chapter 63). We must never allow SCVS to become an emergency. The progressive appearance of the symptoms, the convenience of having a histological diagnosis, and the different therapeutic attitude according to the etiology require a programmed treatment without rushed actions. There are only two situations that call for an emergency intervention: acute obstruction of the airway and brain edema from vascular congestion.

Radiotherapy is the basis of the palliative treatment. Usually it requires the administration of 5–10 fractions over 1–2 weeks. The dose to be used and the response will depend on the histological type. Improvement can show even in the first 48 hours in the case of lymphomas, germinal tumors, or small cell lung cancer. The duration of the response will depend on the histological type but it frequently lasts longer than 3 months.

Spinal cord compression

Spinal cord compression is a real medical emergency since the possibility of the patient having an autonomous life will depend upon its immediate treatment. Treatment must be set up right away. The first step is the administration of corticoids even if the diagnosis has not yet been confirmed.

Surgical treatment with laminectomy is indicated in the following situations: unknown primary tumor, great lack of stability in the spinal cord, relapse already irradiated or with little radiosensitivity, high level of compromise, infantile tumors with severe compression, uncertain diagnosis.

In all other situations surgical treatment can be avoided, since several studies show that its effect is the same as when only radiotherapy is applied. Furthermore, whenever a decompressive laminectomy is carried out, it is necessary to associate it to a later radiotherapy. Radiotherapy must start within the 24 hours following the diagnosis of medullar compression. Usually high doses per fraction (4–8 Gy) are used and the fractionation is lowered in the following days, especially in the cases of lymphomas and leukemias. In chemosensitive tumors such as lymphomas or germinal tumors, an early administration of chemotherapy may improve the symptoms. However, the need to obtain a quick response implies the need to use radiation as the main therapeutic weapon, even in the case of these tumors.

The therapeutic result of the medullary compression is directly related to the speed in administering the treatment. If paraplegia is already present when the patient is treated, then only 10% of the patients will walk again, as opposed to the 80% who recover ambulatory skills when there is only paraparesis or radicular pain.

Other indications of palliative radiotherapy

Choroidal metastases are rare (mainly in breast cancer) and may be bilateral. The treatment of choice that may be beneficial is radiation therapy. Three out of four patients experience sight improvement.

Radiation therapy has a decompressive effect because it reduces the size of the tumor, and thus is indicated with nodes in cervical areas or inguinal masses that provoke limb lymphedema.

Intraoperative radiation therapy can be used with palliative intention in a single session, given at the time of surgery with electrons from a linear accelerator. It may be the best symptomatic treatment to relieve pain from an advanced and unresected tumor in the pancreas, sometimes until death.

Other situations that can receive relief from radiation therapy are the dysphagia due to esophagal tumors or mediastinal nodes, and meningeal carcinomatosis. The last one needs complex irradiation and requires good general status and the full cooperation of the patient during several weeks of treatment.

Conclusion

Radiotherapy, as a palliative treatment, achieves a successful relief of symptoms in more than 75% of cases. It usually does so through short treatments, which are well tolerated and not very aggressive for the patient. In the case of tumors that are locally advanced or recurrent, palliative radiation not only improves the symptoms, but it also increase the survival and the quality of life of the patient. The complexity of the treatments will be determined by the general state of the patient, the state of the tumor, and the existence of alternative treatments with a similar effectiveness to radiotherapy. Under no circumstances should the lack of availability to carry out a treatment with ionized radiation limit its utilization if it is thought to be the most efficient treatment for the patient. An effective palliative treatment must not be evaluated outside the clinical context of the patient.

Acknowledgement

The authors greatly appreciate the assistance from Professor Juan Antonio Santos-Miranda, M.D., Ph.D., Marañón University Hospital, Madrid, Spain, as reviewer of the original manuscript and from Beatriz Centeno, Pennsylvania University at State College, USA, in the translation of this paper.

Box 4.1 Radiotherapy for palliation of symptoms – summary

Many patients with advanced disease and distressing symptoms, more than usually expected, can often be relieved with simple procedures from radiation therapy. An effective palliative treatment must not be evaluated outside the clinical context of the patient.

Radiation therapy can be used to relieve pain not only from the bones, as usually is known, but also from visceral or neuropathic mechanisms, in several situations.

External radiation therapy is the treatment of choice to provide pain relief for localized painful bone metastases due to its high efficacy and excellent tolerance. It can be administered in only a single fraction.

Reirradiation can be performed if bone pain recurs, as can other techniques for multiple metastases as half-body irradiation or intravenous administration of strontium 89.

Whole brain irradiation is the standard palliative treatment for patients with brain metastases. Around 80% of patients obtain an important relief of the symptoms.

In brain metastases there are other specific situations that can be relieved with surgery and stereotaxical procedures. These always need complementary whole brain irradiation.

Chest symptoms such as dyspnea, vena cava syndrome and hemoptysis are effectively palliated with simple techniques of radiation therapy. Bronchial obstruction can be relieved with external or specific procedures.

Other symptoms such as hemorrhage, choroidal metastases, dysphagia, and meningeal carcinomatosis may also benefit from palliative radiotherapy.

Radiotherapy, as a palliative treatment, achieves a successful relief of symptoms in more than 75% of cases and it usually does so through short treatments, which are well tolerated and not very aggressive for the patient.

BIBLIOGRAPHY

Sentinel articles

Blitzer PH. Reanalysis of the RTOG study of the palliation of symptomatic osseous metastasis. *Cancer* 1985;55:1468–72.

Bone Pain Trial Working Party. 8 Gy single fraction radiotherapy for the treatment of metastatic skeletal pain: randomised comparison with a multifraction schedule over 12 months of patient follow-up. *Radiother Oncol* 1999;52:111–21.

Cole DJ. A randomized trial of a single treatment versus conventional fractionation in the palliative radiotherapy of painful bone metastases. *Clin Oncol R Coll Radiol* 1989;1:59–62.

Herranz R, González C. Radioterapia en el tratamiento del dolor canceroso. *Revisiones en Cáncer* 1992;1149–56.

Hoskin PJ, Ford HT, Harmer CL. Hemibody irradiation for metastatic bone pain in two histologically distinct groups of patients. *Clin Oncol* 1989;1:67–9.

Lablaw AD, Laperriere NJ. Emergency treatment of malignant extradural spinal cord compression: an evidence-based guideline. *J Clin Oncol* 1998;16:1613–24.

Leibel SA, Pajak TF, Msullo V et al. A comparison of misonidazole sensitized radiation therapy to radiation therapy alone for the palliation of hepatic metastases: results of a RTOG randomized prospective trial. *Int J Radiat Oncol Biol Phys* 1987;13:1057–64.

McQuay HJ, Collins SL, Carroll D, Moore RA. Radiotherapy for the palliation of painful bone metastases (Cochrane Review). In *The Cochrane Library 1, 2001*. Oxford: Update Software.

Niewald M, Tkocz HJ, Abel U et al. Rapid course radiation therapy vs. more standard treatment: a randomized trial for bone metastases. *Int J Radiat Oncol Biol Phys* 1996;36:1085–9.

Nightengale B, Brune M, Blizzard S et al. Sr^{89} for treating pain from metastatic bone disease. *Am J Health Syst Pharm* 1995;52:2189–95.

Okawa T, Kita M, Goto M, Nishijima H, Miyaji N. Randomized prospective clinical study of small, large and twice-a-day fraction radiotherapy for painful bone metastases. *Radiother Oncol* 1988;13:99–104.

Phillips MH, Stelzer KJ, Griffin TW, Mayberg MR, Winn HR. Stereotactic radiosurgery: a review and comparison of methods. *J Clin Oncol* 1994;12:1085–99.

Price P, Yarnold JR, Easton D, Austin D, Palmer SG. Randomised comparison of single and multifraction radiotherapy schedules in the treatment of painful bone metastases. 3rd European Conference on Clinical Oncology and Cancer Nursing, 1985, p. 63. Stockholm, Sweden.

Rasmusson B, Vejborg I, Jensen AB et al. Irradiation of bone metastases in breast cancer patients: a randomized study with 1 year follow-up. *Radiother Oncol* 1995;34:179–84.

Ratanatharathorn V. Bone metastasis: review and critical analysis of random allocation trials of local field treatment. *Int J Radiat Oncol Biol Phys* 1999;44:1–18.

Serafini AN. Current status of systemic intravenous radiopharmaceuticals for the treatment of painful metastatic bone disease. *Int J Radiat Oncol Biol Phys* 1994;30:1187.

Steenland E, Leer J, van Houwelingen H. The effect of a single fraction compared to multiple fractions on painful bone metastases: a global analysis of the Dutch Bone Metastasis Study. *Radiother Oncol* 1999;52:101–9.

Tong D, Gillick L, Hendrickson FR. The palliation of symptomatic osseous metastases: final results of the study by the Radiation Therapy Oncology Group. *Cancer* 1982;50:893–9.

Vermeulen SS. Whole brain radiotherapy in the treatment of metastatic brain tumors. *Semin Surg Oncol* 1998;14:64–9.

Yarnold JR, on behalf of the Bone Pain Trial Group. Bone Pain Trial: a prospective randomised trial comparing a single dose of 8 Gy and a multifraction radiotherapy schedule in the treatment of metastasic bone pain. *Br J Cancer* 1998;78(Suppl. 2):6.

Review articles

Anderson P, Coia LR. Fractionation and outcomes with palliative radiation therapy. *Semin Radiat Oncol* 2000;10:191–9.

Chenal C. Irradiations palliatives. In *Radiothérapie Oncologiquer*, ed. JP LeBourgeois, J Chavaudra, F Eschwege, pp. 519–24. Paris; Hermann editeurs des sciences et des arts, 1992.

Hoegler D. Radiotherapy for palliation of symptoms in incurable cancer. *Curr Problems Cancer* 1997;1:218–63.

Hoskin PJ. Radiotherapy in symptom management. In *Oxford Textbook of Palliative Medicine*, ed. D Doyle, GW Hanks, N MacDonald. Oxford: Oxford University Press 1993:117–29.

Rose C, Kagan R. The final report of the expert panel for the radiation oncology bone metastasis work group of the American College of Radiology. *Int J Radiat Oncol Biol Phys* 1998;40:1117–24.

Internet sites

Radiotherapy for the palliation of painful bone metastases (Cochrane Review)
http://www.update-software.com/abstracts/ab001793.htm

Center Watch: Clinical Trials in Bone Metastases
http://www.centerwatch.com/patient/studies/cat348.html

Samarium SM–153 in bone pain
http://www.quadranet.com

5

ABCs of clinical trials

J. Lynn Palmer

U.T. M.D. Anderson Cancer Center, Houston

What should a physician know about clinical trials, and why?

First, knowledge of the basics of a clinical trial is important since this type of research highly affects the options that are available to physicians to treat an individual
patient. A physician who reviews journal articles to learn about new options also
needs to have some understanding of the designs and methodology used in the research described by the journal article, and also to have some fundamental knowledge in order to be able to evaluate the appropriateness of the study that was used.
The basic terms and definitions included here will aid in that understanding.

What is a clinical trial?

A clinical trial is defined as a prospective study in human beings that evaluates the
safety or effectiveness of a new intervention or drug regimen, or that compares
the effectiveness of the new intervention to that of current best practice (or other
control group). The details of the particular intervention used (a specific dosage
schedule given in a specific manner to a specific type of patient) is summarized in
a written document called a *research protocol*.

Why use clinical trials?

A clinical trial is an effective tool in determining whether or not an intervention
actually does have the beneficial results that have been hypothesized. Given the
variability of human subjects and the uncertain knowledge of the course of most
diseases, it would be extremely difficult or impossible to determine the specific effect
of an intervention on the outcome of the disease course if an uncontrolled trial was
used. Complicating the matter is that most interventions include some negative side
effects in addition to their beneficial effects. The carefully described plan outlined
in a research protocol enables researchers to weigh information about the benefits

of an intervention and its possibly unwanted effects in order to decide whether, and under what circumstances, the use of the intervention should be recommended.

The *research protocol* includes the study objectives; a scientific background section that justifies the study; patient eligibility criteria; clearly defined criteria for response and toxicity; methods of drug administration, treatment, and data collection; statistical considerations; and an informed consent. This research document should be self-contained and include all information necessary for the conduct of the study.

Through the use of this research protocol, the very human possibility for bias is eliminated or greatly reduced. Bias occurs when patient outcomes associated with one intervention group receive an unfair advantage over the other group. For example, if only the healthiest cancer patients were given the new intervention and a higher proportion of them improved, it might be concluded that the new intervention is much better than current best practice, although this may not be the case. If disease outcomes of two groups of patients are being compared, one group given the intervention and one not, the two groups should be as similar as possible at the beginning of the study. The use of randomization (by chance alone assigning patients to a treatment group) is the best method of ensuring this similarity, and therefore of reducing potential bias.

There are different types of clinical trials

In a hospital setting, usually three types of clinical trials are seen. These are called Phase I, Phase II and Phase III trials and are conducted in sequence to learn more about a given intervention. Several steps or phases of clinical research must occur before a large-scale, randomized Phase III study is implemented. A Phase IV trial will not be discussed at length, but it is a long-term surveillance of an intervention that was found to be effective.

Phase I trials are the initial clinical trials in humans. Although useful preclinical information may be available from animal models or from in vitro studies, the first step in clinical trials is to determine whether the intervention can be tolerated in a small number of individuals. The major objective of a Phase I trial is to evaluate the safety of a new intervention, including excess toxicity and side effects. In many cases, the goal is to estimate how large a dose of the drug can be given before unacceptable toxicity is experienced by patients. This dose is usually referred to as the maximally tolerated dose or MTD. Typically, a small number of patients, usually three, are treated at the same dose. Depending on the number of patients who experience toxicity, the dose for the next three patients is then either escalated, remains the same, or the study is stopped and an MTD is declared for use in the next phase of study. Phase I studies may utilize other, more complicated, statistical methods of determining MTD. Alternatively, the objective may be to determine the dose at which an optimal biological response is seen, although the criteria for measuring this response can be difficult. Phase I trials usually include less than 20 patients.

The objective of a Phase II trial is to determine whether a specific intervention or dosage regimen is effective enough to warrant further study. This would occur if the regimen appeared potentially better than the existing best treatment. The new regimen may also be of interest if it had a lower effectiveness but could be useful after failure of the existing best treatment or as part of a combination treatment. The hypothesis is usually stated that the proportion of patients who improve (also called "response rate") exceeds some prespecified value, usually the response rate for current best practice. The Phase II trial is also relatively small, usually 30 or fewer patients. Phase II trials are frequently designed to occur in more than one stage, so that the trial could be stopped early in case of a relatively ineffective response in patients or unexpected high levels of toxicity. Phase I and Phase II trials are not randomized; in each of these trials the only group studied is the group of patients given the new intervention.

A Phase III trial is usually a randomized trial, comparing a new regimen versus current best treatment (or other control group). Such a trial can be quite large, including 100 patients or more, and could take place at several different centers. Randomization is used to ensure that patients given different interventions are as alike as possible, the only difference between them being the intervention they are given. The Phase III trial is much more definitive due to the larger number of patients and due to the randomization process.

Another technique used to reduce bias in Phase III trials is not to inform patients as to which drug regimen they are receiving. This is called a *blinded study*. Patients know in advance that they will be randomized to one of two drug regimens and agree in advance that their group assignment will be unknown to them until after the study is completed. Blinding of the patients to the treatment group they are assigned is typical in Phase III trials. When both the patient and the researcher (medical practitioner) do not know which group the patient is assigned, this is called a double-blinded study.

What about statistical considerations?

Statistical considerations are vital to any clinical trial or research protocol. The biostatistician ensures that the design of the study is appropriate to meet the objectives of the study. The statistical considerations section also clearly describes in advance the statistical methods that will be used to analyze the data, such as a binomial comparison of response rates, a *t*-test for continuous data, or survival analysis.

The *statistical considerations* also ensure that a sufficient number of patients are entered into a clinical trial to answer its primary objective, but not so many that patients might be subjected unnecessarily to an inefficient treatment or that the study would be conducted over an unnecessarily long period of time. Phase II and Phase III trials will have clearly specified hypotheses about the expected response rates of the current best practice and of the proposed new intervention. Hypotheses could be stated such as: we expect that 40% of patients will respond to the current best practice in this study; we expect that 60% of patients who receive the new drug regimen will respond; and we want to be 80% certain that we can detect this difference in response rates between groups at a significance level of 5% or smaller. The level of certainty (or power) is the probability that the difference will be declared statistically significant if it truly exists at the value stated. The significance level is the (small) probability that a difference will be declared statistically significant when in fact the difference between the groups is smaller than is stated. The number of patients necessary to be entered and evaluated in a study is determined by the difference in response rates to be detected, the power (level of certainty), and significance level required. Detecting a smaller difference in response rates of the two groups requires more patients, holding power and significance level constant.

Outcomes other than response can also be used: examples include survival, disease-free survival, or quality-of-life outcomes, such as pain, nausea, or appetite. Response itself may also be defined as complete response, partial response, no response, or progressive disease, with each of these categories defined as clearly as possible in advance based on tumor size, white blood cell count, or other quantifiable criteria.

Other parts of a protocol

There is also an informed consent included as part of a research protocol that describes the study in terms the patient can understand. The patient signs the informed consent and agrees to be entered into a specific clinical trial.

Who conducts clinical trials?

A medical faculty member is usually the principal investigator of a clinical trial. In addition, some clinical trials may be sponsored by pharmaceutical companies.

What is the process of submitting a clinical trial proposal?

Each clinical trial goes through an official evaluation process. For example, at an academic institution such as M.D. Anderson Cancer Center, there is initially an internal process within the department of the Principle Investigator; the protocol is then submitted to the Office of Protocol Research and a copy is sent to three to five faculty members not associated with the protocol for formal, written review.

Usually two reviewers are medical doctors, one reviewer is a biostatistician, one reviewer is a pharmacist, and another reviewer is a nursing practitioner or other healthcare researcher. If the protocol's primary outcomes are clinical, the protocol is then discussed at a Clinical Research Committee meeting. Protocols with behavioral outcomes, such as quality-of-life, proceed through the same procedure but instead are reviewed at the Psychosocial, Behavioral and Health Services Research Committee. At either committee meeting, the protocol is discussed for scientific merit and for the ability of the protocol to meet its scientific objectives. After discussion, a vote of committee members is taken, and the protocol is either approved, approved with contingencies (changes that must be made before approval), deferred, or disapproved. If the protocol is approved, it is then discussed at an Internal Review Board meeting – a committee whose primary function is to assure the protection of human subjects. If the protocol is approved at this committee, the protocol can then begin accrual of patients.

Where can I learn more about clinical trials?

More information is available in many textbooks such as Friedman et al., or journals such as *Statistics in Medicine*. An especially valuable resource is to work with an individual who has successfully designed, conducted, and completed his or her own clinical trial. And finally, but definitely not of the least importance, talking with a biostatistician about the specifics of your study can be invaluable in helping clarify how the objectives of your study can be met using quantifiable methods.

BIBLIOGRAPHY

Sentinel articles

Altman DG, Schulz KF, Moher D et al. The revised CONSORT statement for reporting randomized trials: explanation and elaboration. *Ann Intern Med* 2001;134:663–94.

Korn EL, Arbuck SG, Pluda JM et al. Clinical trial designs for cytostatic agents: are new approaches needed? *J Clin Oncol* 2001;19:265–72.

Therasse P, Arbuck SG, Eisenhauer EA et al. New guidelines to evaluate the response to treatment in solid tumors. *J Natl Cancer Inst* 2000;92:205–16.

Review articles

Eisenhauer EA, Dwyer PJ, Christian M et al. Phase I clinical trial design in cancer drug development. *J Clin Oncol* 2000;18:684–92.

Friedman LM, Furberg CD, DeMets DL. *Fundamentals of Clinical Trials*, 3rd edn. New York: Springer, 1998.

6

Principles of cancer rehabilitation

Ki Y. Shin

U.T. M.D. Anderson Cancer Center, Houston

Principles of cancer rehabilitation

An impairment is the result of a loss of physiologic structure or function. These are the clinical features or manifestations of a disease. Examples may be weakness or confusion from a brain tumor.

A disability is the lack of ability to perform a task or activity within the normal range. This is the functional consequence of an impairment. An example may be the inability to walk from the weakness resulting from a brain tumor.

A handicap occurs when the interaction of a person with their environment leads to a disadvantage in performing a role otherwise normal for an individual. An example would be the inability to continue work as a mail carrier due to inability to walk from a brain tumor.

Cancer and its treatments often result in deficits in mobility, self-care, or cognition, which can lead to impairment, disability, or handicap.

Cancer rehabilitation strives to minimize disability from the impairments of cancer by maximizing patient function and quality of life.

Quality of life is defined by each individual but usually includes a sense of dignity. Dignity may simply be using a commode rather than a bedpan, being able to dress oneself, or being able to get from bed to chair with little assistance. Cancer rehabilitation attempts to make patients into people again by preserving respect and dignity.

Lehmann et al. in 1978 identified multiple problems in the cancer patient population, which could be improved by rehabilitation measures (Table 6.1). Primary barriers to delivery of rehabilitation care were (1) the lack of identification of patient problems which could be helped by rehabilitation and (2) the lack of appropriate referral by physicians unfamiliar with the concept of rehabilitation.

It is important for healthcare professionals to be aware of the benefits of rehabilitation as early as possible in the course of disease. However, unlike diseases and

Table 6.1. Remediable rehabilitation problems

Psychological/psychiatric impairments
Generalized weakness
Activities of daily living impairments
Pain
Impaired gait/ambulation
Disposition/housing issues
Neurologic impairments
Vocational assessments
Impaired nutrition
Lymphedema management
Musculoskeletal difficulties
Swallowing dysfunction
Impaired communication
Skin management

injuries traditionally seen in rehabilitation medicine, cancer can be progressive in nature. Medical interventions may be ongoing, necessitating ongoing rehabilitation for the cancer patient.

In cancer rehabilitation it is important to know of further planned cancer treatments because these can impact the patient's condition and functional abilities. Chemotherapy can result in fatigue, decreased nutritional intake, and immunosuppression, which can limit function as well as participation in a rehabilitation program. Oftentimes it may be advantageous to delay intensive rehabilitation until these treatments are completed. In addition, surgery to debulk or remove tumor can often lead to neurologic and musculoskeletal deficits which can cause further functional deficits. If major surgery is planned for the near future, therapy for current functional deficits may not address future deficits acquired after surgery.

Cancer rehabilitation must balance the benefits of continued rehabilitation therapies with the physiologic effects of tumor progression and treatments. With advanced cancer patients, further therapies may not make appreciable differences in function, and actually prevent patient activities by using limited patient time and energy resources. Therefore, similar to many other treatments for cancer, it is important to recognize when "enough is enough."

Cancer rehabilitation with its focus on quality of life and function, can often give an objective view of the advanced cancer patient through their functional abilities and endurance, providing primary oncologists and others with important information for palliative care-type decisions.

Cancer rehabilitation addresses complex medical, physical, social, financial, and emotional issues and is most easily facilitated by a comprehensive interdisciplinary team. Effective communication and teamwork is essential in formulating and carrying out plans to achieve successful rehabilitation outcomes. Team members may include a physiatrist or Physical Medicine and Rehabilitation specialist, the primary oncologist, surgeon, radiation oncologist, physical therapist, occupational therapist, speech therapist, case manager, social worker, nutritionist, rehabilitation nurse, and chaplain.

Knowledgeable primary care physicians, oncologists, or surgeons are often able to coordinate appropriate rehabilitation care for their cancer patients, however, the time and resources necessary to put together the appropriate rehabilitation team are not available. Rehabilitation for complicated inpatient cancer patients and advanced cancer patients may require a rehabilitation physician combined with the efforts of a comprehensive interdisciplinary team.

In cancer patients with palliative care needs, the same interdisciplinary team can help teach family members and caregivers how to move and care for the patient, allowing the patient to spend quality time in familiar surroundings. End-stage cancer rehabilitation can occur in the rehabilitation unit, palliative care unit, or hospice. At any stage of disease, quality of life is the goal of cancer rehabilitation, and cancer rehabilitation can be arranged at home as long as it is safe for the patient and family.

Cancer rehabilitation should occur throughout the continuum of disease course to lessen and prevent disability. A rehabilitation program can be prescribed prior to surgery or treatment to improve conditioning and endurance to better tolerate the treatment. Specific therapies may be prescribed to maintain strength or range of motion in an area which may be adversely affected by proposed treatments. Many times, a rehabilitation program is initiated during active ongoing treatment to limit the adverse physical affects of the treatment and also provide the patient an active role he or she can play in the recovery process. Rehabilitation frequently occurs after surgery, radiation therapy, or chemotherapy when the effects of disease and treatment have led to deconditioning or specific functional deficits. Rehabilitation for advanced cancer patients with significant tumor burden can occur with the focus of therapies on improvements in basic mobility and self-care. Finally, rehabilitation for terminal cancer patients can occur with the focus on family training for basic caregiving, bowel and bladder issues, skin care, pain control, and palliative care measures. Cancer rehabilitation ideally should be an ongoing process beginning with diagnosis and continuing throughout the course of the patient's disease.

Rehabilitation issues at the end of life

End-of-life rehabilitation emphasizes symptom control, maximizing quality of life, and family education, which are principles shared with palliative care medicine.

Rehabilitation at the end of life is similar to palliative care, dealing with many of the same issues, and relying on many of the same healthcare professionals.

The framework for rehabilitation interventions is similar to palliative care, utilizing a multidisciplinary team to adequately assess and treat the patient, with emphasis not only on the disease process, but also on the physical symptoms and limitations of the patient, and how to improve or relieve them. The importance of including the family in patient care, providing family support and education is a vital component of both palliative care and rehabilitation.

In rehabilitation, functional goals are used to guide therapies and measure benefits in quality of life. Appropriate rehabilitation goals in the palliative care setting are needed to balance therapies with the need for energy conservation during the terminal stages of life. According to Cheville, patients differ in their level of disease acceptance, expectations for the future, willingness to persevere in aggressive anti-cancer therapy, and in the dimensions of life that are meaningful to them. A combination of these factors can affect the degree in which patients participate in the rehabilitation process. Rehabilitation can allow patients to take an active role in goal setting, and also allow them to see how their own actions and participation in therapy can improve side effects and symptoms.

Yoshioka documented improvements in patient mobility, self-care, and satisfaction with hospice care after a rehabilitation program. Rehabilitation procedures included: (1) positioning techniques to maximize patient comfort and decrease pain; (2) therapeutic exercise to improve muscle strength, range of motion, and balance; (3) activities of daily living (ADL) exercises to help patients function with more independence; (4) endurance training to increase pulmonary and cardiovascular function; (5) chest physiotherapy; (6) swallowing exercises to improve dysphagia; (7) intermittent pneumatic compression for edema; (8) physical modalities to treat pain; (9) acupuncture to treat pain; and (10) bracing and splinting to relieve pain and assist with mobility. Yoshioka felt that active patient care participation by family members released the family members from the frustration that there is nothing left to be done, and left them with feelings of having shared in the process of providing sufficient care.

Similarly, Mackey & Sparling stated education in caregiving techniques such as transfer training and positioning can decrease family stress of providing care and patient concerns about being a burden. Family members' patient care concerns can include: (1) fear of hurting the patient physically by moving them; (2) fear of hurting themselves when moving or transferring the patient; (3) being overprotective in order to protect the patient from further injury or discomfort. With palliative rehabilitation, family members can be reassured that they will not be asked to do any more than they are physically or emotionally capable of doing, and that with proper education, they will be taught how to safely care for and move the patient.

Table 6.2. Common rehabilitation interventions

Physical therapy for strengthening, range of motion exercises, gait training

Occupational therapy for training in activities of daily living such as bathing, grooming, dressing, toileting

Speech therapy for cognitive assessment and training, swallowing evaluation and treatment

Orthotic devices for functional assistance and pain control

Pharmacologic treatments for pain, spasticity, bowel and bladder control

Joint injections, trigger point injections, botulism toxin injections for symptom control

Marcant & Rapin stated some areas addressed by rehabilitation efforts in the palliative care setting include: respiratory function, analgesia, autonomy, and relaxation. Respiratory management can be assisted with percussion, vibration, bronchial postures, and assisted cough. Symptom control measures used by rehabilitation therapists include modalities such as heat, cold, and TENS, for pain alleviation. Physician interventions for symptom control can include joint and soft tissue injections, as well as injections and medical treatment for spasticity (Table 6.2).

Summary

Patient care at the end of life, whether called cancer rehabilitation or palliative care, focuses on issues of symptom control and quality of life. Rehabilitation care also emphasizes patient autonomy and patient safety as long as one is associated with the other. Once family or caregiver assistance is the only alternative for basic activities, cancer rehabilitation can provide the education needed to accomplish this in the home setting.

BIBLIOGRAPHY

Cheville AL. Cancer rehabilitation and palliative care. In *Syllabus of the CME Activity Memorial Sloan–Kettering Cancer Center*, ed. RR Payne, AL Cheville, Course Directors, pp. 125–8. New York: Memorial Sloan–Kettering Cancer Center, 1999.

Lehmann JF, DeLisa JA, Warren CG, deLateur BJ, Bryant PL, Nicholson CG. Cancer rehabilitation: assessment of need, development, and evaluation of a model of care. *Arch Phys Med Rehabil* 1978;59:410–19.

Mackey KC, Sparling JW. Experiences of older women with cancer receiving hospice care: significance for physical therapy. *Phys Therapy* 2000;80:459–68.

Marcant D, PTR, Rapin CH. Role of the physiotherapist in palliative care. *J Pain Symptom Management* 1993;8:68–71.

World Health Organization. *International Classification of Impairments, Disabilities, and Handicaps.* Geneva: WHO, 1980.

Yoshioka H. Rehabilitation for the terminal cancer patient. *Am J Phys Med Rehabil* 1994;73: 199–206.

Internet sites

http://palliative.mdanderson.org

www.oncologypt.org

7

Principles of palliative nursing

Nessa Coyle

Memorial Sloan—Kettering Cancer Center, New York

Leaders in end-of-life care recently developed a set of precepts for palliative care:

palliative care refers to the comprehensive management of the physical, – psychological, social, spiritual and existential needs of the patient, in particular those with incurable, progressive illnesses. Palliative care affirms life and regards dying as a natural process that is a profoundly personal experience for the individual and family. The goal of palliative care is to achieve the best possible quality of life through relief of suffering, control of symptoms and restoration of functional capacity while remaining sensitive to personal, cultural and religious values, beliefs and practices[1]

The following two case reports illustrate the acute and chronic nature of palliative care in cancer nursing. They also demonstrate that relationships, trust, and continuity are important, and that a full and "human" assessment of the patient and family is critical if their needs are to be met.

CASE 1 RG is a 45-year-old man who was diagnosed with advanced gastric cancer one month prior to admission to the cancer center. He is divorced, has two adult daughters, three grandchildren, and lives with his fiancée who is 5 months pregnant. He has a recent history of drug abuse including opioids and crack cocaine, and had been in a methadone maintenance program. On admission to the cancer center he was cachectic, had severe abdominal pain, gross ascites, early satiation, nausea and vomiting, insomnia, fatigue, and general irritability.

RG was not a surgical candidate but was offered chemotherapy, which he accepted. During the 2-week hospital admission he had his ascites drained, a PEG feeding tube inserted, a PORT placed for central venous access, and was started on a parenteral infusion of morphine sulfate for pain.

RG was referred to the Pain and Palliative Care Service for ongoing management of his pain and other symptoms as he continued with palliative chemotherapy. In addition, the Service was asked to help design a "safe" discharge plan and continued follow-up at home. Continuity of care was identified as an essential element to providing effective care for this complex patient.

CASE 2   FT is a 33-year-old man with an 11-year history of a recurrent primary brain tumor. He has
been treated with multimodal therapy including surgery, radiation therapy, and both conventional and experimental chemotherapy. He is bed and wheelchair bound, with marked
cerebellar ataxia, diplopia and loss of peripheral vision, profound hearing loss, chronic
headaches, periodic auditory hallucination, and impaired swallowing. In addition he is
steroid dependent and severely osteoporotic resulting in compression fractures of the thoracic spine and recurrent infections. He has a tracheotomy, a central venous access line and
a PEG feeding tube.

FT is cared for at home by his parents. His daily physical care involves intermittent tracheotomy suctioning with skin care and dressing change, PEG tube feedings, care of the central venous access line, hanging intravenous fluids and intravenous antibiotics as needed,
administering multiple medications via his PEG feeding tubes 3–4 times daily, monitoring
his pain and administering opioid analgesics, bathing, toilet care, skin care, and assisting in
his transfer from bed to wheelchair.

Daily telephone contact with the palliative care nurse has become the primary mode of
monitoring and support for FT and his parents, enhanced by the use of a telecommunication
system. Although community nursing is available to make home visits, this family's strong
bond and sense of continuity with the palliative care oncology nurse has facilitated his
remaining at home. He has been followed for the past 5 years.

The complex and multidimensional needs of the two patients and their families
described above, exemplify the training, skills, compassion, and art required in
palliative care nursing. Assessment skills are critical (Table 7.1).[2] Palliative care is
incorporated into every aspect of cancer nursing, starting from time of diagnosis

Table 7.1. Assessment of patient and family in palliative nursing care. (These questions have specific
correlates to the patient and families illness experience. They provide the clinician with specific
information about how best to deliver effective and compassionate palliative care. Further in-depth
exploration of a particular domain – physical, psychological, social, spiritual – occurs as needed)

The patient
1. Who is the patient and what is his/her social context (e.g., family, work, social network, hobbies)? Ask
   them about their life before the illness and their life now.
2. What is the patient's illness and where is the patient in the natural history of the illness?
3. What is the patient's understanding of their illness and the extent of their illness?
4. What is the patient's understanding of the goals of care (specific and general)? Is this understanding the
   same as the medical goals of care (specific and general)? If not, how do these goals differ?
5. What are the physical consequences of the illness (e.g., effects on physical status (KPS), ability to think
   clearly, ability to take care of basic needs, effects on independence, presence of distressing symptoms)?
   How are these physical consequences of illness being addressed? Is the current approach(es) effective?
   If not, why not?
6. How does the patient rate their overall quality of life? What three factor(s) are most influencing their
   present quality of life either positively or negatively?

Table 7.1. (*cont.*)

7. Is the patient depressed, anxious? Are they able to sleep at night? What are their thoughts at night when all is quiet?

8. Psychologically, how is the patient dealing with their illness? Is this the most stressful time of their life? If not, what was and how did they deal with that?

9. How has the current illness impacted on the patient's life, goals and hopes for the future? How have their hopes and goals changed? What are their worries and fears? Ask the patient if they are depressed.

10. Are there financial concerns?

11. How is the patient dealing with the current situation? What are their support systems, both internal and external? Who/what do they turn to in times of distress (e.g., an individual, God, prayer, meditation)? How does the patient make sense/meaning of what is happening to them?

12. Is there one major area of concern to the patient right now? If so, what is it?

13. What future problems can be anticipated for this particular patient?

The family

1. Who is the family (significant other) and what is their social context (e.g., work, social network, hobbies)? Ask them about their life before the illness and their life now.

2. What has been the impact of the patient's illness on their day-to-day life, and on other members of the family?

3. What has been the biggest area of stress for them throughout the course of this illness?

4. How do they rate their own present overall quality of life? What three factor(s) most influencing their present quality of life either positively or negatively?

5. Are they depressed, anxious? Are they able to sleep at night? What are their thoughts at night when all is quiet?

6. What is their understanding of the patient's illness, its expected course, and goals of care? Have they had experience with a similar illness before? If so, what was that experience like? How does it affect their current experience?

7. Is this the most stressful situation they have ever been in? If not what was? How did they deal with that situation?

8. Who/what do they turn to in times of distress (e.g., an individual, God, prayer, meditation)? How do they make sense/meaning of what is happening?

9. What do they anticipate for the future, for the patient? For themselves?

10. Do they feel able to be a presence and or physically take care of the patient throughout the course of the illness?

11. Do they have a medical condition of their own that may affect their ability to be a presence for the patient during the course of the illness?

12. Do they have one major area of concern/worry? If so, what is it?

and continuing throughout the course of the disease including care of the dying and bereavement follow-up.[3] The patients and their families are as varied as the setting in which the care is provided. Always, the trigger for palliative care in cancer nursing is patient and family need rather than prognosis. However, the palliative care needs of cancer patients and their families invariably become more acute and pronounced as the disease advances. Ineffective curative or life-prolonging treatments may be discontinued, and palliative treatments focusing on symptom control and the psychological, social, and spiritual aspects of quality of life come to the fore.

This is a time when the patient's life as a whole is put into perspective, and the patient and family strive to incorporate the current situation into the broader schema of their life. The meaning of hope may be redefined and that redefinition incorporated into the goals of care for the patient and family. The field of palliative care in cancer nursing has built on the long tradition of hospice care – attention to detail, management of pain and other symptoms, continuity of care, remaining open to exploration of existential issues and suffering, and addressing the needs of the family.

The setting(s)

Palliative nursing care in the oncology population is usually provided within the framework of an interdisciplinary team approach. The composition of such teams varies enormously depending on the needs of the patient and the resources available.[4] Regardless of the specific type of palliative care team it is the nurse who serves as the primary liaison between the team and the patient and family and brings the team plan and requisite teaching to the patient's bedside, as was the case in the patients described above. This plan of palliative care may occur in many different settings: a cancer center, a palliative care unit, a general hospital with oncology beds, a long-term care facility, a nursing home, the patient's home, or an oncology outpatient clinic. In an inpatient setting the palliative care nurse is often a resource for physicians and nurses throughout the institution on symptom management, facilitating changes in goals of care, facilitating communication in family meetings, orchestrating care of the dying, and facilitating bereavement follow-up. In the home and community the palliative care required by advanced cancer patients and their carers becomes largely a nursing responsibility with medical backup.[5]

Referrals

Patients are usually referred to a palliative care nurse in the setting of advancing disease, poorly controlled pain and other symptoms, a fatigued family, evidence of psychosocial distress and multiple telephone calls to the physician. The goals of the palliative care nurse are: (1) to organize a system of care to meet the needs of the patient and family; (2) to collaborate with the team in providing symptom control; (3) to ensure that the patient and family understand that their primary physician is still in control and that the palliative care nurse is working very closely with that physician to coordinate their care and manage their symptoms; and (4) to provide continuity of care for the patient and family.

Nursing education in palliative care

Palliative care education for nurses is being implemented at both an undergraduate and graduate level. Several master's degree programs and nurse practitioner programs have been developed in palliative nursing. In addition, a variety of continuing education approaches have been used in order to reach nurses already in practice. This educational focus is essential as (1) all nurses care for patients with palliative care needs at some point in their career and (2) nurses are increasingly being asked to assume leadership and consultation roles in palliative care both in the hospital setting and in home care. In February 2000 a major initiative to enhance nursing education in palliative care was begun. The project, End of Life Nursing Education Consortium (ELNEC), is cosponsored by the American Association of Colleges of

Table 7.2. End-of-Life Nursing Education Consortium (ELNEC): content of teaching modules

1. Nursing care at the end of life – goals of care, cost issues in palliative care, use of aggressive interventions, personal death awareness, broad review of end-of-life care to encompass all age groups and across various disease trajectories or acute illness
2. Pain management – assessment, pharmacological, and nonpharmacological/complementary therapies
3. Symptom management – assessment, pharmacological, and nonpharmacological/complementary therapies
4. Cultural consideration in EOL care – cultural assessment, beliefs regarding death and dying, afterlife and bereavement
5. Ethical and legal issues – assisted suicide, euthanasia, advanced directives, decision making, advance care planning
6. Communication – breaking bad news, communicating with other disciplines, interdisciplinary collaboration
7. Grief, loss, bereavement – assessment, interventions, nurses' experiences with cumulative loss and grief
8. Preparation and care for the time of death – nursing care at the time of death, including physical care, support of family members, saying goodbye
9. Achieving quality of life at the end of life – including physical, psychological, social, and spiritual well-being and discussion of needs of special populations

Source: Sheehan D, Ferrell BR. Nursing education. In *Textbook of Palliative Nursing*, ed. BR Ferrell, N Coyle, pp. 690–700. Oxford: Oxford University Press, 2001.

Nursing and nurse investigators from the City of Hope National Medical Center, and is funded by the Robert Wood Johnson Foundation (Table 7.2).[6]

Summary

Palliative care in cancer nursing is a complex and enormously rewarding field. The importance of acquisition of assessment and communications skills, as well as a firm foundation in the use of appropriate technology, stands high in the requisite preparation for work with advanced cancer patients who have multiple needs, and their families. The ethical principles of palliative care (relief of suffering, control of symptoms, restoration and maintenance of functional capacity where feasible, and focusing on the patient as a unique individual with important spiritual, cultural, and personal needs) are the essential underpinnings of the humane and humanistic endeavor, which we in the field of palliative care undertake in our daily work.

However, it is important to acknowledge that there are circumstances where the patient and family needs have been accurately assessed but it is not possible to access resources to meet these needs. By that I mean we cannot manufacture a caring and stable family, we cannot always create a supportive community environment, we cannot always provide sufficient help in the home to relieve family caretaker burden unless the family has independent means, and we cannot always satisfy the desires of the dying or advanced cancer patient however hard we try. This raises many questions and underscores the need for political and social awareness. There are chronically ill and dying patients who are underserved and their families unsupported. Patient and family advocacy with all its ramifications is an integral part of palliative nursing.

REFERENCES

1 Last Acts Task Force. *Principles of Palliative Care*. Princeton, NJ: Robert Wood Johnson Foundation, 1997.

2 Cherney N. Principles of assessment for palliative care. In *Concise Oxford Textbook of Palliative Care*, ed. R Dunlop, RK Portenoy, N Coyle, C Davis. Oxford: Oxford University Press, 2001.

3 Super A. The context of palliative care in progressive disease. In *Textbook of Palliative Nursing*, ed. BR Ferrell, N Coyle, pp. 27–36. Oxford: Oxford University Press, 2001.

4 Coyle N, Ingham J, Altilio T. Care of the terminal patients' physical and psychosocial needs. In *Oncology Nursing: Assessment and Clinical Care*, ed. C Miaskowski, P Buchsel, pp. 359–82. St Louis: Mosby, 1999.

5 Milone-Nuzzo P, McCorkle R. Home care. In *Textbook of Palliative Nursing*, ed. BR Ferrell, N Coyle, pp. 543–55. Oxford: Oxford University Press, 2001.

6 Sheehan D, Ferrell BR. Nursing education. In *Textbook of Palliative Nursing*, ed. BR Ferrell, N Coyle, pp. 690–700. Oxford: Oxford University Press, 2001.

Internet sites

Oncology Nursing Society (ONS): http://www.ons.org

City of Hope Pain/Palliative Care Resource Center: http://prc.coh.org

Hospice and Palliative Nurses Association: http://www.HPNA.org

Last Acts: http://www.lastacts.org

8

Ethics of decision making towards the end of life

Christopher K. Daugherty

The University of Chicago, Chicago, IL

Introduction and background

For the more than 500 000 cancer patients who eventually die each year in the US,[1,2] one of their most meaningful options for care is for them to receive state-of-the-art palliative care without receiving any further cancer-remitting therapy. Such state-of-the-art palliative care for the dying can be made available through use of formal hospice services. For advanced cancer patients to receive formal hospice care in the US, through Medicare and insurance hospice benefits, they must be documented by their physician as having a prognosis of 6 months or less. Given that most cancer deaths come with significant advance knowledge, it is clear that a substantial proportion of individuals within this population have a prognosis which qualifies them to receive formal hospice care. However, it is also clear that hospice care, while it is widely available within third-party payer systems in the US, remains underutilized for advanced cancer patients. Although geographic variation exists, and estimates of utilization vary, 20–50% of the otherwise eligible cancer patient population dies each year while receiving formal hospice care.[1,3,4] While these statistics could lead one to believe that hospice care is utilized for many appropriate patients, reviewed Medicare data have shown that the median survival of cancer patients in hospice is only on the order of 2–3 weeks at best, with many dying within days of referral.[3] Some cancer patients even die between the actual time of referral and the provision of services, i.e., literally within hours of the referral.

Perceived dilemmas as obstacles to hospice referral

Because of the complexities in predicting and communicating time to death in those with advanced cancer, and given the short survival time of cancer patients in hospice, oncologists would appear to continue to have difficulty in knowing if referral to hospice is appropriate, or if they should continue with anticancer therapy (even including the use of experimental agents).[5–10] It has been argued that one of the significant obstacles to providing appropriate palliative care, most notably as available in hospice, is a result of physician inaccuracy in predicting time to death.[11,12] As argued by others, because of overestimation of their patients' survival time, oncologists either refer their patients to hospice too late to receive meaningful end-of-life care, or do not refer them at all.[12] However, while oncologists' inability to recognize a terminal prognosis undoubtedly plays some role in many physicians' hesitancy, and even unwillingness, to refer cancer patients to hospice, it does not provide a complete explanation for hospice underutilization. From an oncologist's perspective, it is not an issue of a physician's *knowledge* of a cancer patient's terminal prognosis that creates barriers to palliative care as much as it is their actual *perceptions* and attitudes (as well as those of the involved patients and families) regarding how and when prognoses should be communicated.

Explanation for the hesitancy and unwillingness of oncologists to refer advanced cancer patients to hospice can be found not only by examining oncologists' perceptions regarding the method and timing of communicating a terminal prognosis to patients and families, but also by examining their concerns regarding whether hospice care can provide sufficient clinical resources to care for their more advanced disease patients. From a cancer physician's viewpoint, such perceptions may be best viewed as overt ethical dilemmas. As discussed below, these include: (1) dilemmas related to a physician's ability to effectively communicate a terminal prognosis to cancer patients (and their families) and still facilitate the maintenance of hope; (2) dilemmas relating to carrying out an ethically appropriate informed consent process for hospice care when patients and families remain unwilling to accept a terminal prognosis; and (3) dilemmas surrounding patient fears of abandonment and physician concerns regarding loss of control over their patients' medical care. Finally, the mechanism by which the vast majority of hospice care is both provided and paid for in the US, while certainly increasing access to home hospice for many, has also created ethical dilemmas for many cancer physicians and hospices. More specifically, dilemmas may develop for cancer patients who are believed by their physicians to require clinical services that a hospice is perceived to be unable, or unwilling, to provide because of the hospice's inability to be reimbursed for these services.

Communicating terminal prognoses and maintaining hope

Physician concerns about damaging a patient's and/or family's hope in the face of providing factual information about a terminal prognosis remain matters of concern among many cancer clinicians. Many clinicians may believe that to effectively communicate a terminal prognosis to a patient and/or their family is essentially to destroy the patient's hope.[11,13–16] Undoubtedly, through compassionate and sensitive communication, an individual with advanced cancer can be appropriately and effectively informed of their life-ending diagnosis. Yet, based on their clinical experiences, regardless of the method of communication of a terminal prognosis, some physicians may still maintain that if the facts about the life-ending nature of a patient's prognosis are effectively communicated, the ability of some patients to continue to maintain any meaningful hope is severely limited.[13,14] Such clinical experiences may often be the result of poor or ineffective communication practices on the part of oncologists and their inability to redirect patients' and family members' hopes toward more achievable and realistic outcomes, e.g., death at home and without suffering. In fact, there is little doubt that many oncologists could improve upon their communication practices. However, it must also be recognized that for many patients and families to accept a terminal prognosis is, for them, to give up hope for the only outcome they persist in viewing as meaningful, i.e., hope for continued survival and even cure. For some patients and families, discussions about redirecting hope away from such seemingly unrealistic expectations may only serve to irritate them. Such discussions may even motivate them to aggressively seek out alternatives of care that are more consistent with their own goals.[17–21] In this setting, it may become inappropriate, even unethical, for healthcare providers to continue with their attempts at providing their own rationale for why end-of-life care is recommended. As a result of direct experience, some cancer physicians recognize this and – due to either fatigue, lack of effective communication support resources, or simply their belief that they are doing the right thing – accede to patients' or families' demands for further anticancer therapy.[22]

Given cancer physicians' concerns about destroying or reducing patients' hopes as a result of direct communication of terminal prognoses, and the role these concerns play in creating barriers to appropriate and timely referral to hospice, some specific aspects surrounding the hospice benefit should be kept in mind by cancer clinicians and others. As noted, in order for patients to receive hospice benefits, they must be documented by their physicians as having a prognosis of 6 months or less. As well, there is an obligation to communicate this documented prognosis to patients in order for an ethically appropriate decision to be made to receive hospice care. However, hospice prognosis documentation (and communication) does not require that the prognosis be accurate, i.e., it does not require that patients die within the 6-month prognostic milestone. While this may seem obvious and should go without saying, there exists a great deal of uncertainty about what prognosis documentation means in regard to qualifying for hospice benefits.[1] Practically speaking, for those with a specific advanced cancer diagnosis, prognosis documentation in this setting commonly means that there is some significant likelihood of death occurring from cancer over the next 6 months. The actual likelihood is left to the interpretation of the involved clinicians. Thus, for a cancer patient to be eligible to receive hospice services, a cancer clinician need only believe and recognize that the patient has *some significant chance*, or reasonable possibility, of dying from their disease within 6 months, as opposed to believing that their deaths will come with *absolute certainty* within the next 6 months. If an advanced cancer patient should happen to live longer than 6 months, presumably they have not proven to have no need for hospice care. Rather, if anything, their prognosis is even more grave and they continue to be very appropriate candidates for hospice services. It is the rare cancer patient who would ever be denied continued hospice care because they outlived the 6-month prognostic milestone. If cancer physicians were to keep these issues regarding prognosis documentation in mind when communicating with their patients about hospice care, physicians may find discussions about hospice much more acceptable to patients. Within such a framework, physicians could more openly and comfortably discuss, and patients may more readily accept, the potential benefits of hospice if physicians are specifically communicating about the *possibility* of death within the next 6 months, rather than the *certainty* of death.

Consent for hospice and willingness to accept a terminal prognosis

In consenting to receive hospice care, a patient (or family member) is typically asked to sign informed consent forms that document that the terminal prognosis has been disclosed (even understood) and that they wish to receive no further cancer-remitting therapy. In addition, they are typically asked to sign an advance directive specifically stating that they wish no life-saving interventions, e.g., cardiopulmonary resuscitation or mechanical ventilation, be used in their care. Aware that such consent processes need to be carried out, some cancer physicians may perceive that such formal (even forceful) disclosure of a terminal prognosis (and the emotional difficulties potentially associated with signing such forms) may severely damage a patient's and family members' hopes. They may also believe, with patients and family members often sharing this belief, that to agree to such care is to essentially "give up."[12–14,22] Thus, they will shy away from such discussions or delay them past the point in time when more meaningful hospice care could have been provided. Further, it is recognized and accepted that some patients simply deny their terminal prognoses.[23,24] This may even happen in the face of explicit physician disclosure about a terminal prognosis.[21,22,24] In some circumstances, an occasional patient may even *knowingly choose* to deny their life-ending prognosis in the face of explicit physician disclosure. If this is the case, it obviously becomes quite difficult to refer such patients to hospice who simply and adamantly choose not to accept their terminal prognoses. Some might argue that this lack of acceptance might be overcome with the passage of time and/or ongoing, compassionate, and respectful communication. However, to put forth such an argument may speak to a lack of respect for many oncologists' forthright and honest attempts at prognosis communication. In addition, it may even be disrespectful of the values and preferences of the patients themselves. In this setting, one may ask, if it is even ethical to refer such patients to hospice or other traditional palliative care services.

Physicians should realize that many hospice care providers share their experiences in terms of dealing with prognosis communication and patient denial (or lack of acceptance) of disclosed terminal prognoses. Practically speaking, many sophisticated hospice providers and palliative care professionals are aware that patient and family acceptance of a terminal prognosis is not a one-time, static process. Acceptance (and denial) are ongoing processes that wax and wane over time. Thus, it is often not the case that patients must accept their terminal prognosis in order for them to enter hospice. Many hospices are actually quite experienced in appropriately negotiating conversations and consent discussions surrounding decisions to receive hospice care. In certain circumstances, despite well-intentioned policies, some hospice care providers may even appropriately defer some aspects of the prognosis communication and informed consent procedures for hospice, e.g., the signing of an advance directive. With the overall goal of relieving suffering in all its physical, psychological, spiritual, and emotional forms, some hospices may recognize that to belabor the point of prognosis disclosure to the point of full and explicit *documented* understanding on the part of the patient oftentimes only serves to increase such suffering. Many hospices have become experienced in obtaining appropriate and ethical consent for hospice from patients while, at the same time, allowing them to believe (if they choose to do so) that they are not going to die. Given this, physicians would do well to call upon hospice care providers early in the course of such prognosis discussions with patients and even to allow more sophisticated and trustworthy providers to negotiate the consent process in partnership with the physician.

Patient abandonment and oncologists' loss of control

Another obstacle to effective communication and decision making in regard to cancer physician referral of patients to hospice concerns cancer physicians' perceptions of patient fears of abandonment.[22] Such fears may develop in a cancer patient who has been receiving significant amounts of anticancer therapy, e.g., chemotherapy, for several months or years prior to the recognition of the terminal prognosis. Now, with the introduction of the potential for hospice care, the patient (and even physician) perceives radical changes to the care environment. These perceptions are based on the current hospice experience where cancer patients typically no longer receive chemotherapy, undergo laboratory and radiological evaluations, or receive physician and nursing visits. The significance and meaning of some of the aspects of this prior clinical care on patients' lives can be enormous. Thus, to no longer be involved in these types of clinical care experiences understandably prompts feelings of abandonment on the part of the patient. This may be particularly true for selected cancer patients who have received their care almost exclusively at hospitals or medical centers some distance from their home or community. Traditionally, when patients are referred to hospice in the US, they typically have undergone fewer (if any) physician visits in the clinic and receive the vast majority of their care in the home. For many patients, the change in the physical location of their care can encourage or perpetuate these feelings of abandonment. In addition, while some inpatient care may be required for patients once they enter hospice (either for respite care for family members, or as a result of some clinical crisis that cannot be managed within the home), patients will often be admitted to inpatient units or contracted hospice beds at institutions other than the one where they had been receiving their care prior to hospice admission. With cancer physicians aware of these possibilities, and perhaps unable to cope with them, they may become even more hesitant or unwilling to refer a patient to hospice if they perceive any potential for fear of abandonment in the patient or family as a result of potential admission to an unfamiliar healthcare institution.

In addition, although difficult for oncologists to recognize and discuss, knowingly or unknowingly oncologists may have conflicts of interest in their willingness to refer their patients to palliative care and hospice programs. Understandably, these conflicts may be the result of the emotional or psychological attachments that a physician may develop with their patients, particularly for those with whom they have been intensively involved for months or years. Some relationships may be so strong that a physician is unable to break the clinical bonds that have held the relationship together. As shown by Christakis, evidence for this can even be found in the phenomenon where the longer the physician knows a patient, the less accurate they are in predicting time to death.[12] This presumably relates to the strong emotional attachments that develop within the doctor–patient relationship as a result of more meaningful – in this case, longer – relationships. These emotional attachments lead to an unwillingness of physicians to both accept their patients' deaths, and subsequently communicate this to patients in such a way as to allow appropriate decisions for care. While quite understandable, such unwillingness to "let go" only further serves to create barriers to patients receiving adequate and effective palliative and/or hospice care.

Even more difficult to recognize and discuss are oncologists' conflicts of interests as they relate to the loss of medical decision control and, more specifically, the potential for loss of clinical revenue in their patients who are referred to hospice. Presumably, every oncologist would agree that decision making based on potential clinical revenue is unacceptable and oncologists may find it offensive to even suggest that some decisions to not refer patients for palliative care and/or hospice services are the result of concern over losing chemotherapy, or other clinical care, reimbursements. However, it is also many oncologists' anecdotal experience that they can recall at least one occasion in thinking about their oncologist peers where they may have wondered if the clinical decision of another oncologist regarding the use of certain chemotherapy agents was at all related to the potential for financial reimbursement. Thus, oncologists likely have to acknowledge that such decision making plays at least some role in the timing of some oncologists' discussions about palliative and/or hospice care. In this acknowledgement, oncologists must also become fully introspective into their own behavior as well. Although not sufficient in and of itself, such meaningful introspection has the potential to result in some oncologists overcoming some of these potential conflicts of interests.

In addition to thoughtful introspection among cancer physicians toward their own behaviors, dilemmas surrounding patient fears of abandonment and physicians' unwillingness to relinquish clinical decision control could also be addressed through meaningful continuing education efforts that seek to promote increased understanding as to how hospice care is provided in the US. Specifically, cancer physicians need to be better informed as to how the hospice benefit actually allows them to play a continued and significant role in their patients' care after a patient has enrolled in hospice and still be reimbursed for clinical services. For instance, despite a relatively typical pattern of hospice care for cancer patients, those referred to hospice can continue to visit their physician in the outpatient setting as frequently as they and their physician wish. As well, physicians can bill as they normally would for such visits. At the same time, reasonable limitations may need to be placed on certain aspects of hospice patients' care, e.g., in regard to laboratory testing. As well, the clinical reality in many circumstances is also such that many patients are not well enough to travel to an outpatient facility for routine visits. However, much of this clinical reality is currently the result of otherwise delayed patient referral to hospice. If patients were referred to hospice at an earlier point in their clinical course, physicians would actually be even more able to meaningfully see, and interact with, their patients in clinic.

Cancer physicians should also understand that if patients have such significant concerns about abandonment, and fears of receiving care in an institution about which they know little to nothing (for what may likely be the last days or moments of their lives), they can inform their patients that if they require readmission to an inpatient unit they can simply be brought back to their original care institution. In almost all circumstances this will require removing a patient from hospice care for whatever time they are in the hospital. But there are currently no prohibitions or punishments for removing terminally ill patients from hospice services, and such patients can return under the care of hospice when and if they are discharged back out of the hospital. This may create certain inconveniences for the hospices themselves, and some hospices have very justified concerns regarding potential accusations of fraud as a result of recent issues surrounding hospice audits and the discovery of enrollment of otherwise ineligible patients.[1] However, many of these concerns about fraud and abuse among hospices surrounded the enrollment of patients with neurological diseases, dementia, and patients who were in long-term healthcare facilities. Thus, it is not inappropriate to inform advanced cancer patients enrolling in home hospice that they can remain under their oncologists' outpatient care and can even return under their physician's inpatient care if desired and believed absolutely necessary by them or their family. This information has enormous potential to relieve anxiety in patients (and physicians) who are considering hospice referral but remain hesitant because of concerns over placement, i.e., perceived abandonment, in another institution. The benefits of relieving patient and physician anxiety are far greater than any minimal risks to involved hospices for what is likely be an uncommon instance of when a hospice cancer patient or family member will, in the end, need and want frequent readmissions from home to their original care institution. While some hospices may be reluctant to carry out what is essentially a revocation of services for a patient in their hospice, many now recognize the appropriateness of at least discussing this as a possibility. This is particularly the case if these fears of abandonment act as a significant barrier in the decision making, to the point of preventing a patient from receiving effective and meaningful end-of-life care.

Hospice services and per diem reimbursement: sufficient resources for all dying cancer patients?

Another barrier to providing end-of-life care to advanced cancer patients relates to Medicare, Medicaid, and insurance benefits which provide reimbursement for hospice care services in the US.[1] Currently, such care is paid for through a per diem benefit, with the Medicare per diem being approximately $100.00–120.00 a day (the actual amount being dependent on the region of the country).[1,25] While many cancer patients have prognoses which are undoubtedly terminal, they may still have an otherwise adequate (even good) performance status and show continued evidence of benefit from relatively expensive or aggressive palliative interventions, including antibiotics, radiation therapy, and blood transfusions. In these cases, such a per diem would not cover the costs of such care. This also can be viewed as an ethical issue for cancer physicians. Specifically, cancer physicians may not ever refer certain populations of patients to hospice for what they view as *ethical* reasons if they believe that a hospice is unable or unwilling to provide more costly, but believed by the physician to be effective, palliative interventions. Given the known costs of such interventions, they may perceive that hospices are simply not interested in caring for such patients. While such a viewpoint may be ethically justifiable, oncologists should keep in mind that even the most compassionate and resourceful of hospices, in order to continue to maintain its solvency on a rather meager per diem *and* continue to care for its patients, must have some concerns about the relative costs and benefits of certain interventions. They may even extend such concerns to the point of prohibiting them, either explicitly through clinical care policies or implicitly through known practice patterns. For some oncologists who are aware of these implicit or explicit prohibitions, they would understandably be hesitant or unwilling to refer those patients with advanced disease to hospice who are receiving more costly or aggressive interventions. In addition, such awareness may even further limit their willingness to refer other patients who are not receiving these more aggressive interventions out of perceptions that hospices may be "holding back" on certain types of care.

In some of these circumstances where costly or aggressive interventions are still being undertaken with benefit in those with advanced cancer they may, in fact, not be appropriate candidates for hospice. However, if true palliative benefit is being achieved in a patient with a life-ending cancer diagnosis and some significant likelihood of death exists within the next 6 months, hospices do have an obligation to take such a patient under their care and provide services to them. Providing such services may require subcontracting with other healthcare providers who are more readily able to bring the kinds of significant clinical resources that may be required in this setting, e.g., radiation therapy or blood product transfusion support.[26] Of note, as recently funded by the Robert Wood Johnson Foundation, some hospice and palliative care programs have conducted demonstration projects to determine the feasibility of their earlier involvement in the course of advanced cancer care (I. Byock and B. Volk-Craft, personal communications), even to the extent of supporting the administration of chemotherapy (including the use of experimental anticancer agents in some selected settings).[1] In reality, many hospices may be unable to effectively bring such clinical resources to cancer patients. However, even in the absence of these more broadly designed demonstration projects, some hospices may be more than able (even eager) to accept such patients under their care. This willingness to accept such patients is a result of not only their knowledge that it is clinically and ethically appropriate, but also because they believe that it may result in more meaningful relationships developing with the referring clinicians. They realize and expect that these relationships may lead to other hospice-appropriate patients being referred to them for care who have less intensive clinical needs. Thus, before cancer physicians make assumptions about what types of patients a hospice is willing and/or able to care for, they should communicate directly with hospices on a case-by-case basis about the hospice's ability to provide more aggressive palliative interventions to individual patients.

Conclusions

Some of the barriers in providing end-of-life cancer care in the US might be eliminated, or at least reduced in magnitude, by increasing or restructuring the Medicare hospice benefit for both home hospice and inpatient care.[1] However, for palliative and hospice care to become a more meaningful alternative of care for cancer patients, efforts must also be directed toward the cancer physicians and other healthcare providers who are actively involved in the community care of the vast majority of the cancer patient population. For instance, continuing medical education programs that are specifically designed to improve either oncologists' communication techniques or their understanding of how end-of-life care is provided in relation to hospice benefits would be of great value. Thoughtful education efforts aimed at addressing barriers to hospice referral as ethical dilemmas would also undoubtedly serve to improve the ability of cancer physicians to communicate a terminal prognosis without the perceptions, real or otherwise, regarding the destruction of patient and family hope. Such education efforts would also give appropriate respect and recognition to the daily challenges cancer physicians face in attempting to provide palliative care to their patients suffering from cancer-related symptoms. Cancer physicians themselves also need to become more introspective of their own end-of-life care communication and decision-making behaviors, and specific continuing education efforts in this area may be successful in promoting this introspection.[27] Equally important, innovative research efforts examining current communication and decision-making practices among cancer physicians and patients *in the community* should be undertaken to help us more fully understand how certain behaviors, beliefs, or practices act as barriers to patients receiving adequate hospice and palliative care. Rigorous descriptive research involving individuals with expertise from the social and behavioral sciences would be of enormous value in this setting, and innovative collaborations with these individuals should be undertaken. Given the limited amount of truly generalizable knowledge in this area, such research is needed before testing potential interventions that might hope to reduce these communication and decision-making barriers. Descriptive research that is well designed is likely to identify certain selected behaviors among cancer clinicians that do, in fact, facilitate clinically and ethically appropriate referral to hospice. Attempts could then be made to replicate these identified behaviors as possible interventions in prospective studies with larger, more generalizeable populations. In the absence of fully successful outcomes from thoughtful, well-designed education and research efforts directed towards the actual cancer clinicians and healthcare providers who currently assume the vast majority of advanced cancer patient care, these perceived ethical dilemmas will continue to create misunderstandings that act as barriers to advanced cancer patients receiving adequate palliative care.

Acknowledgements

Supported in part by a Career Development Award from the American Society of Clinical Oncology and a Faculty Scholar Award from the Soros Foundation Open Society Institute's Project on Death in America.

REFERENCES

1 Foley KM, Gelbard H, ed. *Institute of Medicine Report: Improving Palliative Care for Cancer.* Washington, DC: National Academy Press, 2001.

2 Woolam GL. Cancer statistics, 2000. *Cancer J Clinicians* 2001;51:7–33.

3 Virnig BA, Kind S, McBean M, Fisher E. Geographic variation in hospice use prior to death. *J Am Geriat Soc* 2000;48:1117–25.

4 Christakis NA, Escarce JJ. Survival of Medicare patients after enrollment in hospice. *N Engl J Med* 1996;335:172–8.

5 Reuben DB, Mor V, Hiris J. Clinical symptoms and length of survival in patients with terminal cancer. *Arch Intern Med* 1988;148:1586–91.

6 Forster LE, Lynn J. Predicting life span for applicants to inpatient hospice. *Arch Intern Med* 1988;148:2540–3.

7 Kinzbrunner BM. Hospice: what to do when anti-cancer therapy is no longer appropriate, effective, or desired. *Semin Oncol* 1994;21:792–8.

8 Emanuel EJ. Cost savings at the end of life. *J Am Med Assoc* 1996;275:1901–14.

9 Janisch L, Mick R, Schilsky RL et al. Prognostic factors for survival in patients treated in phase I clinical trials. *Cancer* 1994;74:1965–73.

10 Daugherty CK, Ratain MJ, Banik DM, Janisch L, Siegler M. A quantitative analysis of ethical issues in experimental cancer trials: a survey interview study of 144 terminally ill advanced cancer patients. *Institutional Rev Board* 2000;22:6–14.

11 Christakis NA. *Death Foretold: Prophecy and Prognosis in Medical Care.* Chicago, IL: University of Chicago Press, 2000.

12 Christakis NA, Lamont EB. Extent and determinants of error in doctor's prognoses in terminally ill patients: A prospective cohort study. *Br Med J* 2000;320:469–72.

13 Miyaji N. The power of compassion. Truth-telling among American doctors in the care of dying patients. *Soc Sci Med* 1993;36:249–64.

14 Kodish E, Post SG. Oncology and hope. *J Clin Oncol* 1995;13:1817–22.

15 DelVecchio Good MJ, Good B, Schaffer C et al. American oncology and the discourse on hope. *Cult Med Psych* 1990;14:59–79.

16 Sardell AN, Trierweiler SJ. Disclosing the cancer diagnosis. Procedures that influence patient hopefulness. *Cancer* 1993;72:3355–65.

17 Leyden GM, Boulton M, Moynihan C et al. Cancer patients' information needs and information seeking behaviour: an in-depth interview study. *Br Med J* 2000;320:909–15.

18 Brockopp DY, Hayko D, Davenport W, Winscott C. Personal control and the needs for hope and information among adults diagnosed with cancer. *Cancer Nurs* 1989;12:112–16.

19 Blanchard CG, Labrecque MS, Ruckdeschel JC, Blanchard EB. Information and decision-making preferences of hospitalized adult cancer patients. *Soc Sci Med* 1988;27:1139–45.

20 Eidinger RN, Schapira DV. Cancer patients' insight into their treatment, prognosis, and unconventional therapies. *Cancer* 1984;53:2736–40.

21 Gordon EJ, Daugherty CK. Referral and decision making among advanced cancer patients participating in phase I trials at a single institution. *J Clin Med Ethics* 2001;12:31–8.

22 Gordon EJ, Daugherty CK. "Hitting you over the head:" Oncologists' disclosure of prognosis to advanced cancer patients. *Bioethics* 2003 (in press).

23 Rousseau P. Death denial. *J Clin Oncol* 2000;18:3998–9.

24 Fife BL. The conceptualization of meaning and illness. *Soc Sci Med* 1994;38:309–16.

25 Mara CZ. Hospice: an organizational system model for the integration of acute and long-term care. *J Health Hum Services Admin* 2000;22:416–35.

26 Leland JY, Schonwetter RS. Advances in hospice care. *Clin Geriatr Med* 1997;13:381–401.

27 Baile WF, Lenti R, Kudeka AP et al. Improving physician–patient communication in cancer care: Outcome of a workshop for oncologists. *J Cancer Educ* 1997;12:166–73.

9

Breaking bad news

Walter F. Baile[1] and Robert Buckman[2]

[1] U.T. M.D. Anderson Cancer Center, Houston
[2] University of Toronto Sunnybrook Cancer Center, Toronto

Background

Advances in cancer treatment have resulted in decreases in the incidence of most cancers and also increased patient survival. However, physicians treating cancer patients can expect that, for many patients, the hope of cure, treatment benefit, or sustained remission will not be met. Even for patients who have satisfactory outcomes there are many times during the course of the illness where the physician must undertake the difficult and unavoidable task of conveying unfavorable information about the illness or discussing emotionally charged issues such as

- the diagnosis of cancer (especially when metastatic disease has been found)
- cancer recurrence, spread of disease or failure of treatment to affect disease progression
- the presence of irreversible disease or of serious treatment toxicity
- hospice care and cardiopulmonary resuscitation when no further treatment options exist
- positive results of genetic tests.

Goals of giving bad news

Studies have shown that in Western societies most patients desire to have complete information about their illness, its prognosis, and treatment possibilities.[1-5] Many also wish to participate in the important decisions about cancer treatment.[6] Although bad news often upsets the patient, the physician can move from being the messenger of bad news to actually promoting coping by providing empathic understanding and concern. Employing communication skills in addressing patient's emotional needs are an expression of solidarity and can enhance the patient's trust and confidence in the physician.[7]

What is bad news?

Bad news may be defined as "any information that seriously and adversely affects one's view of the future."[8] This simple definition means, however, that to a great extent bad news is in the eye of the beholder, so that the disparity between the actual medical facts and what the patient believes or understands will determine the "badness" of the bad news and also the patient's reaction to it. An example which illustrates this point is when the patient who attributes a lump in her breast to longstanding fibrocystic disease finds out that the biopsy is positive for breast cancer. On the other hand, a patient with recurrent cancer may be disappointed but less shocked to find out that a treatment for an established disease was not effective in achieving a remission. The caveat to this is that one is not able to estimate the impact of any information that one gives the patient until one understands the patient's current understanding of his or her situation.

Why is giving bad news so difficult?

It has been estimated that, in the course of an average career, an oncologist will conduct as many as 200 000 interviews with cancer patients and/or families.[9] It is reasonable to assume that if 10–20% of these interviews involve the disclosure of unfavorable medical information, then there will be over 20 000 clinical interviews where breaking bad news may be the main focus of the interview. For the bearer of bad news it has been scientifically demonstrated that there is a natural (and understandable) aversion toward disclosing potentially distressing information.[10] In medicine the nature of the relationship with the patient, which is focused on helping, may intensify this reluctance, since giving bad news may be seen by the clinician as doing emotional harm to the patient. That is, it may be disturbing in itself to communicate bad news but then awkward to find a way to support and assist the patient.[11,12] Many physicians have had little or no formal or even informal training in communicating unfavorable information. Physicians recognize that cancer patients already experience a great deal of anxiety and uncertainty and have real concerns. They are legitimately concerned about psychologically harming the patient with unfavorable information, destroying hope, or are fearful of being blamed by the patient or family. They may feel helpless to deal with a patient's disease or their emotional reactions or uncomfortable with their own emotional expressions, such as deep sadness for the patient.[12] Physician stress may be unusually high when the patient is young, the prospects for treatment are limited, the physician has had little experience in breaking bad news or has been unsuccessful in treating the patient.[13]

Do patients want the truth?

In the past, concern about causing patient distress was often used as a reason for not disclosing the cancer diagnosis to patients.[14,15] Between 1950 and 1970 several surveys of practicing physicians revealed that many did not tell patients when they had cancer. In a 1961 study of Chicago doctors by Oken,[16] the percentage was reported as 90%. Evidence soon emerged that this practice was not in accord with what patients actually wanted. In 1982 Louis Harris and associates conducted a survey of 1251 Americans for the President's Commission for the Study of Ethical Problems in Medicine and Biomedical Research (reported by Morris and Abram).[17] They asked a hypothetical question regarding preferences for information disclosure if the person questioned were to be found to have cancer. The researchers reported that not only did 96% of those surveyed wish to be told if they had a diagnosis of cancer, but that in cases of grave prognosis 85% wished to be given a realistic estimate of how long they had to live. Physician's behavior was also shown to have changed by then. When Novack et al. repeated Oken's study in 1979, nearly 98% of physicians indicated that it was their policy to inform patients of their diagnosis.[18]

European patients' wishes were found to be similar to the North Americans'.[19,20] A study on 2331 patients in the UK found that 98% wanted to know if their illness was cancer and 87% wanted all possible information, both good news and bad.[20]

Are we obligated to tell the truth to patients?

Not only do the results of other studies over a period of many years indicate that the great majority of patients do wish to be told if the news is bad, but legal as well as ethical obligations now demand that the physician tell the patient, if that is what the patient wants. These obligations have their roots in the principles governing informed consent for treatment and in the concept of patient autonomy in decision making regarding medical treatment.[21] In the United States and Canada medical legal practice has enshrined the patients' rights to truth, not only in the codes of ethical practice but in case law.[22] Yet mandating truth disclosure without regard to the manner in which it is told or to the obligation of the physician to support the patient and assist him or her in decision making can be as upsetting as lying to the patient. As has been aptly suggested, centuries of systematic insensitive deception cannot instantly be remedied by a new routine of systematic insensitive truth telling.[23,24]

Cultural issues

The right of the patient to make autonomous decisions about medical care is an important principle governing information disclosure, particularly in Western societies. However, it is by no means universally practiced. In some cultures medical practice may follow different moral and ethical principles. Rather than patient autonomy which predominates Western medicine, protection of the sick from unfavorable information may determine to a great extent what the patient is told about the illness in non-Western cultures. Thus physicians may withhold bad news from patients under the justification that they are preventing psychological harm and families may insist that they make the decisions as to how much information is given to the patient. For example, in Japan the patient is often excluded from the discussion of how much information should be disclosed, including the diagnosis of cancer. Thus it has been reported that only 30% of cancer patients are told their diagnosis.[25] When understood in its cultural context, this low rate of disclosure can be explained by the fact that in Japan isolation from the group caused by the stigma of cancer is an occurrence which can cause great distress in a country which values maintaining good relations with one's peers.[26] Even in the US some groups may shun information. Thus, among the Navajo Indians there is a belief that giving bad news can actually make it happen[27] and certain cultural groups may prefer that decision making be left to others.[28] A recent survey showed that among 48 members of the medical staff of a hospital in Mexico City, 96% of nurses and 35% of doctors did not use the word cancer in discussions with oncology patients.[29] Other studies have shown a disclosure rate as low as 3% in Egypt[30] and 25% in Italy.[31] In Spain only 32% of incurable cancer patients knew their diagnosis.[32] Among French gastroenterologists, in the case of incurable disease, the spouse or family was more likely to be told than the patient.[33] As the influence of Western medicine and availability of cancer-related information spreads, more information is being given to patients in non-Western cultures.[34] However, a method for giving bad news must take cultural issues into account. By determining exactly how the patient wants bad news handled and how much he or she would like the family or others involved in decision making, one can respect both patient autonomy and cultural values.

How can knowing bad news help the patient?

Many patients today wish to be informed of treatment options and incomplete information will thwart their wishes to be involved in decision making and treatment planning. Studies indicate that the manner in which bad news is disclosed may affect the patient's satisfaction, level of hopefulness, and subsequent psychological adjustment.[35–40] Despite these important outcomes, patients still experience significant information gaps in their basic understanding of their disease status prognosis and purpose of their treatment.[41–47] The idea that the unfavorable information can do psychological harm is unfounded.[48] In fact, a multicentered study on patient preferences for end-of-life discussions revealed that patients are more concerned about having accurate disease-related information than being given an unrealistic expectation of treatment outcome.[49] When a physician is uncomfortable in discussing palliative care with the patient, it may also result in the patient receiving anticancer treatment beyond the point where it is still therapeutic[50] and delay referral to hospice.[51]

Can a plan or strategy for breaking bad news help the clinician?

Curricula for training in oncology have not traditionally included communication skills as part of the curriculum,[52] although resource manuals are now beginning to become available.[53] Learning how to break bad news by observing experienced clinicians or by trial and error seems to be the predominant method by which physicians learn this task. However, this does not guarantee that the observer will acquire a method that will be helpful to the patient or even comfortable for him or herself. Breaking bad news almost always precipitates anxiety in the physician.[13] Misguided attempts to allay that anxiety may lead the physician to control the amount and tone of the bad news message.[23,54–56] However, camouflaging the bad news with false or premature reassurance, avoiding discussing prognosis, or disclosing only the less unpleasant aspects of the clinical situation, may reduce physician stress in the short term but less than full disclosure may leave patients feeling that their physician has been less than honest with them. On the other hand, taking the time to listen, address patient concerns and involve them in treatment decisions are steps likely to result in high patient satisfaction. Physicians who are comfortable in breaking bad news may have reduced stress and burnout.[57]

Several recent review papers have concluded that interviews about breaking bad news should include a number of key elements which facilitate the flow of information.[58–61] These recommendations are reflected in a practical step-by-step technique to offer specific practical advice as to how to mobilize hope or manage the patient's emotional reaction to the bad news, situations which many physicians find to be the most difficult aspect of breaking bad news.

A six-step approach to breaking bad news – SPIKES

The act of actually conveying the bad news is only one step in a complex encounter between the physician and patient. This implies that the task of breaking bad news can best be approached by describing the process and individual steps involved in the encounter and applying well-known principles of communication and counseling. The actual process of giving bad news involves four goals: preparation, information gathering, conveying information, and providing support. This process can be broken down into a number of steps which are practical and focus on facilitating information flow based upon the patient's wishes and needs for information. They are incorporated in a protocol called SPIKES, an inelegant but useful acronym which can assist in remembering the steps of breaking bad news.

Goals of the bad news interview

The SPIKES protocol permits the clinician to fulfill the four essential goals of breaking bad news in six steps.[62] The first goal involves gathering information from the patient. The purpose of this is to determine what the patient already knows and their readiness to hear the bad news. In order to gather the information the physician must do two things. First, he must provide a setting which facilitates the transmission and collection of information. Second, he must ask questions in a manner as to maximize the flow of useful information. This task is explained in Steps 1, 2, and 3 of SPIKES. Next, the physician must transmit information, in accordance with the patient's information needs and wishes, in a way that the patient can understand and so that the physician can determine what the patient did and did not understand. This is covered in Step 4 of SPIKES. A third goal of the protocol is to permit the clinician to support the patient through specific verbal techniques designed to reduce the emotional impact and psychological isolation experienced by the patient as a consequence of the bad news. These include making empathic responses, eliciting patient concerns, and validating patient feelings. The final goal is to develop a strategy in the form of a treatment plan with the input and cooperation of the patient. Each of these goals is associated with a specific operationally assigned task and also with associated skills necessary to complete these tasks.

S – Setting up the interview (Step 1)

Sometimes the physical setting causes interviews about sensitive topics to flounder. An inappropriate setting can engender distrust and antagonism in the opening moments of the interview. For example, patients are not likely to react favorably when troubling news is disclosed when they are still waking up from anesthesia and are unable to completely comprehend information and ask questions.[23] The setting and timing are thus of great importance, and although such details may at first seem a little petty, they are crucial to the success of the interview. Unless the setting has a semblance of privacy, and is at least partially conducive to undistracted and focused discussion, the goals of the interview are unlikely to be met. For those reasons, it is worth spending a few minutes setting up the physical context of the interview, optimizing privacy, using appropriate body language, and starting the interview by employing basic listening and facilitation skills.

In addition to arranging the physical setting, the clinician should also prepare himself mentally for the discussion. Because bad news interviews often elicit emotional responses in the patient and/or family member, the clinician should be prepared to respond to them (see Step 4). As the messenger of bad news, it is not unusual for the clinician to feel sad for the patient. While this is often inevitable, it is helpful for the bearer of the bad news to frequently remind himself that he or she is not responsible for it (even in cases where patients may be blameful). This is especially true when the physician has had a long-standing relationship with the patient or when hopes for cure or positive results have been high.

Some of the important guidelines include the following.

Arrange for privacy

If you are going to the patient's room, shut the door and reduce distractions from radio or TV (after you ask the patient's permission).

Involve significant others

Most patients want to have someone with them when bad news is disclosed. When many family members are present, it is helpful to ask the patient to choose a family representative to be present during the discussion. In this way the doctor will be able to direct his attention on the patient.

Sit down

Standing while the patient is sitting or lying is not conducive to information exchange because it is intimidating to the patient and gives the message you may be leaving at any time. Sitting down next to the patient and unbuttoning your jacket or lab coat is an important signal that you have something important to say and is also a sign that you will not be rushed. If the patient is in the hospital, a chair by the bedside is ideal, but if there isn't one, sit on the bed after asking the patient's permission to do so. When you sit, try not to have barriers between you and the patient (including relatives). In an office, set your chair across the corner of the desk near the patient's (rather than directly across the desk). If you have recently examined the patient in clinic, allow them to get dressed before beginning the conversation.

Try to look attentive and calm

Move your chair close to the patient's bedside. Maintaining eye contact may be uncomfortable but it is an important way of establishing a connection with the patient and a sign to the patient that you are listening. It is often helpful to lower your eyes, breaking eye contact, if the patient becomes tearful or angry. Having a box of tissues nearby if the patient becomes upset will allow you to respond to the patient's weeping. Touching the patient during the interview if both you and the patient are comfortable with it (the patient will withdraw if he or she is not) is also a way of connecting with the patient and is an expression of solidarity. It is done on the arm or forearm (or by holding the patient's hand).

Change to listening mode

Many communication skills facilitate dialogue and send the message that you are there to listen (as well as to inform). Most valuable of these are (1) silence, (2) repetition, and (3) acknowledgement. The use of silence simply means that when the patient talks you are careful not to interrupt before the patient is finished. Repetition means using one important word or phrase from the patient's last sentence in your first sentence. Acknowledgement, by nodding your head, making statements such as "I see" or smiling at appropriate points show the patient you are listening.

Management of time and interruptions

Give the patient a clear indication of any time constraints you have and handle interruptions (phones or pagers) without ignoring or snubbing the patient you are with. Putting your pager on silent alarm or asking a colleague to answer pages for you while you are with the patient will prevent undesirable interruptions from occurring.

P – Assessing the patient's Perception (Step 2)

Step 2 and Step 3 are the pivotal points of the interview, when you implement the axiom "before you tell, ask." This means that the clinician needs to gather important information from the patient before he can communicate the bad news. The first piece of information (Step 2) is to gather from the patient a reasonably accurate picture of how the patient perceives the medical situation – what it is and whether it is serious or not, and what their expectations are for treatment. This is particularly important on the first interview since the patient may harbor misinformation, fears, and unrealistic expectations. The exact words used to do this will vary according to your own style and comfort. However, questions should be open-ended to allow the patient to tell things in his or her own words; for example, "What have you been told about your medical situation so far?" or "what is your understanding of the reasons we did the MRI?" As the patient responds, it is important to listen to the patient's vocabulary and level of comprehension. Based on this you can assess how large (or small) is the gap between the patient's expectations and the medical situation (this gap is often unexpectedly wide,[42,43,47]) and formulate your explanation of the illness (see Step 4) in terms the patient will understand. With new patients who have been previously evaluated or treated it can be helpful to have them narrate the history of their illness. This can accomplish the goal of determining if the patient is engaging in any variation of denial: wishful thinking, omission of essential but unfavorable aspects of the illness, or unrealistic expectations of treatment.[63,64]

I – Getting the patient's Invitation (Step 3)

Although, as discussed above, most patients today want full disclosure of information concerning their diagnosis and prognosis, a few do not wish to know the results of tests and laboratory investigations and may prefer that the physician focus on what is to be done next. Shunning information is a valid psychological coping mechanism[65] especially as a cancer progresses.[66] Obtaining overt permission to disclose information respects the patient's right not to know. Permission is best obtained at the time of ordering tests. This will give the physician the opportunity to plan the subsequent discussion with the patient.

As with Step 2, the question concerning disclosure depends on your own style and the connection you and the patient have. Examples: "How would you like me to give you the information about the test results? Would you like me to explain the medical information in some detail or would you rather I sketched out the results and spent more time on discussing a treatment plan? Shall I call you when the information is available or would you like to come in so we can go over the next steps?" If the patient does not want to know the information (a rare event these days), it is a good idea to show that you respect that choice and will answer any questions that the patient might have in the future, and offer to talk to a friend or relative if that is what the patient wants. A second but equally important task is to determine the patient's expectations of treatment. While many patients may hope for a cure they also expect to receive the best treatment available, have good pain control, and have expert consultation when it is needed.[37] Expectations may include finding a cure, effect a remission, freedom from pain, receiving the best treatment possible, or other aspects of quality of life. Unless the physician knows what the patient is hoping for he may tend to assume it is always cure. Knowing early on what the patient expects will allow you to lay out a realistic treatment plan and, in cases of advanced disease, begin to prepare for the possibility of an unfavorable outcome. This strategy of "hoping for the best but preparing for the worst" is usually quite acceptable to patients and allows the clinician to offer encouragement while avoiding creating unrealistic expectations of treatment.

K – Giving the patient knowledge and information (Step 4)

A "warning shot" best precedes transmission of negative information that alerts the patient to the arrival of bad news.[67] This strategy of warning allows the patient to psychologically begin to make the transition to being less well.[68] Examples of warning shots include "Unfortunately, I've got some bad news to tell you" or "I'm sorry to tell you that . . . ."

Giving medical facts, the one-way part of the clinician–patient dialogue, may be improved by a few simple guidelines: start at the level of comprehension and vocabulary your patient demonstrated earlier in the interview (a technique sometimes called aligning); always use nontechnical language, and avoid scientific (and there-fore esoteric) jargon. "Medspeak," the clinical language all of us use, is an effective and highly compressed medical language, but it is often unintelligible to everyone else. Try and use words such as "spread" instead of "metastasized" and "sample of tissue" instead of "biopsy." Give information in small chunks. Pause every three or four sentences and check whether the other person understood what you said (for example, punctuate the information with phrases like "Do you see what I mean?" or "Am I making sense?" "Is this making clear so far?" "Do you follow me?" Tailor the amount and rate of information giving to the patient's response and understanding. If he or she clearly understands what you are saying, move on. If not, go over the ground again. As reactions and emotions arise in response to what you are saying, acknowledge and respond to them. This should be an invariable part of information giving, but may be thought of as a separate step (Step 5) in the protocol. When the patient's prognosis is poor, phrases such as "there is nothing more we can do for you" or "we have nothing more to offer you" should be avoided. These phrases are correct if the only goal of treatment is cure or remission of disease. They are inconsistent, however, with the desire of many patients for pain relief, symptom control, and reassurance that they will not suffer even if no cure is available.[69]

E — Addressing the patient's Emotions with empathic, validating, and exploratory responses (Step 5)

Responding to the patient's emotions is one of the most difficult challenges of break-ing bad news. As previously mentioned, physician anxiety or unpleasant feelings can be a powerful deterrent to full disclosure of information.[12]

Empathic and validating statements provide the physician with a strategy to counterbalance the awkward or uncomfortable feeling associated with being the messenger of bad news. When the physician demonstrates solidarity with and sup-port for the patient, it reduces the psychological isolation of the person who is receiving the negative information.[70] An empathic response consists of three steps. First, listen for and identify emotions. Whenever there are emotions expressed an empathic response is indicated. Second, identify the emotion experienced by the patient by naming it to oneself. Third, identify the reason for the emotion. This is usually connected to the bad news. If you are not sure, ask the patient and then let the patient know that you have connected the two by making an empathic statement. An example:

Doctor: Unfortunately your tumor is at a very advanced stage and the likelihood of our getting a cure at this point is very unlikely.
Patient: How could this be? I've always taken care of myself. No one in my family ever had cancer!
Doctor: I know that this is very difficult for you to believe, especially since you've always been healthy.

Until an emotion is cleared it will be difficult to go on to discuss other issues. Another important aspect of the empathic response is that clinicians can also apply it to themselves ("I also wish the news were better"). Empathic responses do not mean that you need to be in the patient's shoes and experience his or her emotions. An empathic response indicates your perception of the patient's emotion, not your experiencing of it. It is useful to follow the empathic response with a validating response, such as "it's understandable that you would feel that way," which lets the patient know that his or her feelings are legitimate. When patients feel embarrassed by their own emotional reactions, letting them know that it is normal to feel the way they do is a show of support.

Sometimes emotions may be clearly expressed, such as when the patient cries. At other times they may not be expressed, such as when the patient is silent. This latter situation requires that the physician make an exploratory response before he can make an empathic reponse ("Can you tell me what you are thinking?"). Sometimes emotions may be subtle or indirectly expressed or disguised, as in thinly veiled disappointment or anger: "I guess this means I'll have to suffer through chemotherapy again."

Combining empathic, exploratory, and validating statements is one of the most powerful ways of providing support for the patient. It allows the patient to feel less isolated, that the doctor is aware of the patient as a person and that he or she recognizes that their feelings or thoughts are normal and to be expected.[71,72]

S – Strategy and Summary (Step 6)

A crucial element of the breaking bad news interview is the discussion of a clear plan for dealing with the medical problem. Patients who have a clear plan for the future are likely to be less anxious and uncertain. However, patients may be in a state of shock, anxiety, or dissociation immediately after hearing the bad news and therefore they may not be prepared to hear or discuss the treatment plan at that time. Here the axiom "before you tell, ask" is again pertinent. That is, it is important to ask the patient if they are ready to discuss a plan or if they would like to return. Many oncologists in fact routinely schedule a separate visit to discuss details of further treatment, especially in newly diagnosed patients.

The discussion of a treatment plan is also an opportunity for the physician to present treatment options. Many cancer therapies involve choices and most patients wish to be informed about them.[19,20] In some cases, such as the choice of treatment for some forms of breast cancer, there is actually a legal mandate to explain treatment options to the patient.[22] For some physicians the discussion of treatment options may be an uncomfortable departure from their view of themselves as the experts. Others may feel that they know the patient well enough to know the treatment that he or she would choose. However, discussing options with the patient fulfills the ethical (and sometimes legal) requirement to ensure patient autonomy and informed consent in decision making. Explaining treatment options to the patient is likely to establish the perception, in the patient's mind, that the physician regards him or her as a partner in the relationship and that the patient can trust that the physician regards their wishes as important. Checking the patient's understanding of your explanation is also important, as patients may overestimate the efficacy of treatment and the chances of survival and misunderstand the purpose of treatment, be it curative or palliative.[64] They also may distort statistics, as in the wife of a patient with malignant glioblastoma who, when told that they were able to remove about 75% of the tumor, later reported that her husband had a 75% chance of a cure.

In cases where the treatment for the particular cancer is not associated with a high probability of cure or remission, the physician can introduce the idea of palliative care as opposed to more aggressive anticancer treatment. Although a good proportion of patients will choose aggressive treatment, this strategy will make having a subsequent discussion about hospice with the patient less stressful. The physician who takes total responsibility for treatment decisions is more likely to feel he has disappointed the patient when treatment is not effective and the patient's disease progresses. This may be especially true when he has been overly optimistic about the outcome of the therapy he is proposing. A patient with Stage 3 lung cancer reported that his physician told him that he was going to make him the "poster boy for lung cancer." While there is no way of knowing whether this is exactly what was said, the interaction created unbridled optimism in the patient, which was later dashed when the patient failed to respond to treatment.

In following a strategy, check frequently with the patient about his or her understanding of the information provided, making sure that the patient comprehends your explanation.

Finally, give a brief summary of the ground covered in the interview, and before closing give the patient an opportunity to identify any issues that have not been discussed. If you do not have time to discuss these now, you will at least have created the opening agenda for the next interview.

Do clinicians find the SPIKES protocol useful?

In a survey of participants at a workshop at the Annual Meeting of the American Society of Clinical Oncology in 1998, we asked respondents (there were 500) if they felt the SPIKES protocol would be useful in their practice. Ninety-nine percent of those attending found that the SPIKES protocol was practical and easy to understand. They reported, however, that using empathic, validating, and exploratory statements to respond to patient emotions would be the greatest challenge of the protocol.[62]

Does the SPIKES protocol reflect the consensus of experts?

A recent review of the literature showed that very few studies have sampled patient opinion as to their preferences for disclosure of unfavorable medical information.[13] However, of the scarce information available, the content of the SPIKES protocol closely reflects the consensus of cancer patients and professionals as to the essential elements in breaking bad news.[6,13,58,73]

Does the SPIKES protocol reflect patient preferences for receiving bad news?

In a recent study,[74] we showed that cancer patients were able to identify three essential factors which defined their preferences for how bad news should be delivered: content: what information is given; facilitation: how the information is given; support: how the physician addresses the emotional and other concerns the patient may have. Although these findings are preliminary, the steps of the SPIKES protocol can be said to be "patient-focused" in addressing areas which patients themselves feel are important in this important area of communication.

How should the SPIKES protocol be taught?

It should be obvious from the discussion above that the SPIKES protocol represents a process of giving bad news which consists of a number of steps. It would be unrealistic to expect that clinicians master all of these steps at once. The aspect of SPIKES likely to be found to be most difficult is handling patient emotions[62] because it requires practice to master the techniques of making empathic responses, asking about patient concerns, and validating their statements. It also requires that the clinician reflect on his own feelings of helplessness and perhaps desire to make things better for the patient by downplaying the bad news. The SPIKES protocol has been incorporated into filmed scenarios which appear as part of two CD–ROMs on physician–patient communication which readers may find a useful self-instruction tool.[75,76]

At the University of Texas M.D. Anderson Cancer Center we used the SPIKES protocol and the CD–ROMs to teach how to break bad news in workshops for oncologists and oncology fellows. The workshops had a didactic component in which the steps were formally presented and demonstrated followed by a practical component in which clinicians worked with simulated patients or role-played, portraying patients whom they had found it difficult to break bad news to in their practice. We evaluated the participants of two of these workshops attended by 29 oncology faculty members and fellows. Those attending reported increased confidence in carrying out a number of verbal and nonverbal tasks associated with breaking bad news.[77,78] Others in different teaching settings have also found the workshop format to be useful.[79–81]

Summary

In medicine the ability to communicate effectively with patients and families can no longer be thought of as an optional skill. It will in fact soon become a required skill for those wishing to recertify in internal medicine. It is an essential tool in conveying disease-related information to the patient and is important in facilitating patient participation in important decisions. Communication skills can be taught and retained. The SPIKES protocol for breaking bad news is a specialized form of skill training in doctor–patient communication, which is employed in teaching postgraduate doctors communication skills and gives the clinician a step-wise strategy, which can be practiced until it is comfortable: it is also brief and easy to remember. Furthermore, it focuses on the patient's own particular state at the time – first in ascertaining what the patient knows and wants to know, and then by addressing the patient's particular set of worries and questions. The subsequent use of empathic responses gives the physician a strategy for handling strong emotion through the use of empathic, clarifying, and validating responses. These responses form the basis for patient support, an essential psychological intervention for distress.

We are currently in the process of determining whether the SPIKES protocol can reduce the stress of breaking bad news for the physician, and also improve the interview and the support as experienced by the patient. We are further investigating patient preferences for bad news disclosure across a variety of disease sites and by age, gender, and stage of disease. We are also conducting long-term follow-up of workshops in which the protocol has been taught to oncologists and oncology trainees to determine empirically how it is implemented.

REFERENCES

1 Cassileth BR, Zupkis RV, Sutton-Smith K et al. Information and participation preferences among cancer patients. *Ann Intern Med* 1980;92:832–6.

2 Blanchard CG, Labrecque MS, Ruckdeschel JC et al. Information and decision-making preferences of hospitalized adult cancer patients. *Soc Sci Med* 1988;27:1139–45.

3 Davison BJ, Degner LF, Morgan TR. Information and decision-making preferences of men with prostate cancer. *Oncol Nurs Forum* 1995;22:1401–8.

4 Sutherland HJ, Llewellyn-Thomas HA, Lockwood GA et al. Cancer patients: their desire for information and participation in treatment decisions. *J R Soc Med* 1989;82:260–3.

5 Meredith C, Symonds P, Webster L et al. Information needs of cancer patients in west Scotland: Cross sectional survey of patients' views. *Br Med J* 1996;313:724–6.

6 Benbassat J, Pilpel D, Tidhar M. Patients' preferences for participation in clinical decision-making: a review of published surveys. *Behav Med* 1998;24:81–8.

7 Caplan G. *Principles of Preventive Psychiatry*. New York: Basic Books, 1964.

8 Buckman R. *Breaking Bad News: A Guide for Health Care Professionals*. Baltimore: Johns Hopkins University Press, 1992.

9 Fallowfield L, Lipkin M, Hall A. Teaching senior oncologists communication skills: results from phase I of a comprehensive longitudinal program in the United Kingdom. *J Clin Oncol* 1998;16:1961–8.

10 Tesser A, Rosen S, Tesser M. On the reluctance to communicate undesirable messages (the MUM effect). A field study. *Psychol Rep* 1971;29:651–4.

11 Tesser A, Conlee MC. Recipient emotionality as a determinant of the transmission of bad news. *Proc Annu Conv Am Psychol Assoc*, 1973;247–8.

12 Buckman R. Breaking bad news: why is it still so difficult? *Br Med J (Clinic Res Edn)* 1984;288:1597–9.

13 Ptacek JT, Eberhardt TL. Breaking bad news. A review of the literature. *J Am Med Assoc* 1996;276:496–502.

14 Fitts WT, Ravid IS. What should physicians tell patients with cancer? *J Am Med Assoc* 1953;153:901–4.

15 Friedman HS. Physician management of dying patients: an exploration. *Psychiatry Med* 1970;295–305.

16 Oken D. What to tell cancer patients: a study of medical attitudes. *J Am Med Assoc* 1961;175:1120–8.

17 Morris B, Abram C. *Making Healthcare Decisions. The Ethical and Legal Implications of Informed Consent in the Practitioner–Patient Relationship*. Washington, United States Superintendent.

18 Novack DH, Plumer R, Smith RL et al. Changes in physicians' attitudes toward telling the cancer patient. *J Am Med Assoc* 1979;241:897–900.

19 Degner LF, Kristjanson LJ, Bowman D et al. Information needs and decisional preferences in women with breast cancer. *J Am Med Assoc* 1997; 277:1485–92.

20 Jenkins V, Fallowfield L, Saul J. Information needs of patients with cancer: results from a large study in UK cancer centers. *Br J Cancer* 2001;84:48–51.

21 Annas G. Informed consent, cancer, and truth in prognosis. *N Engl J Med* 1994;330:223–5.

22 Goldberg RJ. Disclosure of information to adult cancer patients: issues and update. *J Clin Oncol* 1984;2:948–55.

23 Lind SE, DelVecchio GM, Seidel. Telling the diagnosis of cancer. *J Clin Oncol* 1989;7: 583–9.

24 Holland J. Giving bad news. Is there a kinder, gentler way? *Cancer* 1999;86:738–40.

25 Koinuma N. An international perspective on full disclosure. In *Proceedings of the Second International Congress of Psycho-Oncology*, Kobe, Japan, October 19–22, 1995, p. 84.

26 Uchitome Y, Yamawaki S. Truth-telling practice in cancer care in Japan. In *Communication with the Cancer Patient. Information and Truth*, ed. A Surbone, M Zwitter. *Ann NY Acad Sci* 1997;809:290–9.

27 Carrese JA, Rhodes LA. Western bioethics on the Navajo reservation. *J Am Med Assoc* 1995;274:826–9.

28 Blackhall LJ, Murphy ST, Frank G, Michel V, Azen S. Ethnicity and attitudes toward patient autonomy. *J Am Med Assoc* 1995;274:820–5.

29 Torrecillas L. Communication of the cancer diagnosis to Mexican patients. *Ann NY Acad Sci* 1997;809:188–96.

30 El-Ghazali S. Is it wise to tell the truth, the whole truth and nothing but the truth to a cancer patient? *Ann NY Acad Sci* 1997;809:97–108.

31 Grassi L, Messina EG, Magnani K, Valle E, Cartei G. Physicians' attitudes to and problems with truth-telling to cancer patients. *Support Care Cancer* 2000;8:40–5.

32 Centano-Cortez C, Nunez-Olarte JM. Questioning diagnosis disclosure in terminal cancer patients. A prospective study evaluating patient's responses. *Palliat Med* 1994;8:39–44.

33 Adenis A, Venin P, Hecquet B. What do gastroenterologists, surgeons and oncologists tell patients with colon cancer? Results of a survey from the Northern France area. *Bull Cancer* 1998;85:803.

34 Sorbone A. Truth telling to the patient. *J Am Med Assoc* 1992;268:1661–2.

35 Ford S, Fallowfield L, Lewis S. Doctor–patient interactions in oncology. *Soc Sci Med.*

36 Butow PN, Dunn SM, Tattersall MH. Communication with cancer patients: does it matter? *J Palliat Care* 1995;11:34–8.

37 Sardell AN, Trierweiler SJ. Disclosing the cancer diagnosis. Procedures that influence patient hopefulness. *Cancer* 1993;72:3355–65.

38 Roberts CS, Cox CE, Reintgen DS et al. Influence of physician communication on newly diagnosed breast cancer patients' psychologic adjustment and decision-making. *Cancer* 1994;74:336–41.

39 Slavin LA, O'Malley JE, Koocher GP, Foster DJ. Communication of the cancer diagnosis to pediatric patients: impact on long-term adjustment. *Am J Psychiatry* 1982; 139:179–83.

40 Last BF, van Veldhuizen AM. Information about diagnosis and prognosis related to anxiety and depression in children with cancer aged 8–16 years. *Eur J Cancer* 1996;32:290–4.

41 Eidinger RN, Schapira DV. Cancer patients' insight into their treatment, prognosis and unconvential therapies. *Cancer* 1984:53:2736–40.

42 Mackillop WJ, Stewart WE, Ginsberg AD, Stewart SS. Cancer patients' perceptions of their disease and its treatment. *Br J Cancer* 1998;58:355–8.

43 Quirt CF, McKillop WJ, Ginsberg AD et al. Do doctors know when their patients don't? A survey of doctor–patient communication in lung cancer. *Lung Cancer* 1997;18:1–20.

44 Siminoff LA, Fetting JH, Abeloff MD. Doctor–patient communication about breast cancer adjuvant therapy. *J Clin Oncol* 1989;7:1192–200.

45 Weeks JC, Cook Ef, O'Day SJ et al. Relationship between cancer patients' predictions of prognosis and their treatment preferences. *J Am Med Assoc* 1998;279:1709–14.

46 Haidet P, Hamel MB, Davis RB et al. Outcomes, preferences for resuscitation, and physician-patient communication among patients with metastatic colorectal cancer. SUPPORT investigators. Study to understand prognoses and preferences for outcomes and risks of treatment. *Ann Intern Med* 127:1–12.

47 Chan A, Woodruff R. Communicating with patients with advanced cancer. *J Palliat Care* 1997;13:29–33.

48 Cassem NH, Stewart RS. Management and care of the dying patient. *Int J Psychiatry Med* 1975;6:293–304.

49 Pfeiffer MP, Sidorov JE, Smith AC et al. The discussion of end-of-life medical care by primary care patients and physicians. A multicentered study using structured qualitative interviews. *J Gen Intern Med* 1994;9:82–8.

50 Mayer RJ, Cassel C, Emmanuel E. Report of the task force on end of life issues. Presented at the Annual Meeting of the American Society of Clinical Oncology, Los Angeles California, May 16, 1998.

51 Emanuel EJ, Yinong Young-Xu, Ashe A et al. How much chemotherapy are patients receiving at the end of life. *Proc Am Soc Clin Oncol*, 2001; Abstract 953.

52 American Society of Clinical Oncology. Training resource document for curriculum development in medical oncology. *J Clin Oncol* 1998;15:372–9.

53 Optimizing patient care: the importance of symptom management. *Am Soc Clin Oncol*, 2001.

54 Maguire P. Barriers to psychological care of the dying. *Br Med J (Clin Res Edn)* 1985;291: 1711–13.

55 Buckman R. Breaking bad news: why is it still so difficult? *Br Med J (Clin Res Edn)* 1984; 288:1597–9.

56 Taylor C. Telling bad news: physicians and the disclosure of undesirable information. *Sociol Health Illness* 1988;10:120–32.

57 Ramirez AJ, Graham J, Richards MA et al. Burnout and psychiatric disorder among cancer clinicians [see comments]. *Br J Cancer* 1995;71:1263–9.

58 Girgis A, Sanson-Fisher RW. Breaking bad news: consensus guidelines for medical practitioners. *J Clin Oncol* 1995;13:2449–56.

59 Donovan K. Breaking bad news (I). *World Health Organization Monograph 93e-2B*, 3–14, 1993.

60 Premi JN. Communicating bad news to patients (2). *World Health Organization Monograph 93.2BV*, 15–24.

61 Girgis A, Sanson-Fisher RW. Breaking bad news I: current best advice for clinicians. *Behav Med* 1998;24:53–9.

62 Baile WF, Buckman R, Lenzi R, Glober G, Beale E, Kudelka AP. SPIKES – A six-step protocol for delivering bad news: application to the patient with cancer. *Oncologist* 2000;5:302–3411.

63 Lubinsky MS. Bearing bad news: dealing with the mimics of denial. *J Genet Counsel* 1999;3: 5–12.

64 Gattellari M, Butow PN, Tattersall MH, Dunn SM, MacLeod CA. Misunderstanding in cancer patients: why shoot the messenger. *Ann Oncol* 1999;10:39–46.

65 Miller SM. Monitoring versus blunting styles of coping with cancer influence the information patients want and need about their disease. Implications for cancer screening and management. *Cancer* 1995;76:167–77.

66 Butow PN, Maclean M, Dunn SM, Tattersall MH, Boyer MJ. The dynamics of change: cancer patients' preferences for information, involvement and support. *Ann Oncol* 1997; 8:857–63.

67 Maguire P, Faulkner A. Communicate with cancer patients: 1. Handling bad news and difficult questions. *Br Med J* 1988;297:907–9.

68 Maynard DW. How to tell patients bad news: the strategy of "forecasting". *Cleve Clin J Med* 1997;64:181–2.

69 Greisinger AJ, Lorimor RJ, Aday LA, Winn RJ, Baile WF. Terminally ill cancer patients: their most important concerns. *Cancer Pract* 1997;5:147–54.

70 Suchman AL. A model of empathic communication in the medical interview. *J Am Med Assoc* 1997;277:678–82.

71 Matthews DA, Suchman AL, Branch WT. Enhancing the therapeutic potential of patient-clinician relationships. *Ann Intern Med* 1993;118:973–7.

72 Novack DH. Therapeutic aspects of the clinical encounter. *J Gen Intern Med* 1987;2:346–55.

73 Girgis A, Sanson-Fisher RW. Breaking bad news 1: Current best advice for clinicians. *Behav Med* 1998;24:53–9.

74 Parker P, Baile WF, Lenzi R, DeMoor C, Cohen L. Breaking bad news about cancer: patient preferences for communication. *J Clin Oncol* 2001;19:2049–56.

75 Buckman R, Korsch B, Baile WF. *A Practical Guide to Communication Skills in Clinical Practice* (4 CD–ROM set). Toronto: Medical Audio-Visual Communications, 1998.

76 Buckman R, Baile WF. A Practical Guide to Communication Skills in Cancer Care (3 CD–ROM set). Toronto: Medical Audio-Visual Communications, 2001.

77 Baile WF, Lenzi R, Kudelka AP et al. Improving physician–patient communication in cancer care: outcome of a workshop for oncologists. *J Cancer Educ* 1997;12:166–73.

78 Baile WF, Kudelka AF, Beale EA et al. Communication skills training in oncology: Description and preliminary outcomes of workshops on breaking bad news and managing patient reactions to illness. *Cancer* (in press).

79 Vaidya VU, Greenberg L, Kantilal MP, Strauss L, Pollack MM. Teaching physicians how to break bad news. A 1-day workshop using standardized patients. *Arch Pediatr* Adolesc Med 1999;153:419–22.

80 Garg A, Buckman R, Kason Y. Teaching medical students how to break bad news. *Can Med Assoc J* 1997;156:1159–64.

81 Maguire P, Fairbairn S, Fletcher C. Consultation skills of young doctors: I – Benefits of feedback training in interviewing as students persist. *Br Med J (Clin Res Edn)* 1986;292:1573–6.

10

The use of complementary/alternative medicine

Mary Ann Richardson

The National Center for Complementary and Alternative Medicine, Bethesda

Introduction

Complementary and alternative medicine (CAM) or integrated therapies range from drug-like interventions with single herbs to complex herbal formulas, high dose vitamins and supplements, mind–body–spiritual interventions, physical approaches, energy-based therapies, and multifaceted treatment regimens. The lack of standardized products, the complexity of multiple regimens, and individualized treatments pose challenges to evaluation by researchers. Despite the lack of evidence to support efficacy, many patients with advanced cancer seek these approaches. As interest in CAM therapies continues to rise with growing public concerns about appropriate end-of-life care, this chapter presents a rationale for discussing CAM with patients and exploring the potential role of these therapies in conventional oncology care.

Palliative care has been described as "...care that takes place in a context where...cure is no longer possible and disease modification provides diminishing returns."[1] The goal of palliative care is to provide for any unmet physical, psychosocial, and spiritual needs of terminally ill patients and their families.[2] The most important concerns expressed by hospice patients are the existential, spiritual, familial, physical, and emotional aspects of illness; however, these concerns have rarely been the focus of care at the end of life.[3,4] When cure is not an option, maintaining quality of life and controlling symptoms are more appropriate than potentially distressing treatments associated with limited improvement but physical and emotional suffering. Social and cultural forces are demanding a more holistic approach[5] to convey empathy and compassion[6] and support the dignity and quality of life in the final days.[7] The palliative care community acknowledges that therapies beyond technologic approaches are needed to improve quality of life and relieve suffering[8] and recognizes the need for education about CAM.[9] Many patients allocate their limited resources and time on CAM therapies in search of hope, whether they have refused or failed conventional treatment, or simply wish to complement conventional treatment. Therefore, oncologists should be willing to discuss these approaches and their potential role.[10]

Use of complementary/alternative medicine by advanced cancer patients

CAM are healthcare practices that are not an integral part of conventional medicine and are grouped into five major domains by the National Center for Complementary and Alternative Medicine (NCCAM): (1) alternative medical systems (traditional Chinese medicine, homeopathy); (2) mind–body interventions (meditation, imagery, relaxation); (3) biologically based treatments (melatonin, herbals, mushrooms, vitamins); (4) manipulative and body-based methods (yoga, massage); and (5) energy therapies (QiGong, therapeutic touch).[11] The definition of CAM is continually changing as research determines approaches to be safe and efficacious, and thus integrates them into mainstream medical practices.

CAM is used at various stages along the disease continuum by approximately 31.4% (range 7–64%) of cancer patients worldwide[12] and by upwards of 70% in cancer research and treatment centers in the US.[13] Among patients with advanced disease, prevalence of use ranges from 7% (70% would have used it if available)[14] to 26% and 60% in Canada,[15–17] 63% to 64% in Hong Kong[18] and Taiwan,[19] to 61% in Austria,[20] 58% in Germany[21] and 42% in Norway.[22] Use does not differ for men and women,[16,18,19] but is higher among younger patients.[16,19]

Herbs and herbal teas (Essiac, echinacea, traditional Chinese medicine) are used predominately,[16,18] but patients often cannot identify the herbs or pills and refer to them as medications not prescribed by their doctor.[14,19] Other commonly used agents are vitamin and mineral supplements (beta carotene, vitamin C, melatonin, enzymes, hydrazine sulfate, coenzyme-Q10),[16,17] mind–body approaches (imagery/visualization, faith healing, meditation),[17] and biologics (cartilage and mushrooms).[17] Most patients use a modality for less than 3 months[16,18] and seek more aggressive therapies in the later stages of disease.[20]

When the prognosis is dismal and mainstream medicine has nothing further to offer, patients want hope.[10] Hope may be the single greatest reason cancer patients seek CAM therapies and includes hope for disease control, cure, and survival; relief of pain and symptoms; and quality of life.[16–19,23] Among patients with metastatic disease, 60% believed the CAM treatments could control their disease, and 37% believed it would provide a cure.[14] Similarly, patients are willing to accept conventional treatments that offer minimal benefits.[24]

In a large cohort of terminally ill cancer patients, those who believed they would survive for at least 6 months were more than twice as likely (odds ratio = 2.6;

95% confidence interval 1.8, 3.7) to favor aggressive, life-saving treatments than patients who believed they had a small chance (as little as 10%) of not surviving for 6 months.[25] Among 1063 patients with colon and lung cancer, preferences shifted to comfort rather than life-extending care as their health declined; however, more than 40% died in pain and 28% in severe confusion.[4] Patients with advanced disease need expanded choices for less damaging and more supportive palliative treatments to address their emotional, social, cultural, and spiritual needs when quality of life is the therapeutic endpoint.

Potential role for CAM therapies

Many CAM therapies are noninvasive and possible options for the clinical setting to offer comfort and hope to patients. Although a review of the CAM research field is beyond the scope of this chapter, a growing body of literature suggests that music, aromatherapy, massage, and therapeutic touch may comfort patients with advanced disease and improve their life quality.[26–28] A recent systematic review of CAM for palliation of pain, dyspnea, and nausea associated with cancer and chronic obstructive pulmonary disease (COPD) identified 15 studies with cancer patients.[29] Interventions included a range of approaches: transcutaneous electrical nerve stimulation (TENS); acupuncture and acupressure; massage either alone or combined with aromatherapy, psychological approaches, music, hypnosis; and breathing, coping, and counseling approaches. Only seven of the studies were randomized controlled trials (RCTs); sample sizes ranged from nine patients in a case series evaluating music therapy to 239 patients in an RCT evaluating acupuncture. The researchers concluded overall that relaxation techniques, acupuncture, and TENS may improve intractable pain in dying patients. The authors also suggested that acupuncture and breathing retraining for patients with chronic obstructive pulmonary disease might be generalizable to cancer patients.

A second review of eight studies published between 1982–1995 evaluated relaxation and imagery for cancer pain, but was not limited to end-of-life care.[30] Sample sizes were small, and study designs were limited. However, studies with 20 or more subjects found that CAM interventions were associated with reduced pain. In contrast, studies with less than 20 subjects were negative. Despite the paucity of published research and the need for more rigorous designs and adequate power, these researchers concluded that the meager evidence suggests that CAM approaches, specifically cognitive and behavioral approaches, may benefit the sensory experience of cancer pain. Less evidence exists for improvement in affective states and functional status.[30]

Some hospice settings are incorporating CAM modalities into their clinical practice. For example, the San Diego Hospice has an Integrative Palliative Care program that is part of the medical division. In this setting, traditional Chinese medicine along with massage, music, energy, aromatherapy, and contemplative practices of meditation and prayer are offered to patients as part of integrative, comprehensive palliative care.

Discussing CAM therapies and resources

Oncologists are becoming increasingly aware that patients use CAM, yet few discuss these therapies with patients.[31–35] Such discussions are important, especially for herbals and biopharmacologic therapies, since they are widely used and have been associated with adverse events[36,37] and interactions with conventional treatment.[38]

In the palliative care setting, communications with patients who have refused curative cancer therapies for CAM may be challenging. Several case reports provide examples.[39] In one case, a 27-year-old man refused massive head and neck surgery in favor of a complex treatment of nutrition, herbs, and imagery provided in Mexico. In a second instance, a 36-year-old woman refused surgery for early stage disease that progressed to invasive cervical cancer. She subsequently refused a radical hysterectomy and lymph node dissection and relied on faith healing. In both of the cases, the palliative care team respected the belief systems of these patients, accommodated their needs by allowing requests such as for special foods, and communicated in a nonconfrontational manner. These interactions allowed patients the time necessary to adjust and accept their palliative treatment options.

In order to communicate with patients about CAM therapies, physicians and nurses must have some understanding of these approaches and access to reliable information. Resources such as searchable databases, systematic reviews and summaries, and books are available to provide this information (Table 10.1).

Summary

The spiritual, emotional, and physical needs of terminal cancer patients must be addressed and the role of CAM therapies in addressing these needs examined. Public awareness of the limitations of end-of-life care and the possible role of CAM therapies was highlighted in October, 1999 at Congressional hearings entitled "Improving Care at the End of Life with Complementary Medicine." In September 2000, a television documentary and subsequent media coverage focused our nation on the issues of end-of-life.[40,41] The following month, an End of Life Research Interest Group at the National Institutes of Health (NIH) hosted the first open forum at NIH to explore a research agenda. In January 2001, the National Center

Table 10.1. Resources for information about CAM

American Cancer Society	Comprehensive summary of CAM therapies *American Cancer Society's Guide to Complementary and Alternative Cancer Methods*, 2000 http://www.cancer.org
Longwood Herbal Taskforce	Quality scientific information to physicians, pharmacists, nurses and other healthcare professionals about herbals http://www.mcp.edu/herbal/
National Center for Complementary and Alternative Medicine	CAM on PubMED 220 000 CAM related bibliographic citations from Medline http://nccam.nih.gov/
National Cancer Institute	Physician Database Query (PDQ) has summaries of seven CAM therapies www.cancer.gov/cancerinfo/pdq/cam
University of Texas – Center for CAM	Systematic reviews of over two dozen CAM agents are reviewed with other resource links http://www.mdanderson.org/departments/cimer

for Complementary and Alternative Medicine (NCCAM) released a request for applications to evaluate CAM for patients with cancer and HIV/AIDS who are at the end of life.

The limited research suggests that some CAM approaches may benefit patients (music, mind–body, acupuncture, TENS). Many agents remain untested in the US (biopharmacologics, herbals, and traditional Chinese medicine regimens) and therefore, scientific testing is a logical next step. Rigorous research is needed to assess CAM's role in managing or reducing the symptoms associated with the conditions of end-stage disease, preventing or reducing side effects of conventional medications, and enhancing psychological, social, and spiritual well-being and quality of life. If CAM can improve quality of life or modify the disease course, oncologists should not feel threatened to practice side by side with these therapies.[42]

Advancing the level of scientific investigation of these approaches will benefit the patients ultimately, as information becomes more reliable. This is the time to build bridges, not moats, between thoughtful and careful science and CAM therapies.[43,44] The oncology community must be willing to educate themselves so they can responsibly communicate with patients about CAM, support research that investigates CAM approaches, tolerate treatments that are harmless, and integrate those that prove to be safe and beneficial.

39 Jenkins CA, Scarfe A, Bruera E. Integration of palliative care with alternative medicine in patients who have refused curative cancer therapy: a report of two cases. *J Palliat Care* 1998;14:55–9.

40 Committee on Government Reform Hearing, 106th Congress. *Improving Care at the End of Life With Complementary Medicine.* Washington, DC: US Government Printing Office, 1999.

41 Cloud J. Society: a kinder, gentler death. *Time* 2000:61–74.

42 Stoll BA. Can unorthodox cancer therapy improve quality of life? *Ann Oncol* 1993;4:121–3.

43 Hoey J. The arrogance of science and the pitfalls of hope. *Can Med Assoc J* 1998;159:803–4.

44 Jonas WB. Alternative medicine – learning from the past, examining the present, advancing the future. (editorial). *J Am Med Assoc* 1998;280:1616–18.

11

Understanding "hospice"

Vincent Hsieh and Jane Ingham

Georgetown University Medical Center, Washington, DC

Introduction

"Hospice" is a philosophy of care, the goal of which is to assist patients who are nearing the end of life to be pain free, comfortable, and to live with dignity.[1] Hospice programs exist in many countries, however, the spectrum of services that they offer varies widely. When the word "hospice" is used, it often refers to a program, or even an institution, that espouses the "hospice" philosophy. Hence, in some countries the word "hospice" is used to refer to programs that focus predominantly on care in the home, and, in others, it refers to facilities that provide inpatient care at the very end of life. In many countries "palliative care" has emerged as a philosophy and a programmatic approach to care for those living with advanced, life-threatening illness. Palliative care programs have similar aims to hospice programs but extend the reach of the "hospice" philosophy from a sole focus on the end and very end of life to patients who are living with advanced, life-threatening illness. Many such patients may still be seeking life-sustaining or even curative therapies. Finally, in many countries physicians, nurses, and family caregivers, who face health systems without "systems" or "programs" specifically designed to care for those at the end of life, attempt to put together care systems that address the "hospice" or "palliative care" related needs of patients who are nearing the end of life.

Simply put, "hospice care" is a component of "palliative care" which is itself a component of optimal care. As health professionals strive to ensure that those with advanced, life-threatening illness receive optimal care, they need, firstly, to have an understanding of what constitutes "optimal care." To deliver such care, it is crucial that there is an understanding of the patient's goals, the spectrum of his or her needs, and the needs of the family and caregivers. In this setting, health professionals usually need to assist the patient and family to find ways to address an array of needs and to access appropriate palliative or hospice care. To understand specifically how "palliative care" or "hospice" can assist in a particular patient's

care, health professionals must have an understanding of the array of services that exist within the palliative care or hospice programs in the region in which the patient resides. If such programs do not exist, there are still an array of needs that can often be addressed if careful thought is given to matching the patient's and family's needs with existing, nonprogrammatically based services and supports. This chapter will, in a brief overview, provide a framework for health professionals to begin to consider these issues.

What are goals of optimal care?

"Optimal care" is a concept that simply conveys a goal to deliver the best possible care throughout the course of illness and includes the following.[2–4]

- Patients and their families must be provided with a sufficient understanding of the prognosis for their condition, and the risks and benefits of their treatment options, to make treatment decisions.[3]
- As a part of the care process, clear and informed treatment goals should be developed and, if appropriate, altered over time as transitions occur in the disease state and prognosis. If there is difficulty establishing treatment goals all involved should have access to approaches to addressing this problem.[3]
- Care should feature medical interventions and service delivery that address, and are consistent with, patient's and family's goals of care.[5]
- Care should be directed towards the needs of the patient, the family, and the caregivers.[2]
- Care should emphasize and promote quality of life, with practical, emotional, and spiritual support, and minimization of symptomatic distress.[5] This aspect of care is often referred to as "palliative care."

If care at the end of life is to be optimized, it is critical that these goals are integrated *throughout* the process of care, particularly in the setting of life-threatening illness.

What are the core principles of "palliative care" and what is needed to ensure and promote optimal care and quality of life towards the end of life?

Palliative care was defined, in its early development, as "the active total care of patients whose disease is not responsive to curative treatment."[2,4] More recently, there has been recognition that many aspects of palliative care should be applied throughout the course of life-threatening disease. Those who are near to the end of life should not be the only population who receive care with an intensive focus on symptom management and psychosocial and spiritual support. In addition, those patients who elect life-sustaining therapies and/or experimental therapies should not suffer as a consequence of having limited, or no, access to such support. The

Canadian Palliative Care Association has long been an exponent of this concept and has defined palliative care as "the combination of active and compassionate therapies intended to comfort and support individuals and families who are living with, or dying from, a progressive life-threatening illness, or are bereaved."[6] Embedded within this definition is a recognition that the concerns of patients who are living with incurable, life-threatening illness are similar to the concerns of those who have life-threatening but potentially curable illness. In the US, the Last Acts Task Force defined palliative care as "the comprehensive management of the physical, psychological, social, spiritual and existential needs of patients," and further stated, "it is especially suited to the care of people with incurable, progressive illnesses."[5]

As alluded to above, care should always seek to honor the preferences of the patient and family with particular emphasis on their needs, values, and goals. Especially towards the end of life, it is common for the illness to change or progress and for patients to go through transition periods where changes occur and goals need to be reconsidered. Goals that may have once been achievable may become unrealistic. When this occurs it may be that the patient is "obviously" more ill or indeed there may not be any visible clinical change. Discussions about goals and interventions need to reflect recognition of the realities of the prognostic change. Assuming such discussions take place, patients and their families can proceed to develop "a sufficient understanding of the prognosis for their condition, and the risks and benefits of their treatment options, to make treatment decisions." These decisions may shift the goals from curative or life-sustaining goals to comfort and quality of life as the *only* priorities. It should not, however, be this "shift" that prompts a "shift" to careful attention being paid to the following core principles of palliative care. These principles should be an integral part of care *throughout* illness.

In summary, the following are principles that are integral to palliative care.[2,4-6] Palliative care:

- seeks to provide comprehensive care with practical and meticulous physical, psychological, social, and spiritual support. Within this there must be an intense focus on the prevention and minimization of distress and the promotion of "good health" in its most broad sense within the context of illness.
- can be complementary to other disease-specific therapies and should be available throughout the illness and bereavement trajectory and to those of all ages, including children, with life-threatening illness.
- should be sensitive to personal, cultural and religious values, beliefs, and practices.
- should respect the identified goals of care, preferences, and choices.
- utilizes the strengths of interdisciplinary resources.
- acknowledges and addresses caregiver concerns, both for professional and non-professional caregivers.
- builds systems and mechanisms of support for patients and families.

What are the core principles of hospice, and what role can hospice have in the delivery of optimal palliative care?

As mentioned above, the core principles of hospice interface closely with the core principles of optimal care and palliative care. Hospices worldwide, however, do tend to offer care only to those who are near to the end of life and have shifted their goals to a single focus – comfort and quality of life. Although hospices in some countries offer services to those who still have some "life-sustaining" goals, the majority of programs offering such would describe themselves as "palliative care" programs.

Unfortunately, in the US, the Medicare Hospice Benefit has come to be viewed *as* "hospice" and to define its "core principles." It is important to understand, however, that "hospice" is *not* a government-defined benefit, with, for example, a 6-month prognosis criteria for eligibility. "Hospice" is a philosophy of care that is essentially very similar to the philosophy of palliative care. Although "palliative care" is somewhat broader in its reach, extending into earlier phases of illness, "hospice" embraces all of the principles of palliative care with the exception of the principle related to the delivery of care *"throughout"* the course of illness. Figure 11.1

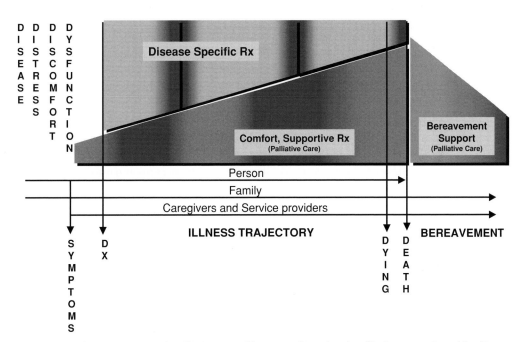

Figure 11.1   The continuum of palliative care illustrates the role of palliative care alongside disease-specific treatment and into the bereavement period. Reproduced with permission from *Palliative Care: Towards a Consensus in Standardized Principles of Practice. First Phase Working Document*, ed. F Ferris, I Cummings, p. 13. Ottawa: The Canadian Palliative Care Association, 1995.

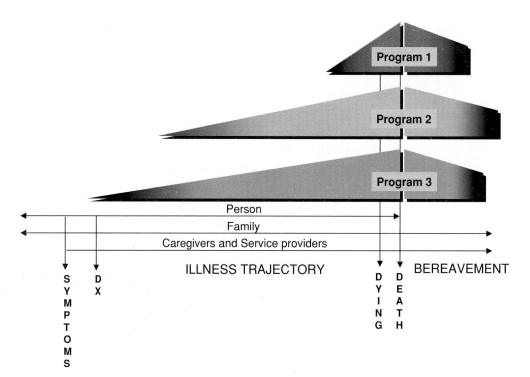

Figure 11.2 The continuum of palliative care programs illustrates the types of palliative care programs that can offer care alongside disease-specific treatment and into the bereavement period. Reproduced with permission from *Palliative Care: Towards a Consensus in Standardized Principles of Practice. First Phase Working Document*, ed. F Ferris, I Cummings, p. 13. Ottawa: The Canadian Palliative Care Association, 1995.

provides an illustration of this concept with palliative care being available throughout the course of illness, alongside life-sustaining treatments and into bereavement.[6] Figure 11.2 illustrates some programmatic responses to the delivery of palliative care with "Program 1" on this figure being that which most commonly corresponds to "hospice care."[6] Programs 2 and 3 reflect broader programmatic approaches to palliative care. In summary, hospices most commonly restrict the care they offer to patients whose focus is on optimizing quality of life – to those who are not seeking, and unlikely to benefit from, life-sustaining treatments.

The core principles of "hospice" are as follows.

- Hospice care aims to help patients to be pain free, comfortable, and to live with dignity towards the end of life. Hospice strives to improve the quality of life, in general accord with patients' and families' wishes, by preventing or diminishing distress and suffering. Particular emphasis is placed on preventing or minimizing physical distress while preserving as much lucidity as possible.
- Efforts are made to promote quality of life for patients, their families, and their caregivers, all of whom are considered to be part of the "unit of care."

- Hospice programs assemble and coordinate interdisciplinary teams of professionals capable of providing continuous and comprehensive care that addresses the physical, psychological, social, and spiritual needs of the patient and family.
- Generally, hospices offer care to patients who have reached a point where their disease is not responsive to curative treatment, and, within that context, have abandoned attempts to sustain life with therapies directed towards curing or prolonging life (e.g., therapies such as chemotherapy). Hospices generally provide care for those who have focused their goals predominantly on comfort and quality of life.

Who might benefit from palliative and, specifically, hospice care?

Throughout the course of any illness, health professionals should address the physical, psychological, social, and spiritual concerns that arise as a consequence of illness. In addition, especially in the setting of life-threatening illness, the needs of the family and caregivers should be considered important by the healthcare team. Thus, all patients with difficult illness should have access to "palliative care."

The potential benefit from an intense focus on quality of life is especially great for patients who are faced with advanced, life-threatening illness. In this setting, and in the setting of clearly incurable illness, when the patient's and the family's needs are often intensifying and the burden of illness increasing, optimal care mandates that consideration should be given to approaches to care that optimize the delivery of the palliative aspects of care. Approaches to addressing symptoms and assisting with psychological and spiritual concerns of the patient and family should be implemented as needed. Examples of such approaches may include, among many others, a pain treatment regimen, specialist advice about difficult symptoms and distress, spiritual and chaplaincy support, and home care support with 24-hour access to care or back-up support in the home (the latter is especially important if the patient's goal is to stay at home).

In the setting of advanced life-threatening illnesses or clearly incurable progressive illness, it is important for patients to, at a minimum, "regroup" regarding goals of care. If the patient has been informed about the prognosis for the condition, and the risks and benefits of the treatment options, the goals can be established and physicians can advise the patient and family about approaches to appropriate services including, if needed, home care support. When goals are focused solely on comfort and quality of life a palliative or hospice approach to care should be considered, and depending on the country or region, a hospice program as the system of care is likely to be most appropriate. If goals include some "life-sustaining" goals, hospice may or may not be an accessible system for the patient and the physician should explore options for palliative care.

Of note, although with some illnesses it is common for physicians to recognize a poor prognostic situation and to see obvious needs, with other illnesses a less predictable trajectory and less "visible" needs contribute to a lower likelihood of a "palliative" or "hospice" approach being considered.[7] Function and symptoms for those living with serious chronic illness at the end of life generally follow one of the following trajectories: (1) a short period of obvious decline at the end, which is typical of cancer, although sudden death can also occur in this condition; (2) long-term disability, with periodic exacerbation, and unpredictable timing of death, which characterizes dying with chronic organ system failure; or (3) self-care deficits and a slowly dwindling course to death, which usually results from frailty or dementia.[8] An example of a disease that may have a "somewhat" unpredictable decline is advanced cardiovascular disease. A variety of different trajectories can occur during the latter stages of this condition, including sudden deterioration, for which patients and families may be ill prepared. For such illnesses, one useful approach that has been suggested for physicians considering the care needs of chronically ill patients is for them to consider the question "would you be surprised if your patient died in the next 6–12 months?"[8] A negative response should trigger consideration of the likely end-of-life needs of the patient and family. If this is undertaken certain issues can be considered well in advance including, for example, living wills, advance directives, and family plans.

How do I understand what hospice can offer a particular patient?

While the core principles of hospice are similar internationally, specific features of hospices and the services that they deliver may vary at national and regional levels. Below is a list of questions that should be asked when considering the possible contribution that a hospice program can offer to the care of the patient and family. Due to space constraints, the examples below illustrate some of the contrasting features of hospice programs in the US and the UK. The important point, however, is that when considering the referral of a patient to a hospice program *in any country* these are the crucial issues that health professionals should understand or ask about.

Where will care take place?

In the US, most hospice care takes place at the patient's home with regular visits by nurses, home health aides, social workers, and trained volunteers. In contrast, hospices in the UK are more commonly residential facilities for those who are nearing the final days of life.

Who will coordinate the care?

In the US, hospice home care is usually coordinated by a hospice nurse who visits the patient in the home. Hospice care may also be brought into nursing homes or other long-term facilities through visits by hospice nurses. In contrast, in the UK end-of-life home care is usually coordinated by the patient's local physician – often a general practitioner with the support of local community nursing services. If the patient is in an inpatient hospice facility, the inpatient hospice team usually coordinates care.

Who will provide medical care?

In the US, while the patient's primary care physician is responsible for all medical decisions, registered nurses who may visit the patient daily, weekly, or as needed, commonly discuss the medical situation with the patient's physician and may make recommendations about medical therapies to that physician. It is not uncommon in the US for homebound patients on hospice *not* to have face-to-face interactions with a physician. In some countries and some regions in the US, primary care physicians provide direct home care.

What types of services will be provided?

The services listed below (examples of US hospice services) may *not* be offered by all hospices worldwide; however, access to many of these services is *essential* if quality of life in the setting of advanced life-threatening illness and at the end of life is to be optimized. In caring for patients with such illness, physicians should be asking "how can my patient address his/her needs in a manner that is in keeping with his/her goals and access to these types of services?" Oftentimes a hospice program is the best, most comprehensive, and cohesive way to access these services and to address the patient's and family's needs. Importantly, however, if the patient is seeking life-sustaining therapies or wishes to be transferred to a hospital in the event of deterioration, then this issue will need to be specifically discussed with the hospice program – many hospice programs do *not* provide this type of support. In addition, physicians should be aware that in many developed health systems the services below can be accessed without having palliative care or hospice programs formally involved; however, this route risks being less cohesive and coordinated than it could be via "program-based" mechanisms.

In the US the following services are *mandated* by the Medicare Hospice Benefit.

- Regular home visits by registered/licensed nurses and home nursing visits as needed for emergency care.
- 24-hour on-call nursing advice for emergencies in the home.
- Home health aide visits.
- Social work/counseling.
- Medical equipment/supplies.
- Medications for symptom control/pain relief.
- Volunteer support.

- Spiritual/chaplaincy support.
- A physician medical director must oversee the delivery of hospice care. These physicians are not always involved in the day-to-day care of each patient. The hospice nurse usually undertakes this latter task in collaboration with the patient's primary physician. (Optimally patients should have access to physician support in the home if needed.)

In the US *some* of the following services *may* be offered by hospice programs.

- Physical therapy, speech therapy, occupational therapy, and dietary counseling *may* be available.
- Inpatient hospice beds *may* be available in the US, but there are commonly limits on the length of time that a patient can stay in such a facility. Usually patients are eligible for such if acute symptom-related needs are present but are not eligible if the need is only for intensified nursing care or "custodial" care.

In the US the following services are *less or not likely* to be covered by hospice programs.

- Life-sustaining interventions such as total parenteral nutrition, dialysis, chemotherapy, and surgery (in the US patients either do not enroll in a hospice program, or occasionally even "sign-off" hospice, if they have a need for such services). There are some exceptions to this and physicians are advised to discuss these issues with the individual hospice program.
- Symptom management and palliative care in the hospital setting where patients are receiving life-sustaining treatments. It is in this setting that palliative care programs have developed in a number of countries (Canada, Australia, Britain, and Italy to name a few) and are developing in the US.

Will hospice services be provided after-hours?

To ensure the comfort of patients who elect to stay at home at the end of life, an approach to covering after-hours needs must always be considered. Approaches to this vary worldwide, but in the US most hospices offer 24-hour on-call nursing advice for emergencies that occur in the home. In other countries, family physicians may directly provide the after-hours support.

Is my patient eligible for hospice services and how long will they receive these services?

Clearly, eligibility criteria for hospice may differ internationally as well as regionally. In the US the majority of patients 65 years and older are eligible for the Medicare Hospice Benefit which currently covers two initial 90-day benefit periods followed by unlimited 60-day benefit periods. The patient must be "re-certified" by a physician as being likely to have less than 6 months to live before entering each benefit period. Psychological and social support for the bereaved is typically offered for 1 year. To assist US physicians establish a prognosis (a requirement for hospice eligibility), the National Hospice Organization has developed a useful set of guide-lines.[8] Services may vary for patients who have a type of medical coverage other than Medicare.

What are the barriers and problems that might be encountered in regard to hospice care?

Delayed admission to hospice

Although patients suffering from advanced stages of illness in the US are theoreti-cally eligible for hospice 6 months before death, the typical patient begins receiving hospice home care services only 25 days before death (median length of stay in 1999).[1]

Among many factors contributing to the delay are:

- A patient attitude that is simply explained by the phrase, "I'm not ready for that," accompanied by a desire to continue with life-sustaining treatments.
- Difficulties in providing the 6-month prognosis that is a US Medicare requirement.[9]
- Physician reluctance to "give up" or to broach discussions about the "end of life" with patients.
- Lack of patient and/or physician understanding about hospice services.

Limits in services offered by hospices

Some hospices may be seen as underutilizing certain services, such as important physician input, and some are limited in the care that they offer. The common focus on "end-of-life care" versus "life-sustaining care" may present a limit for some patients. These limits have many reasons behind them, including financial, regulatory, and philosophical issues. At a given time in a given region, some of these limits may be surmountable and others may not. There is tremendous variability in these limits, and physicians should explore these with local hospice programs.

Many other barriers to effective hospice and palliative care exist

These include those at the levels of patient/family, the health professional, the healthcare system, and the society.[10] Examples of such barriers include, among many others:

- Patient and family hesitation and fear in recognizing that options may be limited for life-sustaining therapies.
- Lack of information resources for the public dealing with palliative and end-of-life care; fears related to the use of opioids for pain.
- Limited palliative care educational opportunities for nurses and physicians.
- Disparities in care in ethnic and socio-economic segments of populations.

- Attitudes that result in a failure to prioritize palliative care.
- National healthcare policies that impede or do not attend to end-of-life care as a priority.

The pediatric population

In the pediatric population with life-threatening illness all of these barriers apply, along with additional problems that relate to the comparative rarity of childhood death and the unfamiliarity of many health professionals with death occurring in childhood.

Conclusion

This brief overview of hospice and palliative care has been provided as a practical guide to the key issues that should be considered when physicians and other health professionals are considering how they can provide optimal care for patients and families in the setting of advanced, life-threatening illness and towards the end of life. Historically, hospice programs have pioneered many of the "core principles" that we now see as crucial parts of palliative and optimal care.[11] These principles include meticulous attention to pain and symptom management, care directed towards the patient *and* family, and the interdisciplinary team approach to care. In many countries, hospice services are significantly underutilized, and although hospice programs may not always provide the spectrum of services needed to meet each patient's goals, many times they do. Certainly the "philosophy" of hospice advocates for, and many individual hospices offer, an excellent and high-quality array of services for patients who are nearing the end of life. Given that it is widely recognized that patients and families often do not access optimal end-of-life care, patients, families, and health professionals should give careful consideration to the potential role of hospice care in the care of all patients who are nearing the end of life.

REFERENCES

1 National Hospice and Palliative Care Organization web site, http://www.nhpco.org.

2 World Health Organization Expert Committee. *Cancer Pain Relief and Palliative Care. Report of a WHO Expert Committee.* World Health Organization Technical Report Series, 1990;804: 1–75.

3 The American Academy of Neurology Ethics and Humanities Subcommittee. Palliative care in neurology. *Neurology* 1996;46:870–2.

4 World Health Organization. *Cancer Pain Relief and Palliative Care in Children.* Geneva: World Health Organization, 1998.

5 Ferris F, Cummings, I. (ed.) *Palliative Care: Towards a Consensus in Standardized Principles of Practice. First Phase Working Document.* Ottawa: The Canadian Palliative Care Association, 1995.

6 Last Acts Palliative Care Task Force. *Precepts of Palliative Care*, 1997. Last Acts Organization web site: http://www.lastacts.org

7 Field MJ, Cassel EK. (ed.) *Approaching Death: Improving Care at the End of Life*, p. 437. Washington, DC: National Academy Press, 1997.

8 Lynn J. Perspectives on care at the close of life. Serving patients who may die soon and their families: the role of hospice and other services. *J Am Med Assoc* 2001;285:925–32.

9 The National Hospice Organization. Medical guidelines for determining prognosis in selected non-cancer diseases. *Hosp J*, 1996;11: 47–63.

10 Foley K, Gelband H. *Improving Palliative Care for Cancer.* Washington, DC: Institute of Medicine, Commission on Life Sciences and National Research Council, 2001.

11 Saunders C. Foreword to Oxford Textbook of Palliative Medicine. In *Oxford Textbook of Palliative Care*, ed. D Doyle, GWC Hanks, N MacDonald, pp. v–ix. New York: Oxford University Press, 1998.

12

Practical aspects of home care

Anna Wreath Taube

University of Alberta, Edmonton

Introduction

Palliative care of a cancer patient at home can be one of the most meaningful and rewarding life experiences possible for both the relatives or significant others in the patient's life and for involved professionals. In many poorer parts of the world, of course, there never has been an alternative care setting, but the custom of home care of the advanced cancer patient declined sharply after the mid-twentieth century in much of the industrialized world. In recent years, both patient quality of life issues and government attempts to download costlier acute care medical services to the less costly community setting have encouraged reconsideration of home care of advanced cancer patients as a viable alternative to hospital, or even hospice, care in the Western world.

For family or other lay caregivers, despite the desire to do so, the task is often challenging, emotionally and physically exhausting, and potentially financially costly. Given the exponential advances in palliative medical/radiation oncology and palliative medicine, the terminal phase of many cancer illnesses is now considerably prolonged and families face extended periods of much more complicated cancer home care than in earlier eras. The specifics of home care in any given community may obviously vary considerably, depending on local medical practices and socio-economic, political, and cultural factors. The following considerations are offered as general suggestions for approaches and resources to facilitate home care of the advanced cancer patient.

General considerations

1. In the vast majority of communities successful long-term home care of the advanced cancer patient depends on lay caregivers. Even when palliative home-care services are available, the responsibility for the majority of minute-to-minute bedside nursing and medication administration usually falls on lay caregivers.

Teaching these caregivers, monitoring their stress levels and needs, providing emotional and practical support and, at times, managing family dysfunction is time-consuming and requires considerable patience, sensitivity, and skill on the part of involved professionals.

2. Both patient and lay caregivers must desire the home setting. If either party does not support the goal of care in the home, the chances of achieving this are much diminished.

3. Involved professionals optimally will have an adequate comfort level in providing care in a setting much less controlled than the institutional setting.

4. Communication between all players, including the patient as appropriate, but especially between all lay and all professional caregivers must be thorough and timely. A formalized home chart system is one excellent option to achieve this, but frequent telephone, faxed, or computerized communication is often necessary.

5. Management should be kept as simple as possible. Minimize polypharmacy. Keep medication times and route of administration as simple as possible. Use controlled-release products when available and appropriate (controlled-release analgesics are not appropriate when pain is inadequately controlled). As possible, utilize the easier subcutaneous rather than intravenous route when oral hydration and medication administration are no longer viable.

6. Establish and document the patient's Do Not Resuscitate (DNR) status as soon as is medically and psychosocially appropriate, since accurate prediction of time of death is notoriously difficult. See # 7 in "Other valuable resources" below.

7. Institutional admission is not lay caregiver failure. When patient symptomatology is complex or caregiver burnout is a reality, admission may be very much in the patient's better interest.

8. Appropriate physician and other professional discipline remuneration for the time-consuming assessment and supportive care of both patient and lay caregivers, as well as travel time (unfortunately rarely reimbursed), will encourage professional involvement in home patient care. In the author's community, the government-financed physician remuneration program provides time-based physician palliative fee schedules.

Caregiving and medical resources

1. A committed, knowledgeable, attending physician who provides home visits, 24 hours per day/7 days per week ("24/7") coverage, and proactive care is paramount. Many crises such as severe uncontrolled pain, agitated delirium, severe nausea/vomiting from constipation (all common events, common, severe stressors for patient and families, and common reasons for emergency department usage) are preventable if skilled proactive physician monitoring is

the norm. The higher the number of medical crises in the home, the less optimal the chances of prolonged patient care in this setting.

2. The availability of at least two lay caregivers who, practically and emotionally, can devote themselves to patient bedside care is recommended. It is very difficult for one lay caregiver alone to provide "24/7" care for any extended period of time.

3. The availability of "24/7" funded multidisciplinary palliative home-care service is invaluable. Although most such services do not supply "24/7" bedside nursing care, they often provide some hours of nursing respite to lay caregivers. More importantly, they provide another resource for proactive monitoring, teaching, counseling, and access to around the clock advice in emergency situations, as well as home physiotherapy/occupational therapy service. Additionally, many professional home-care services offer "24/7" technical help, such as changing subcutaneous needle sites or administering enemas, tasks that lay caregivers may be reluctant to assume. Prolonged home care of the advanced cancer patient is most viable if medical and nursing advice is available on a "24/7" basis.

4. A palliative community consulting team furthers facilitates home care of the advanced cancer patient, especially if available "24/7."

Other valuable resources

1. Laboratory home blood collection service.
2. Portable home radiology service.
3. "24/7" community pharmacy service. An alternative for off-hour pharmacy needs is an "Emergency Drug and Supply Kit," possibly made available, for example, through the palliative consult team.
4. Pharmacy home delivery.
5. Other convenient pharmacy services, such preloaded medication syringes or syringe-drivers, or pre-programmed pumps.
6. Home paracentesis availability, such as may be offered by a palliative consult team.
7. Available medical examiner office (or equivalent) registration of possible home death. If congruent with the community's legal system, such predeath registration may allow removal of the body from the home without an in-the-home signed death certificate. In the author's community this is the case and the attending physician is not legally required to visit the home to sign the death certificate immediately following the death. This practicality may encourage more primary care physicians to attend home palliative patients.
8. Available emergency response department registration of patient "DNR" status. In the author's community an emergency call from the home to ambulance, fire,

or police departments in the event of a patient's death will lead to full resuscitation measures, if such notification is not in place prior to the call or documentation of the patient's DNR code status is not present in the home. When resuscitation is inappropriate but the community's legal requirement necessitates such measures if DNR code status is not registered or documented in the home prior to death, such procedures can be devastating to the family.

Consideration of potential costs to patient/family

Financial costs

Coverage for costs such as medications, medical equipment, or privately hired nursing services varies extensively. If coverage is not available, or not in place even if available, the patient/family expenses for care at home may be astronomical. In the author's setting, the province of Alberta provides a premium-free, co-payment (lifetime maximum of Canadian $ 1000.00) Palliative Drug Benefit Plan for palliative home patients, covering supplies such as those for subcutaneous hydration and bowel care that are often not covered by other available insurance plans.

If the patient requires ambulance transportation to and from an acute care setting for day procedures that cannot be done in the home, ambulance insurance coverage may not be in place. In the author's setting, most patients do not have this coverage, resulting in very significant out-of-pocket costs if such transportation is needed.

Further significant financial cost may be incurred if lay caregivers must take unpaid leave in order to provide bedside nursing care. Professionals and patients and/or families must be aware of and patients/families able to sustain such potential out-of-pocket costs.

Patient/lay caregiver loss of privacy and control

Even when patients and lay caregivers appreciate the home care offered by professionals, multidisciplinary professional visits are often time-consuming, many in number, and necessarily done, to some extent, at the convenience of the professional. This may lead to feelings of loss of both control and privacy on the part of patient and lay caregivers, causing further sources of stress and/or distress to them. Involved professionals must be sensitive to this phenomenon.

Conclusion

This chapter has attempted to outline the most critical considerations and community resources necessary to facilitate care of the advanced cancer patient in the home.

BIBLIOGRAPHY

Doyle D. Domicillary palliative care. In *Oxford Textbook of Palliative Medicine*, 2nd edn, ed. D Doyle, G Hanks, N MacDonald, pp. 957–73. Oxford: Oxford University Press, 1998.

Macmillan K, Peden J, Hopkinson J, Hycha D. *A Caregivers's Guide: a Handbook about End of Life Care*. Edmonton: The Palliative Care Association of Alberta, 2000.

Mount BM. *The ACP Home Care Guide for Advanced Cancer*. American College of Physicians. Web site: www.acponline.org/public/h_care/contents.htm

13

Cultural differences in advanced cancer care

Juan M. Núñez-Olarte

Hospital General Universitario Gregorio Marañón, Madrid

Introduction

Culture could be defined as that complex whole which includes knowledge, belief, art, morals, law, custom, and any other capabilities and habits acquired by man as a member of society. The influence of culture is very pervasive, it is not restricted to religious rituals, and can be detected in several aspects of advanced cancer care.

Traditional issues in advanced cancer care related to culture

Traditionally culture has been associated with some issues considered to be relevant in the setting of advanced cancer:

- Rituals of dying and death.
- Manners of grieving and the grieving process itself.
- Gender roles and family systems.
- Emotional expression and sharing.
- Dietary requirements and use of alternative therapies.
- Beliefs about causation of illness.

New issues in advanced cancer care related to culture

There are several "new" issues emerging in the care of advanced cancer that are related to culture:

- Terminal sedation versus euthanasia.
- Last 48 hours of life versus traditions of *Agonía*.
- Definition of "terminality."
- Hospice versus nonhospice traditions.
- External versus internal *locus of control* and acceptance of death.
- Perceived value of disclosure and cognition.
- Communication – diagnosis disclosure – truth-telling.

Diagnosis disclosure

The last decade has witnessed a transition in health professionals in the UK and USA from "full open disclosure" to "conditional disclosure" of terminal diagnosis and prognosis when confronting dying patients. Simultaneously, research in countries such as Spain, Italy, Japan, Greece, Portugal, Israel, France, Colombia, and the Philippines has prompted the review of the long-held assumption that diagnosis disclosure is always in the best interest of the patient. There are different cultural reasons in every country or region that support its degree of commitment to "truth-telling," as studies in minorities within the USA, UK, and Australia clearly indicate.

With the available evidence it is difficult to support the "open awareness" approach that has been so prevalent in the early literature in palliative care. Some recent studies are starting to tackle the difficult issue of communication styles and their impact in advanced cancer patients. Some authors are suggesting the use of advance directives in communication given the fact of the perceived complexities. But there are even deeper levels of analysis suggesting that breaking bad news is part of a "ritual" in the process of adapting to terminal disease.

Influence of culture on patients' pain perception and treatment

Certain cultural traditions hold the view that reality is not completely controllable, as humans can control only certain aspects of their environment and life. North American researchers tend to see this as a passive and pessimistic attitude, whereas Hispanic and Latin American researchers view it as realistic. The psychological construct known as locus of control (LOC) style helps to frame these differences. When viewed as ideal types, an internal LOC style involves a reported perception that life events and circumstances are the result of one's own actions, whereas an external LOC style includes the perception that they are beyond one's own control, in the hands of fate, chance, or other people.

Research has shown that cultural background is significantly related not only to differences in response to chronic pain, but also to differences in reported pain perception of total pain intensity and in pain described in both sensory and affective terms. Minority patients have been found to receive inadequate pain treatment, and better assessment is certainly needed. Nevertheless, stereotyping patients from certain ethnic groups is inappropriate as there are always significant interindividual variations.

Influence of culture on physicians' attitudes

There is some evidence up to now on the following:
- Ethnicity and attitude towards patient autonomy and end-of-life care.
- Race, age, and gender and attitudes towards end-of-life decisions.

- Culture and attitudes towards advance directives.
- Culture and attitudes and beliefs regarding communication.
- Opioid and psychotropic prescription.

Practical recommendations for the clinician

- Evaluate the preference in communication and decision-making style of your patient and his/her family.
- Do not generalize or stereotype according to ethnic or cultural background.
- Be open to different approaches from minority groups within your culture, or from patients coming from other cultures.
- Consider the information regarding your own and other cultures as essential for the well-being and optimal care of your patients.
- Be aware of the role, and potential influence, of the translator when needed.

Conclusion

Research in this sensitive area is badly needed in advanced cancer care. The health professional working in the field is usually not equipped with the knowledge, or has the availability of advice from human sciences. Nevertheless, and in spite of these shortcomings, there is an ethical imperative to try to expand current knowledge in this field in order to better serve the needs of patients and families. There is always the danger of oversimplification and/or an early generalization of the results of the studies. An unbiased, honest, unprejudiced, and as scientific as realistically possible approach to this type of research is essential for its success.

Cultural diversity is not a threatening phenomenon. It is certainly a challenge, because it introduces another level of complexity in our decision-making process, but simultaneously it exposes us to the full richness of the suffering human being.

BIBLIOGRAPHY

Bates MS, Edwards WT, Anderson KO. Ethnocultural influences on variation in chronic pain perception. *Pain* 1993;52:101–12.

Bruera E, Neumann C, Mazzocato C, Sala R, Stiefel F. Attitudes and beliefs of palliative care physicians regarding communication with terminally ill cancer patients. *Palliat Med* 2000;14:287–98.

Cleeland CS, Gonin R, Baez L, Loehrer P, Pandya KJ. Pain and treatment of pain in minority patients with cancer. *Ann Intern Med* 1997;127:813–16.

Fainsinger RL, Waller A, Bercovici M, Bengston K, Landman W, Hosking M, Núñez-Olarte JM, de Moissac D. A multi-centre international study of sedation for uncontrolled symptoms in terminally ill patients. *Palliat Med* 2000;14:257–65.

Latimer EJ. Cultural dimensions. In *A Guide to End-of-Life Care for Seniors*, ed. Fisher R et al. Toronto: Sunnybrook Health Sciences Center, 2000.

Neuberger J. Introduction. Cultural issues in palliative care. In *Oxford Textbook of Palliative Medicine*, 2nd edn, ed. D Doyle et al. Oxford: Oxford University Press, 1998.

Núñez Olarte JM, Fainsinger RL, de Moissac D. Influencia de factores culturales en la estrategia de tratamiento. *Med Paliat* 2000;7:76–7.

Núñez Olarte JM, Gracia Guillén D. Cultural issues and ethical dilemmas in palliative and end-of-life care in Spain. *Cancer Control* 2001;8:1–9.

Oliviere D. Culture and ethnicity. *Eur J Palliat Care* 1999;6:53–6.

Poulson J. Impact of cultural differences in care of the terminally ill. In *Palliative Medicine: A Case-based Manual*, ed. N MacDonald. Oxford: Oxford University Press, 1998.

Tylor EB. *Primitive Culture*. London: John Murray, 1971.

Internet site

See also most of the issues of *Innovations in End-of-Life Care*, an on-line journal and international forum.

Web site: www2.edc.org/lastacts

Print excerpts in every issue of *Journal of Palliative Medicine*. Compendia volumes 1 & 2, ed. MZ Solomon et al. Mary Ann Liebert Pub, 2000, 2001.

14

Implementing social services

A. Marlene Lockey

U.T. M.D. Anderson Cancer Center, Houston

Introduction

Advanced cancer brings intense psychosocial distress to both patient and family. No area of a patient's and family's life is untouched by cancer, and unmet needs in any area of life become magnified as the disease progresses. Family members or designated caretakers are an essential part of the care team, and they affect the quality of care the patient receives. Consequently, attention to family issues arising from the patient's diagnosis is part of the patient's treatment. The family's distress is the patient's distress and meeting nonmedical needs and addressing family concerns will relieve tensions that affect the patient's physical symptoms. As family members or other nonmedical caretakers provide more technologically complex care for longer periods of critical illness, the medical team must be mindful of the burden carried by these partners in care.

This chapter provides indicators for medical providers' ongoing evaluation of the well-being of patient and family. These indicators are based on information provided by patients concerning their needs and on issues delineated by medical practice as important to patients and their families. By knowing objective indicators, medical providers can reassess psychosocial components of treatment plans and implement services to address nonmedical and subjective problems that may be exacerbating the patient's suffering.

Needs identified by patients

The concerns of patients with advanced-stage cancer are typically more psychosocial than medical. Even a medically oriented need like symptom management has emotional and social components that require intervention, not only for the patient but for the family and nonmedical caretakers. Feeling emotionally overwhelmed, poorly supported, and fatigued is common among family caretakers. Their anxiety and depression as a result of the patient's diagnosis may be greater than the patient's. Impaired family function impedes treatment. Providing support may involve enlisting the services of family practitioners, social workers, chaplains, psychologists, and other specialists on the multidisciplinary treatment team and in the community.

Common concerns identified by patients, in order of frequency, are:

- Changes in functional status or level of activity.
- Role changes in the patient's life and family.
- Symptoms, particularly pain.
- Responses of family and significant others to the stresses of illness.
- Increasing loss of control over more areas of life.
- Financial burden on patient and family.
- Ambivalence regarding full medical disclosure and fear of bad news.

Some of these concerns emotionally engage patients, family caretakers, and medical team members more than others. Seldom does one concern exist without the presence of others. A father may, for example, express grief over being unable to attend his child's soccer games. This concern requires supportive counseling and an emotional assessment. If the change is caused by a recent decline in activity, further inquiry should be made regarding other functional and coping needs. Is additional supervision or assistive medical equipment required? Has the decline affected income? If so, what have been the consequences to the family and medical needs? How are the caretaker and other family members coping? If this father's physical decline included incontinence, he might be ashamed to talk about his need for toileting equipment and assistance, yet emotions about loss of personal dignity are as profound as the inability to attend a child's sporting events.

Asked to identify the most frequently unmet needs, patients narrow the list to psychosocial issues. Although a majority of patients do not report unmet needs, those who do, identify unmet needs in the following areas:

- Activities of daily living, such as housekeeping, meal preparation, transportation.
- Emotional need for support and counseling.
- Physical needs, such as assistance with bathing, walking.
- Insurance or payment for medical care.
- Financial concerns.

These needs do not fall within areas of direct medical care, but if unmet, they may increase a patient's emotional stress and even influence the course of treatment. Although the problems do not always result in noncompliance with treatment, the significance of this list of commonly unmet needs is often seen when reasons for noncompliance are explored. Failure to follow dietary recommendations, for example, may be evidence of a need for help with meal preparation. A patient's reluctance to increase the medication dosage for adequate pain relief may be due to a lack of money. Missed appointments may be the result of transportation problems. Patients hesitate to share financial or other nonmedical worries because they are afraid the medical team might reduce their level of medical care. The medical team's willingness to assist with patients in obtaining resources for their medical care encourages open communication, reduces symptoms that are social in etiology, and attends to a patient's integrity.

Indicators of family needs identified by medical practitioners

The experience of treating patients for advanced cancer has enabled medical teams to recognize signs of increased distress in patients and their families. Mindful of psychosocial dynamics inherent in demographical data and clinical findings, cancer treatment teams approach each appointment aware that the patient and family may need help in coping with illness and are inexperienced in how the medical team can help. If conversation confirms a need, the appropriate team member should be involved to implement and to monitor needed services.

Characteristic indicators of patients and families with psychosocial needs are:
- The cancer is growing or not diminished.
- Due to their roles within families, females are more likely to report a need for psychosocial services.
- Physical deconditioning resulting from either a recent hospitalization or from receiving a combination of cancer treatment therapies.
- Certain cancers require more services. These include lung, bowel, colon, rectum, and brain tumors.
- Information needs are greater in 31–65-year-old patients with parenting and employment responsibilities.

In the presence of a debilitating advanced cancer, patients and their families often confront new problems. Particular characteristics and behaviors distinguish patients who report unmet psychosocial needs. This suggests the need for continuous monitoring of each patient and family to evaluate psychosocial stresses for unmet needs. Indicators for unmet needs are:
- Illness is restricting the patient's activities.
- Patient is submitting application for financial assistance.
- Primary home caretaker is not a spouse or relative.
- Family caretaker is caring for family members in addition to the patient.

A new decline in the patient's level of functioning is the indicator of highest priority. Each decline is accompanied by medical equipment needs, additional family training, greater social restrictions for both patient and caretaker, heightened emotional responses among all family members, increased threat to family income,

Reassess these needs:

Information	Patient supervision	Psychological/counseling
Medical equipment	Family training	Responses to role changes
Medical payment concerns	Extra in-home assistance	Social support
Financial	Transportation	Family coping
	Cultural considerations	Spiritual issues

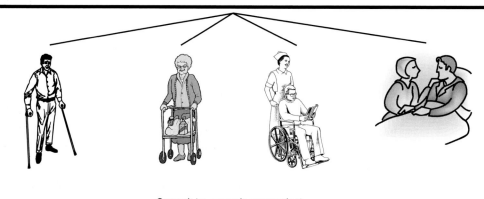

Consult/re-consult appropriate
multidisciplinary team members
as needs are identified

Figure 14.1   Each decline in patient physical, cognitive, or sensory functioning requires reassessment of psychosocial needs.

and spiritual concerns, to name only a few. Figure 14.1 presents a summary of this reassessment process.

Treatment plan: psychosocial focus

Treatment plans are most complete when assessments by multidisciplinary team members are integrated during an interdisciplinary team conference. When this is not possible, a designated team member should assess the global needs of advanced-stage cancer patients, which include psychosocial as well as medical concerns. Social workers are professionally trained to provide psychosocial assessments, and if a part of the medical team, they can evaluate changing needs for both patient and family. Interventions can be provided by specialized team members of the required specialty or through referrals to community services.

To meet the identified needs of both patient and family, treatment plans should address the following main psychosocial areas.

The patient's:

• Functional status.
• Supervision needs.

The patient's and family's:

- Emotional support needs.
- Information needs.
- Financial concerns.
- Cultural and spiritual issues.

Conclusion

Patient and family needs must be assessed and reassessed throughout the duration of illness. Decreasing functional status and prolonged illness bring different needs to the fore; they often drain a family's psychological and financial strengths, and they weaken the family's social life. Studies of unmet needs of cancer patients point primarily to unmet functional and social needs. Patients reference their needs with the medical team member with whom they are most comfortable; this team member is often not the one who can address these needs. A patient who feels comfortable with a nurse or dietician, for example, will talk about financial concerns or a patient will talk about emotional distress with the physical therapist. All team members must be familiar with the indicators of patient and family needs for assistance to be initiated quickly to alleviate or reduce unnecessary despair and suffering.

Box 14.1 Implementing social services – summary

- Patients with advanced cancer typically have more psychosocial concerns than medical concerns.
- Unmet needs in any area of a patient's and family's life will magnify with disease progression.
- Addressing family concerns is part of patient treatment because family functioning affects patient symptoms and quality of care.
- Decline in the patient's physical or cognitive functioning signals a need to reassess the psychosocial components of the treatment plan.
- All members of the multidisciplinary team must know the indicators of psychosocial needs and refer the patient and family quickly to the appropriate team member for intervention.

BIBLIOGRAPHY

Sentinel articles/books

Baider L, Cooper CL, Kaplan De-Nour A. *Cancer and the Family*, 2nd edn. New York: John Wiley & Son Ltd, 2000.

Cassileth BR, Lusk EJ, Strouse TB, Miller DS, Brown LC, Cross PA. A psychological analysis of cancer patients and their next of kin. *Cancer* 1985;55:72–6.

Miller RD, Walsh TD. Psychosocial aspects of palliative care in advanced cancer. *J Pain Symptom Manage* 1991;6:24–9.

Senn H-J, Glaus A, Schmid L. (ed.) *Supportive Care in Cancer Patients.* Series: *Recent Results in Cancer Research*, 108. New York: Springer-Verlag, 1988.

Review articles/books

Berger A, Portenoy RK, Weissman DE. (ed.) *Principles and Practice of Supportive Oncology.* Philadelphia: Lippincott-Raven, 1982.

Glajchen M. Psychosocial consequences of inadequate health insurance for patients with cancer. *Cancer Pract* 1994;2:115–20.

Higginson I, Priest P. (1996). Predictors of family anxiety in the weeks before bereavement. *Soc Sci Med* 1996;43:1621–5.

Holland JC. (ed.) *Psycho-Oncology.* New York: Oxford University Press, 1998.

Kutner JS, Steiner JF, Corbett JJ, Jahniger DW, Barron PL. Information needs in terminal illness. *Soc Sci Med* 1999;48:1341–52.

Maguire P, Walsh S, Jeacock J, Kingston R. Physical and psychological needs of patients dying from colo-rectal cancer. *Palliat Med* 1999;13:45–50.

Nijboer C, Triemstra M, Tempelaar R, Sanderman R, van der Bos GAM. Determinants of caregiving experiences and mental health of partners of cancer patients. *Cancer* 1999;86:577–88.

Payne S, Smith P, Dean S. Identifying the concerns of informal carers in palliative care. *Palliat Med* 1999;13:37–44.

Sanson-Fischer R, Girgis A, Boyes A, Bonevski B, Burton L, Cook P, the Supportive Care Review Group. The unmet supportive care needs of patients with cancer. *Cancer* 2000;88:226–37.

Siegel K, Raveis VH, Houts P, Mor V. Caregiver burden and unmet patient needs. *Cancer* 1991;68:1131–40.

Internet sites

Cancer Care:
   http://www.cancercare.org

Cancer Information Network (CIN):
   http://www.cancernetwork.com/(professional site)

NCI Cancer Information
   http://www.cancer.gov

International Psychosocial Oncology Society (IPOS)/
   American Society of Psychosocial and Behavioral Oncology/AIDS (ASPBOA)
   http://www.ipos-aspboa.org

15

Pastoral care

Derek B. Murray

5 Comely Bank Place, Edinburgh

When a person is diagnosed with serious illness, it is obvious that medical intervention is necessary, if only to describe the condition. In an increasingly secular society, at least in the Western world, spiritual needs may not seem to be so urgent, or indeed to exist at all. Yet while there is a drift away from organized religion there is also a growing realization that humans have spiritual concerns and that along with physical and social pain, there is emotional and spiritual pain. Pastoral care can be described as an integral and necessary part of good palliative care.

Pastoral care has been described thus: *At its most basic, pastoral care is an active and purposeful concern for people within the context of ultimate meaning and value.* This broad definition should cover a wide variety of religious and spiritual practices. Pastoral care is not evangelism. The pastor approaches the sick person at her invitation and seeks to discover specific questions and concerns. He does not seek to impose his own views. Nor is pastoral care to be equated with social work. Pastors have a distinct training and particular gifts to offer, which may include skill in social care matters, but which are specific to those with pastoral training.

Pastoral care will be delivered by clergy but not only by such specially designated persons. Some patients, entering the last phase of their lives, will wish to be visited by their own priest or minister or another person from the worshipping congregation. Many will not have such a relationship with the church, and it is the task of chaplains to be available to all those who need them.

Pastoral care implies *availability*. Those with far-advanced illness do not have the will or the energy to send for a remote person, and the chaplain should be familiar wit other staff, both in a caring unit and in the wider community. Questions may arise which demand instant attention, and an appointment system is scarcely appropriate.

Pastoral care implies *immediacy*. Pastors should not be afraid of touch, of holding the hand or touching the brow. The "laying on of hands" is much more than a churchly rite. It is a recognition of the universal human need to be close to others.

The carer must never appear to withdraw, either in dignity or in revulsion at physical conditions.

Pastoral care demands *flexibility*. There is often no time to learn much about the patient's background. Vocabularies for expressing spiritual and religious concern may differ or indeed scarcely exist. An ability to make a quick translation into terms meaningful to the patient is very important. The pastor's dogmatic views and professional language must not be allowed to get in the way of care.

Pastoral care demands *a listening ear*. It is not always what is said but what is left unsaid or what is implied that matters. Questions are put in allusive ways, and the alert pastor will pick up inner meanings. A pastor must be able to be quiet and listen, and must often escape from the tyranny of words.

Pastoral care demands *a tentative approach*. Pastors do not have all the answers, and often the patient needs only to articulate the question to be helped. It is impossible to judge a person's spiritual position or attitude from an entry in an admission form. Each patient is on a unique journey, and this must be acknowledged.

Pastoral care requires some *knowledge of common spiritual problems*, which affect both the religious and those who would not consider themselves such.

- *Fear of death* as such seems very often to be subsumed in the fear of the dying process. Reassurance and the growth of confidence in the caring staff need to be nurtured. The patient needs to hear the same story repeated by all carers, and should not receive mixed messages, with realism from the doctor and soothing words from the chaplain.

- *Fear of meaninglessness* is deep seated in many people. Has my life amounted to anything? Will anyone remember me kindly? Encouragement to relate a life story can give some meaning to a life which is under examination as death looms. The question "why me?" is naturally often asked, and of course there is no immediate answer which explains why one person and not another has acquired life-threatening disease. This is one of the questions that has to be allowed to be asked, and if the pastor can lead the patient to rephrase it "why not me?" then some good has been achieved. But the transition must be made entirely by the dying person.

- *The fear of anxiety of guilt and condemnation* afflicts many, and leads to a breakdown of faith even in firm believers. Guilt for a past action remembered in the quiet of a hospital room, or a more generalized feeling of unworthiness can be assuaged by the pastor's acceptance, and by telling again the story of the unconditional love of God may help alleviate this fear. If guilt is being projected on others – the doctors, the minister, or God, it is possible to guide the patient through the consequent anger.

Pastoral carers must be aware that they are vulnerable to the same fears and doubts as patients have and must ensure that they are themselves in some sort of community of care, whether that be formal supervision, or an acknowledged membership of a caring team.

What has been said so far might seem to confine pastoral care to interaction between patients in a unit and carers working there. Of course the network is much wider, and those who work in the community are aware of the need for this sort of care to be given and received. Not only patients but also their families and sometimes their neighbors have many questions. Indeed it is often the immediate family whose needs appear greater than the patient's. Pastoral care is involved in the networks of relationships of which the patient is part. So it is needed within the caring team, and support systems of some sort, informal or formal, are a spiritual necessity.

16

Bereavement

Stephen D. King
Seattle Cancer Care Alliance, Seattle

Bereavement is a state of severe loss and deprivation of emotionally invested relationships with, for example, a person, ideal, thing, place, dream, activity, sense
of self, security, or status. Grief is the emotional, mental, physical, behavioral, and
spiritual response to bereavement; it is also the means to healing. This chapter
focuses upon bereavement and grief due to death, attending to their impact upon
healthcare providers; the grief process including nuances peculiar to children; disenfranchised grief; and some guidelines in communicating with others. The content
is limited in that it is primarily from a Western cultural perspective.

Impact of bereavement and grief upon healthcare providers

Bereavement and grief impact healthcare providers in a number of ways. First, we
observe our patients and their loved ones experiencing anticipatory and actual bereavement and grief. In the context of lost health, patients and their families may
experience anew losses from their past – death of a loved one, a broken intimate
relationship. Furthermore, they may experience losses of control, modesty, inno-
cence and security, normal daily routine. In the face of life-threatening illness, they
anticipate the loss of life (i.e., loss of existence, of experiences, of relationships, of
dreams).

Second, we as healthcare providers also experience bereavement and grief. When
a patient dies, we may experience not only the loss of a person with whom we have
worked and for whom we have cared, but we may also experience our own sense of
confidence in our ability to care for and take care of others diminished. Something
in our own history of personal losses may be evoked – the death of a family member,
a previous death of a patient who had been very important to us. In addition, in
the context of changing healthcare, losses of identity, community, and ideal of care
may be experienced.

The grief process

Bereavement is a state. Grief is a process. Elizabeth Kubler-Ross popularized discussion of grief dynamics, but her thoughts often took on interpretations of grief as rigid stages that all persons must pass through in generally similar fashion. Some healthcare providers sought to guide (or force) the bereaved to grieve in a particular way according to a predetermined time frame. But grief is not linear; it moves back and forth through overlapping phases of disorganization and reorganization after initial shock and disbelief. Generally, grief is not pathological but rather a natural, though painful, healing process.

William Worden has identified four tasks in this process: accepting the reality of the loss, living and working through the pain, adjusting to an environment in which the deceased is absent, and emotionally relating to the deceased in a new way as one moves on with one's life. The acceptance of the reality of the loss means accepting not only the fact of the loss but also the meaning and the irreversibility of the loss. A large number of emotional, physical, cognitive, spiritual, and behavioral responses are normal parts of the pain evoked by bereavement. Emotions may include shock, sadness, anger, guilt, anxiety, helplessness, loss of esteem, loneliness, yearning, and relief. The bereaved may experience a hollowness in the pit of the stomach, weariness, oversensitivity to noise, weakness, tightness of the chest or throat. Cognitive responses include times of disbelief, confusion, preoccupation, momentary perception of having seen or heard the deceased, and/or a sense of the presence of the deceased. The bereaved may also experience conflict between personal experience and theological beliefs, experience spiritual confusion and distress, and/or experience increased depth of spirituality, peace, hope, and enrichment of life, meaning, and values. Behavioral changes such as sleeping more or less, eating more or less, social withdrawal, restlessness, tearfulness at even inexplicable times, treasuring objects or places important to the deceased or in relationship with the deceased are possible. These responses may come and go over what seems to be a significant period of time (Table 16.1). This should not be surprising given that in grief, as Freud noted, the world is poorer and bereft of someone very important.

Worden discusses a number of internal and external factors that influence the intensity and duration of the grief process. These determinants include such things as who the deceased was (e.g., one's child), the nature of the attachment (e.g., ambivalent), the mode of death (e.g., sudden and unexpected), historical antecedents (e.g., the bereaved's previous losses), personality variables (e.g., coping capacity, age, ego strength), social variables (e.g., social support, ethnicity), spiritual beliefs (e.g., hope, meaning), and concurrent stresses (e.g., financial crisis).

Grieving is not completed at a funeral. Sometimes it may not even be largely completed after a year of living through the seasons and "first times" after the death.

Table 16.1. Responses to grief

Emotional
  Shock
  Sadness
  Anger
  Guilt
  Anxiety
  Helplessness
  Loss of esteem
  Loneliness
  Yearning
  Relief
Physical
  Hollowness
  Weariness
  Oversensitivity to noise
  Weakness
  Tightness of the chest or throat
Cognitive
  Disbelief
  Confusion
  Preoccupation
  Hallucination
  Perceived presence of the deceased
Spiritual
  Conflict between experience and belief
  Spiritual confusion and distress
  Increased depth of spirituality
  Enrichment of life
Behavioral
  Sleeping more or less
  Eating more or less
  Social withdrawal
  Restlessness
  Tearfulness and emotionally labile
  Treasuring objects or places important to the deceased

In a significant loss there may always be moments of pain in connection with the death. The grieving process is "worked through" when the pain is no longer overwhelming but can be accepted and lived with, when the deceased still has a place in one's life but a different place that can help one live more fully. Klass,

Silverman, and Nickman call this a "continuing bond" with the deceased. As Mitch Albom observed in *Tuesdays with Morrie*, death ends a lifetime, not a relationship.

As noted above, this chapter is written from a Western cultural perspective. Paul Rosenblatt (Parkes et al., 1997) notes that culture impacts what emotions are experienced and how they are expressed and understood. Individuals within a particular culture may be unique as well. Grief can be complicated for bereaved persons living outside their culture of origin. We may help by encouraging them to engage in rituals and emotional expression appropriate to their culture. Outsiders are not expected to engage in insiders' style of grief. "A genuine and caring offer of sympathy, shared tears, or [other expressions of care] may have more meaning than stilted efforts to act [like them]."

Children and death

In addition to differences in grief across cultures, there are differences between children and adults. Children's bereavement and grief depend upon their cognitive and emotional development. We can be guided by some rough generalizations about phases in a child's developmental understanding of death. In general, children

- 2 or 3 to 5 years old do not understand death as permanent or as a regular life process;
- 5 to 7 years old can accept a person has permanently died but may not understand that all people including themselves die and often lack the skills to cope with their cognitions and emotions; and
- 7 years or older begin to understand death as inevitable for all including themselves.

Children may experience many of the same emotions as adults who are grieving. But they may have a different guilt dynamic. Young children have a strong sense of magical power. In their minds, if they wish it, it may happen; if they have misbehaved, there may be a consequence. Thus, if children have wished for the death of someone out of anger or if they have misbehaved and then someone dies, they may believe the death was their fault. Children need reassurance that the death was not their responsibility. Also, a child may have greater extremes in assuming the mannerisms of the deceased, in idealizing the deceased, in having anxieties about having the same illness as the person who died, in anxieties about who will take care of them if a parent dies. Occasionally a grieving child will regress in behavior patterns or have more difficulties at school and at home.

Questions frequently arise as to how to involve children in the illness process. In general, children should be told the truth with openness and honesty but with sensitivity. A child needs to be able to trust the information and the information providers. A young child who wants to go to a hospital room to visit a loved one should be permitted but with adequate preparation about what the child may see and information about those sights. Often, their imagination about what is happening is worse than reality. Children typically do not have problems if they want to visit and if they are prepared. But they may choose to only stay for a moment. The same approach may be taken in regard to funerals.

Disenfranchised grief

The grief process may be complicated by what Kenneth Doka has popularized as "disenfranchised grief," grief in which the relationship, the loss, and/or the grieving "cannot be openly acknowledged, socially validated, or publicly mourned." Relationships of close relatives are acknowledged whereas the relationship of an ex-spouse, secret paramour, or in-law may be overlooked. Losses such as in perinatal demise frequently do not receive full validation. The grief of the very old and the very young are frequently overlooked. Too often care providers focus attention upon the most obvious griever (e.g., spouse, most tearful) to the neglect of the silent sufferer in the corner.

But beyond our patients and their loved ones, healthcare providers are significant victims of disenfranchised grief in response both to the death of our patients and to institutional change. Good care providers do become attached to certain patients and/or their loved ones. The felt experience of the significance of the relationships, which are sometimes the most important dimension of the healthcare we provide, is valid. At other times our need to grieve is invalidated by the demands of our work. For example, Julie died 20 minutes ago but another patient, John, needs attention now. Or perhaps we must cut short our grieving with Julie's family in order to celebrate good news with John about a biopsy result. We may never again bring our grief over Julie to the foreground. Gradually the losses accumulate. Frequently there are inadequate opportunities for grieving at work and we do not attend to grief at home. More attention to peer support, follow-up with bereaved loved ones, and memorial rituals for staff would help the grieving and healing of staff.

Today's healthcare milieu is chaotic. Reimbursement turmoil is changing the way we provide healthcare. Reorganizations of even long-standing healthcare centers as well as downsizing are common. These changes impact the work life of staff. Roles and identities change; long-term teams who enjoy working together and who have a good rhythm for working together are torn apart. Staff grieve the loss of dreams, working relationships, professional identity. But rarely do the staff have a name for this experience. Rarer still is the institution that attends this bereavement and

Table 16.2. Disenfranchised grief

Defined: grief in which the relationship, the loss, and/or
  the grieving "cannot be openly acknowledged, socially
  validated, or publicly mourned."
Realms:
  Within families and friendships
  Between patients/families and healthcare providers
  Between healthcare providers and their work environment

grief. It is neither "openly acknowledged, socially validated, or publicly mourned." Awareness of and attention to this disenfranchised grief would benefit healthcare provision and providers (Table 16.2).

What helps and doesn't help

In communicating with those who are grieving, there are some general ways that are helpful or that are not helpful. In terms of things that are not helpful, it typically does not help someone to tell them what they should do to get through. Although there are general suggestions of what might be helpful, everyone grieves and copes differently. Pushing someone along in the grieving process hurts: "You should get over it; it is time to move on." "Be strong." Theological explanations, such as "It is God's will," are not only potentially bad theology, they can aggravate the grief process of the spirituality of the bereaved. Minimizing the loss by saying, "At least she isn't suffering" or "She is in heaven now," rarely helps. One might get a response like, "No. She isn't suffering now. She is dead. And nothing will bring her back to me and the life she enjoyed."

Generally, the best care is that of being present and listening. Perhaps one can respond with a genuine response, "I don't know what to say; no words seem to be helpful." It is usually helpful to invite conversation about the loss, e.g., "Tell me about..." Through nonintrusive presence one gives permission to grieve in an authentic manner. Consequently, a healthcare provider dropping by the room after the death of a patient to acknowledge the death/loss is a meaningful act. Offering availability to listen and to respond to questions in the future is also helpful (Table 16.3). Always, the agenda is care for the bereaved, not taking care of oneself. Not necessarily at the time of death but during a follow-up contact, the healthcare provider may inquire about how the bereaved is coping, including ways of grieving. If the person seems to be struggling and asking for ideas, the healthcare provider may offer some possibilities of rituals that would be healing.

Table 16.3. Communication guidelines

Do not:
    Tell someone exactly how to grieve
    Push the grieving process
    Theologically minimize the loss and pain
    Minimize the bereaved's loss
Do:
    Be present nonintrusively
    Listen
    Offer genuine responses
    Invite stories and conversation
    Be available – now and later
    Follow-up

Table 16.4. Conclusions

People have the capacity for significant relationships:
    Within families and friendships
    With patients and their loved ones
    With our work environment
Consequently, healthcare providers:
    Observe bereavement
    Experience bereavement
Relationships and bereavement are universal but the
    grief process is complex and may vary.
There are healing responses:
    Sensitivity
    Presence
    Attentiveness
    Sojourning
    Listening
    Ritual

Conclusion

We have a wonderful capacity to form meaningful and significant relationships, not only within families and friendships but also between patients/families and healthcare professionals as well as between professionals and our work world (Table 16.4). Likewise, we professionals are likely to both observe and experience significant bereavement in our lives. Although the relationships and bereavement are universal experiences, the grief response to those may vary in subtle and profound ways that require sensitivity and respect – both for others and for ourselves. Sensitivity, presence, attentiveness, listening, sojourning, and ritual are important healing responses to bereavement and its grief.

BIBLIOGRAPHY

Books and articles

Casarett D, Kutner JS, Abrahm J. Life after death: a practical approach to grief and bereavement. *Ann Intern Med* 2001;134:208–15.

Corr CA. Enhancing the concept of disenfranchised grief. *Omega* 1998–1999;38:1–20.

American Association of Retired Persons. *Customs of Bereavement; A Guide for Providing Cross-cultural Assistance.* Washington, DC: American Association of Retired Persons, 1990.

Doka KJ. (ed.) *Disenfranchised Grief; Recognizing Hidden Sorrow.* Lexington, MA: Lexington Books, 1989.

Hunter RJ. (ed.) *Dictionary of Pastoral Care and Counseling.* Nashville: Abingdon Press, 1990. See entries, "Grief and loss," "Grief and loss in childhood and adolescence," and "Grief and mourning, Jewish care in."

Klass D, Silverman PR, Nickman SL. (ed.) *Continuing Bonds: New Understandings of Grief.* Series in death education, aging, and health care. Washington, DC: Taylor and Francis, 1996.

Parkes CM, Laungani P, Young, B. (ed.) *Death and Bereavement across Cultures.* New York: Routledge, 1997.

Sanders CM. *Grief: the Mourning After; Dealing with Adult Bereavement.* The Wiley series on Personality Processes, ed. IB Weiner. New York: John Wiley & Sons, 1989.

Worden JW. *Grief Counseling and Grief Therapy; a Handbook for the Mental Health Practitioner,* 2nd edn. New York: Springer Publishing Company, 1991.

Internet site

Growth House, Inc. Topic: Grief. Available at: www.growthhouse.org

Part II

Primary tumors

17

Lung cancer

Suzie Whelen and Thomas J. Smith

Department of Medicine and Massey Cancer Center, Virginia Commonwealth University, Richmond

Introduction

Lung cancer remains the leading cause of cancer-related death in North America and Europe, and more people die of lung cancer than colon, breast, and prostate cancer combined. During 2000, there were predicted to be about 164 100 new cases of lung cancer, 89 500 men and 74 600 women.[1] The increase in death rate is slowing, but has not begun to drop.

More than 80% of lung cancer deaths are attributable to smoking, and only asbestos exposure and family history enhance risk substantially. Fundamentally, lung cancer occurs as a result of deregulation of normal gene expression. Molecular changes that have been demonstrated in lung cancer include activation of oncogenes such as ras, myc, bcl-2, and c-erbB-2; loss of tumor suppressor genes such as p53, RB, and p16; and alterations in angiogenesis such as vascular endothelial growth factor (VEGF) overexpression in primary lung tumors. All represent potential therapy targets.

Categories/staging

The diagnosis is established by examination of either cytology or surgical pathology specimens. Lung cancer is rarely if ever treated without a specific tissue diagnosis. The most widely accepted histologic classification for lung tumors is that proposed by the World Health Organization (WHO) and revised in 1999. It includes four major types: squamous cell, adenocarcinoma, small cell, and large cell.

Small cell lung cancer (SCLC) is the more aggressively spreading tumor with neuroendocrine features and accounts for 20% of all lung cancers. Staging of SCLC is either limited to the chest (lung with primary tumor) or extensive with spread outside the chest. Limited disease is often defined as disease that will fit into one radiation port; this often excludes patients with pleural effusions from being staged

Table 17.1. Staging system in current use

	Definition	Comment
Small cell lung cancer		
Limited	Disease confined to one hemithorax	Helpful if disease fits in one radiation port
Extensive	Outside one hemithorax	Malignant pleural effusions may fit here but controversial
Non-small cell lung cancer		
Stage I	A T1NOMO B T2NOMO	No nodes positive
Stage II	A T1N1MO B T2N1MO T3NOMO	N1 nodes are peribronchial or hilar
Stage IIIA	T3N1MO T1N2MO T2N2MO T3N2MO	N2 nodes are mediastinal or subcarinal
Stage IIIB	T1N3MO T4NOMO T2N3MO T4N1MO T3N3MO T4N2MO T4N3MO	Satellite tumor nodules and malignant pleural effusions are T4. N3 nodes are contralateral
Stage IV	Any T, any N, M1	

as limited disease. The distinction is key, as some limited stage patients can be cured.

Non-small cell lung cancer (NSCLC) is divided into three major types: adenocarcinoma (approximately 40%), squamous (30%) and large cell (15%) rate of occurrence. These histologies are classified together because all have the potential for cure with surgical resection and respond to the same chemotherapy drugs. Staging of NSCLC is based on the 1997 revised American Joint Committee on Cancer worldwide TNM (tumor, node, metastasis) system which includes clinical, surgical (via bronchoscopy or mediastinoscopy), and pathologic assessment (Table 17.1). Surgical staging of the mediastinum is considered standard if accurate evaluation of the nodal status is needed to determine therapy. All but stage IV patients can be treated with curative intent.

Stages I and II are surgically resectable tumors. Advanced disease includes stages III (IIIA is to T3N2M0, and IIIB is any T4 or N3) and IV (any M1). Satellite tumor nodules in the same lobe as the primary lesion that are not lymph nodes should be classified as T4 lesions. Tumors of any size with invasion of the mediastinum or involving the heart, great vessels, trachea, recurrent laryngeal nerve, esophagus, vertebral body, or carina or the presence of a malignant pleural effusion are classed as T4 and are unresectable. Metastases may be to ipsilateral mediastinal and subcarinal lymph nodes (N2) or to any contralateral or supraclavicular lymph nodes (N3). Intrapulmonary ipsilateral metastasis in a lobe other than the lobe containing the primary lesions should be classified as an M1 lesion.

Prognosis

The 5-year survival for all stages of lung cancer combined is only 14%. The 5-year survival for NSCLC by stage is approximately: I, 40–60%; II, 25–35%; III, 10–15%; and IV, 5%.[2] If the disease is still localized, 5-year survival is about 49%; however, only 15% of lung cancers are discovered that early.[1] Survival has increased from 34% in 1975 to the current 41% due to improvements in early detection and surgical techniques and possibly adjuvant therapy. The natural history of *metastatic* NSCLC is poor with median survival only 5 to 6 months, and only 10% of patients are alive at one year.[3]

The most important predictor of survival in NSCLC is the TNM stage at diagnosis. Weight loss of 5% of body weight and poor performance status at the time of diagnosis have a significantly negative impact on survival. Patients presenting without symptoms (shortness of breath, cough, hemoptysis, weight loss, fatigue, pain, headache, superior vena cava syndrome, etc.) had a 5-year survival of 74% versus only a 41% survival rate in patients with symptoms.[4] Hypercalcemia of malignancy is associated with a median survival of only one month regardless of stage, and is a contraindication to resection.

SCLC generally has the worst overall survival because of its very aggressive clinical course with frequent widespread metastases (most commonly bone, liver, and brain). Untreated patients with limited-stage and extensive-stage SCLC have a median survival of 3 and 1.5 months, respectively.[3,5] With combination chemotherapy and chest radiotherapy, the median survival is improved to 10–16 months for patients with limited-stage disease, and 6–11 months for patients with extensive disease.

Surgery

Treatment options for lung cancer include surgery, radiation, and chemotherapy, as summarized in Table 17.2. Surgery is the major potentially curative therapeutic option for NSCLC. When the chest tumor is limited to a hemithorax and can be totally encompassed by excision, surgery should be considered. Mortality rates should be < 6%, for pneumonectomy, < 3% for lobectomy, and < 1% for lesser resections.

Table 17.2. Management of lung cancer

	Primary treatment plan	Comment
Small cell lung cancer		
Limited	Chemotherapy with concurrent radiation	Prophylactic cranial radiation for complete responders
Extensive	Chemotherapy alone	
Non-small cell lung cancer		
Stages I and II	Surgery	Mortality less at high volume centers
		No proven role for adjuvant chemotherapy or radiation
Stage IIIA	Induction chemotherapy followed by surgery and/or radiation	
Stage IIIB	Chemotherapy followed by or concurrent with radiation	No proven role for chemotherapy or radiation after resection
		Radiation may prolong disease-free survival if resection incomplete
Stage IV	Palliative chemotherapy or radiation alone	No indication for combined modality therapy
		Possible resection of single metachronous metastases in brain, adrenal gland, liver
		Survival is poor enough to justify referral to hospice at diagnosis for symptom control, if chemotherapy is not successful in prolonging life or reducing symptoms

The role of surgery in stage IIIA NSCLC is controversial but should be explored with each patient. T3 disease indicates a primary tumor with local invasion of surrounding structures that is still completely resectable and thus potentially curable. N2 tumors with ipsilateral mediastinal lymph node involvement are potentially resectable, but only 18% can have complete resection with only a 9% 3-year survival.[6] Preoperative chemotherapy followed by surgery or radiation for stage IIIA NSCLC patients has become routine based on a number of small randomized trials showing small survival benefits.[7] At present, there is no proven role for postoperative adjuvant chemotherapy.[8]

Stage IIIB NSCLC, by virtue of unresectable lymph node spread (N3) to the contralateral mediastinum or supraclavicular nodes or primary tumor invasion of mediastinal structures (T4), is inoperable with a small likelihood of long-term survival following surgical excision. Similarly, lung cancer that has metastasized to distant organs is treated without surgery. Recently, there has been interest in removing the primary tumor as well as a solitary metastatic focus in the brain, adrenal, or other organs for patients with NSCLC. In carefully selected individuals, this may result in long-term disease-free survival. Endoscopic laser ablation can be done as palliative treatment of endobronchial unresectable or recurrent lung cancer.

Due to the systemic nature of SCLC at diagnosis, surgical resection is not an option for these lung cancer patients. If a solitary lung mass is found at resection to be SCLC, it has become standard to administer several cycles of adjuvant chemotherapy with apparent improved survival although this approach has not been proven in randomized trials.

Radiation

Radiation therapy has long been administered in an effort to control NSCLC (Table 17.2). The dose of 60 Gy over 6 weeks was adopted as the standard dose for definitive radiation therapy (RT) despite a 6-year survival of only 5%. New hyperfractionated (two or three smaller fractions a day, for a shorter time course), intensity-modulated radiation therapy, and three-dimensional conformal methods of delivering RT are changing response and adverse effects to treatment. The combined use of chemotherapy and radiation as primary treatment for stages IIIA and IIIB will be discussed in the chemotherapy section below. Radiation can be used neoadjuvantly (or preoperatively) to reduce tumor size for resection in patients with IIIA disease, but this approach has not made substantial gains. It may also be given with chemotherapy (see below section). RT is used adjuvantly (or postoperatively) when known residual disease is present, such as positive microscopic surgical margins and positive lymph nodes and may decrease the local recurrence rate. Multiple randomized prospective trials have failed to show a survival advantage for the administration of adjuvant therapy (radiation or chemotherapy) following complete resection of NSCLC.[9]

The palliative effects of RT are often significant despite poor survival. About 60% or more of patients will have symptom relief, often lasting for months. Newer approaches of hypofractionation (1–4 larger doses) appear to give similar results and are far more convenient for the patient.[10] This hypofractionated approach can be used for the primary tumor, bone, or other metastases, and for the palliation of hemoptysis, where radiation has been shown to be more effective than laser ablation.[10]

For limited stage SCLC, RT is used concurrently with chemotherapy with moderate improvement in survival (5–10 patients of 100 treated) over chemotherapy alone.[1] RT is used only for symptomatic palliation in extensive stage SCLC, as chemotherapy is the primary treatment modality. Patients with SCLC who have a complete response to treatment (complete remission) should be considered for prophylactic cranial irradiation (PCI). Patients whose cancer can be controlled outside the brain have a 60% actuarial risk of developing central nervous system (CNS) metastases after treatment, and PCI can reduce development of CNS metastases by more than 50% and improve survival by about six patients of every 100.[11]

Chemotherapy

Summary recommendations are given in Table 17.2.

Small cell lung cancer

Combination chemotherapy has been the cornerstone of treatment for patients with SCLC for decades.[3] SCLC patients with extensive disease benefit from multidrug regimens of chemotherapy in terms of survival and palliation of symptoms. Doses and schedules used in current programs (cisplatin/etoposide, carboplatin/etoposide, etc.) yield overall response rates of 70–85% and complete response rates of 20–30% in extensive disease.[3] Combination chemotherapy plus chest irradiation (as done in limited stage SCLC) does not appear to improve survival compared with chemotherapy alone in extensive stage disease. A number of new agents with activity in SCLC are currently being evaluated (paclitaxel, topotecan, irinotecan, gemcitabine).

Patients who are medically stable with extensive stage SCLC may be treated with new agents under evaluation (as first-line therapy), with provisions for early change to standard combination therapy if there is no response.

Some patients will present with advanced SCLC and poor performance status due to their bulk of disease. These patients will die within days if not treated with aggressive chemotherapy and often will enter remission and live for many good months if they are treated expeditiously.

Non-small cell lung cancer

More recently, chemotherapy has also become the standard of care for patients with stage III and IV NSCLC.[7,12] Since over two-thirds of NSCLC patients present with stages III or IV disease, or those who relapse after surgery, chemotherapy is now being considered for most patients diagnosed with lung cancer in the US. Because of the poor long-term results, all patients with advanced lung cancer (NSCLC and SCLC) should be considered for treatment on clinical trials (http://cancer.gov/search/clinical_trials/).

Stage IIIA N2 NSCLC patients have a 5-year survival rate of 10–15% overall. With preoperative chemotherapy 65–75% of patients were able to have a resection of their cancer and 27–28% were alive at 3 years. In small studies, median survival was more than three times as long in patients treated preoperatively versus patients treated with surgery but no chemotherapy.[13,14] Unresectable IIIA patients may be treated with combination chemotherapy and RT, chemotherapy or radiation alone depending on symptoms and performance status.

Stage IIIB NSCLC patients with good performance status are best managed by initial chemotherapy or chemotherapy plus radiation. Many randomized studies of unresectable patients with stage III disease show that treatment with neoadjuvant or concurrent cisplatin-based chemotherapy and chest irradiation is associated with improved survival compared with treatment with RT alone; combination therapy resulting in a 10% reduction in the risk of death compared with RT.[7,12,15] The optimal sequencing of modalities such as concurrent versus sequential remains to be determined; however, concurrent therapy may yield more responses with slightly higher toxicity.[16,17]

Stage IV NSCLC patients treated with older chemotherapy regimens gained approximately 6 weeks or 10% improvement in 1-year survival (to about 20%) compared with best supportive care.[1] Newer chemotherapy regimens (with agents such as docetaxel, gemcitabine, paclitaxel, or vinorelbine) suggest median survivals ranging 6–9 months with 1-year survival at 30–40%. No single regimen has been proven superior. Advanced NSCLC patients with poor performance status (PS $\geq$ 2) should generally not be recommended chemotherapy because these patients tend to experience increased toxicity, decreased survival, and no clinical benefit. Newer single-agent regimens such as vinorelbine or gemcitabine alone appear to be safer in such patients and may offer some palliative benefit.[18,19]

Main issues and suggestions for management

Dyspnea is present in 40–60% of lung cancer patients at diagnosis and 70% of all cancer patients.[7] It can result from a variety of causes and is often multifactorial. Causes and treatments are listed in Table 17.3.

Management of dyspnea depends on the underlying cause, and treatment should be sought aggressively as this symptom is extremely distressing to both patients and families. Dyspnea that is new, changed from prior baseline, or worse should be evaluated for treatable causes. Pulse oximetry and chest radiograph often provide

Table 17.3. Causes and treatment of dyspnea in lung cancer patients

Cause	Treatment	Comment
Extensive tumor	Primary treatment	60% will have relief of cough and dyspnea with chemotherapy
Atalectasis/obstruction	Radiation, laser, stents	
Lymphangitic spread	Prednisone 1 mg/kg daily	Treat like bronchospasm
Pleural effusion	Drainage and sclerosis	
Pericardial effusion	Drainage and sclerosis	
Pneumonia	Antibiotics	
Bronchospasm and emphysema	Prednisone and bronchodilators	
Heart failure	Diuretics	Common
Pulmonary embolism	Heparin	Diagnosis with CAT scan is sensitive and specific; lung cancer one of most common hypercoaguable states

Note: CAT, computerized axial tomography.

useful information as oxygen and antibiotics may provide some relief of symptoms. Uncorrectable dyspnea may be treated with morphine or other narcotics such as fentanyl by mouth, nebulizer, or injection titrated to relief. Benzodiazepines may aid the anxiety produced by progressive dyspnea in advanced lung cancer patients (Table 17.4) (see Chapter 44 also).

Cough is the most common symptom reported at presentation by patients with lung cancer, occurring in 45–75% of patients. Because the majority of patients with lung cancer are smokers, most have had a chronic cough as baseline. Treatment of cancer may help relieve cough; however, many patients may need cough suppression with narcotics such as codeine. When hemoptysis occurs, depending on its severity, cough suppression is essential and further therapy may be needed. Hemoptysis manifested as frank blood (often in the range of 5–10 ml per hour), not blood-streaked sputum, may require bronchoscopic or surgical intervention. Radiation therapy is the mainstay of hemoptysis treatment, and hypofractionated schemes are recommended.

Pleural effusion occurs in 15–20% of lung cancer patients and most are found to be malignant although about one-half are cytologically negative. Proper classification of an effusion by thoracentesis can both prevent ineffective local measures such as surgery or RT as well as ensure that resectable patients are not denied the benefits of surgery. The management of the effusion depends on symptoms and performance status. Patients who can tolerate procedures may benefit from

Table 17.4. Common side effects of the disease or treatment, and remedies

Symptom	Treatment	Comments
Dyspnea	Narcotics, e.g., morphine 5–10 mg every 4 hours Benzodiazepines, e.g., lorazepam 0.5–1 mg every 4 hours	Oxygen, although commonly administered, is expensive and not often helpful. Dyspnea and hypoxia have a poor correlation
Cough	As above	
Hemoptysis	Radiation therapy. Cough suppression	
Pleural effusions	Drainage	
Superior vena cava syndrome	Small cell lung cancer – chemotherapy Non-small cell lung cancer – radiation or combined modality treatment.	*Not* an emergency. Role of steroids and warfarin unsettled
Esophagitis	No known successful treatment. Commonly treated with omeprazole, antifungals, symptomatic relief. Carafate worsens symptoms	Commonly due to radiation from 2–6 weeks. More common with combined modality treatment
Paraneoplastic syndromes	Hypercalcemia: pamidronate 90 mg i.v. Hyponatremia: liberal salt intake, restrict water intake, demeclocycline	Hypercalcemia is generally a preterminal event with median survival of 1 month, no long-term survivors even if apparently resectable[24]
Cachexia	Megestrol acetate 200–800 mg or prednisone 10–20 mg daily will improve appetite in one-third of patients	
Brain metastases	Dexamethasone 16 mg daily p.o. or i.v.	Resect single brain metastases if disease otherwise controlled. Role of stereotactic radiation uncertain

video-assisted thoracoscopy and talc insufflation or traditional thoracoscopy tube placement. Patients with advanced disease and poor performance status can have a flexible small-bore catheter placed to allow drainage of the effusion for relief of dyspnea and chest discomfort (see Chapter 62). Patients who do not want any procedures should be treated for the resulting progressive dyspnea.

Superior vena cava (SVC) syndrome is caused 70% of the time by lung cancer.[20] It is usually a consequence of obstruction of the superior vena cava by right paratracheal adenopathy or central extension of a primary tumor in the right upper lobe. The most common symptoms are dyspnea, facial swelling or head fullness, cough, arm swelling, chest pain, neck or chest wall vein distension, dysphagia, or flushing. SVC syndrome, long thought to be a medical emergency, is now recognized as a common and not life-threatening complication; in the largest series, only a handful of deaths in 1800 patients were due to it.[21] For SCLC, combination chemotherapy with or without RT is the standard of care. For NSCLC, RT is the primary treatment. Serial venography and autopsy findings suggest that the symptomatic improvement achieved by RT is not always due to improvement of flow through the SVC, but is probably a result of the development of collaterals after pressure in the mediastinum is eased. SVC syndrome is discussed further in Chapter 63.

Acute *esophagitis* is a common accompaniment of RT and combined modality therapy in lung cancer. The epithelium of the esophagus is a moderately radiosensitive acute-reacting tissue which can generally tolerate conventionally fractionated RT doses in the range of 45–50 Gy. Symptoms of esophagitis include subacute retrosternal, burning chest pain, dysphagia, and odynophagia, usually beginning in the second to third week of therapy, increasing in severity throughout treatment and then subsiding 1–2 weeks after completion of treatment. Patients should be examined for a source of infectious esophagitis such as fungal, viral, or bacterial organisms and treated appropriately with fluconazole, aciclovir, or antibiotics if these exist. Otherwise, there is no standard care for RT-induced esophagitis but patients may be treated symptomatically with antacids, H-2 blockers or proton pump inhibitors, prophylactic fungal treatment such as fluconazole, and pain medications such as narcotics. Carafate worsens esophagitis and should not be used.[22] Advanced NSCLC patients receiving combined modality therapy with chemotherapy and RT concurrently may benefit from prophylactic treatment of esophagitis with omeprazole and fluconazole, but this treatment has not been formally evaluated.

Paraneoplastic syndromes result in organ dysfunction with remote effects of the primary lung cancer. Several different paraneoplastic syndromes are common in 10–20% of patients with bronchogenic carcinoma (PDQ). Some of the more common syndromes associated with lung cancer are as follows: endocrinologic such as hypercalcemia and hyponatremia (syndrome of inappropriate antidiuretic hormone, or SIADH); neurologic such as Lambert–Eaton myasthenic syndrome (LEMS) and peripheral neuropathy; musculoskeletal such as hypertrophic pulmonary osteoarthropathy; hematologic such as anemia, idiopathic thrombocytopenia purpura, leukocytosis, and thrombocytosis; and miscellaneous such as cachexia and fever. In particular, squamous cell carcinoma is the most common histology associated with hypercalcemia, and SCLC is most commonly associated with SIADH and ectopic Cushing's syndrome (ectopic ACTH production). SCLC is also the most common histologic type associated with neurologic paraneoplastic syndromes such as LEMS (proximal muscles weakness, autonomic dysfunction, and paresthesias) and neuropathy. In all the paraneoplastic syndromes, successful treatment of the malignancy usually improves the symptoms. If primary treatment of the lung cancer is not possible, then treatment of the paraneoplastic dysfunction is directed at the resulting symptoms.

Lung cancer is the most common cause of *brain metastases*. Approximately one-half of SCLC patients develop brain metastases during the course of their disease. The manifestations are variable and depend on the location of the lesion and the amount of associated edema or hemorrhage. Symptoms include focal weakness, generalized or focal seizures, confusion or dementia, dysphasia, visual disturbances, or ataxia. Initial management of symptomatic brain metastases is with corticosteroids, initially intravenous then orally. Diphenylhydantoin is not recommended prophylactically but reserved for patients with seizures. Aggressive treatment of brain metastases is usually based on the extent of the primary lung disease and patient performance status; resection of one to three metastatic lesions is reasonable in patients who are in good general condition. Resection followed by whole-brain irradiation results in better long-term control than RT alone.[23] Studies investigating stereotactic radiosurgery (gamma knife) are ongoing but it does not add benefit to whole-brain radiation for most patients. See Chapter 58 for further details.

Acknowledgement

Supported in part by a grant from the Office of Cancer Communications, National Cancer Institute (RFP CO 94388-63), and a Faculty Scholar Award, *Project on Death in America*, Open Society, New York.

REFERENCES

1 American Cancer Society Lung Cancer Resource Center. 2001. Internet Communication.

2 Mountain CF. Revisions in the International System for Staging Lung Cancer. *Chest* 1997;111:1710–17.

3 PDQ cancer net non-small cell lung cancer and small cell lung cancer treatment – Health Professionals. 2001. Internet Communication.

4 Harpole D, Herndon J, Young W et al. NSCLC: a multivariate analysis of treatment methods and patterns of recurrence. *Cancer* 1995;76:787.

5 DeVore R, Johnson D. Chemotherapy for small cell lung cancer. In *Lung Cancer Principles and Practice*, ed. H Pass, JB Mitchell, D Johnson, A Turrisi, J Minna, pp. 923–39. Philadelphia, PA: Lippincott Williams and Wilkins, 2000.

6 Felip E et al. Preoperative high-dose cisplatin versus moderate-dose cisplatin combined with ifosfamide and mitomycin in stage IIIA (N2) NSCLC: results of a randomized multicenter trial. *Clin Lung Cancer* 2000;1:287–93.

7 American Society of Clinical Oncology. Clinical practice guidelines for the treatment of unresectable non-small-cell lung cancer. *J Clin Oncol* 1997;15:2996–3018.

8 Keller S, Adak S, Wagner H et al. A randomized trial of postoperative adjuvant therapy in patients with completely resected stage II or IIIA non-small cell lung cancer. *N Engl J Med* 2000;343:1217–22.

9 Keller S. Adjuvant therapy of NSCLC. *Clin Lung Cancer* 2000;1:269–74.

10 Smith T, von Roehn J, von Gunten C, Loprinzi C. (ed.) ASCO *Curriculum: Optimizing Cancer Care – The Importance of Symptom Management.* Kendall/Hunt Publishing Company, 2001.

11 Arriagada R et al. Prophylactic cranial irradiation for patients with SCLC in complete remission. *J Natl Cancer Inst* 1995;87:183–90.

12 NSCLC Collaborative Group. Chemotherapy in non-small cell lung cancer: a meta-analysis using updated data on individual patients from 52 randomized clinical trials. *Br Med J* 1995;311:899–909.

13 Rosell R et al. A randomized rial comparing preoperative chemotherapy plus surgery with surgery alone in patients with NSCLC. *N Engl J Med* 1994;330:153–8.

14 Roth JA et al. A randomized trial comparing perioperative chemotherapy and surgery with surgery alone in resectable stage IIIA NSCLC. *J Natl Cancer Inst* 1994;86:673–80.

15 Sause W et al. RTOG 88-08 and ECOG 4588: preliminary results of a phase III trial in regionally advanced, unresectable NSCLC. *J Natl Cancer Inst* 1995;87:198–205.

16 Choy H, Akerley W, Safran H et al. Multiinstitutional phase II trial of paclitaxel, carboplatin, and concurrent radiation therapy for locally advanced NSCLC. *J Clin Oncol* 1998;16:3316–22.

17 Johnson D, Turrisi A. Combined modality treatment for locally advanced, unresectable non-small cell lung cancer. In *Lung Cancer Principles and Practice*, ed. H Pass, J Mitchell, D Johnson, A Turrisi, J Minna, pp. 910–20. Philadelphia, PA: Lippincott Williams and Wilkins, 2000.

18 Gralla et al. Vinorelbine in the treatment of NSCLC: studies with single agent and in combination with cisplatin. *Ann Oncol* 1999;10:S41–5.

19 Kelly et al. The role of single-agent gemcitabine in the treatment of NSCLC. *Ann Oncol* 1999;10:S53–6.

20 Yahalom J. Superior vena cava syndrome. In *Cancer Principles and Practice of Oncology* ed. VT DeVita, S Hellman, SA Rosenberg, pp. 2469–75. Philadelphia, PA: Lippincott-Raven Publishers, 1997.

21 Ahmann F. A reassessment of the clinical implications of the superior vena cava syndrome. *J Clin Oncol* 1984;2:961.

22 Martenson J, Bollinger J, Sloan J et al. Sucralfate in the prevention of treatment-induced diarrhea in patients receiving pelvic radiation therapy: a north central cancer treatment group phase III double-blind placebo-controlled trial. *J Clin Oncol* 2000;18:1239–45.

23 Olak J, Ferguson M. Surgical management of second primary and metastatic lung cancer. In *Lung Cancer Principles and Practice* ed. H Pass, J Mitchell, D Johnson, A Turrisi, J Minna, pp. 730–41. Philadelphia, PA: Lippincott Williams and Wilkins, 2000.

24 Ralston S, Gallacher S, Patel U, Campbell J, Boyle I. Cancer-associated hypercalcemia: morbidity and mortality. C experience in 126 treated patients. *Ann Intern Med* 1990; 112:499–504.

18

Breast cancer

Kathy D. Miller

Indiana University School of Medicine, Indianapolis

Introduction

Breast cancer remains the most common non-skin cancer diagnosed and the second leading cause of cancer death (lung cancer now leading) in US women each year. Breast cancer does occur in men but much less frequently, affecting about 1500 men per year. Due in large part to the increased use of mammographic screening and advances in adjuvant therapy, mortality rates from breast cancer have been slowly declining for the last 10 years. Early stage breast cancer is successfully treated in over 90% of patients. Currently only about 10% of patients present with metastatic breast cancer. Of patients with apparently localized disease, approximately one-quarter with lymph-node negative and one-half with lymph-node positive breast cancer will ultimately develop metastatic disease. This means that of the 180 000 women in the US diagnosed with breast cancer each year, the disease proves fatal in ~40 000.

Ductal carcinomas account for about 85% of invasive breast cancers, lobular carcinomas about 10%. Other types of breast cancer including medullary, mucinous, tubular, and colloid are uncommon subtypes of ductal carcinomas with a slightly more favorable prognosis. Though there are some differences in the pattern of recurrence, ductal and lobular cancers are treated similarly. Sarcomas, metaplastic carcinomas, neuroendocrine tumors, and other rare histologic types are treated quite differently and will not be discussed further.

Pattern of spread and recurrence

Breast cancer can spread through either the lymphatic system to the axillary (or less commonly internal mammary) lymph nodes or hematogenously to distant organs. The amount of local disease at diagnosis predicts the risk of distant recurrence. That is to say, patients with larger tumors and more involved nodes are more likely to harbor microscopic distant disease that may ultimately become apparent as overt metastases. Less well-recognized is the impact of tumor size and nodal involvement on the time course of recurrence. The median interval to recurrence is longest in patients with the smallest tumors. Similarly, the median interval to recurrence is over 5 years in patients without axillary node involvement, ~3.5 years for patients with 1–4+ lymph nodes and 2.5 years for patients with four or more involved nodes. Put quite simply, the size and extent of local disease at the time of diagnosis predicts the relative bulk of systemic disease. The more local disease, the more systemic disease and the earlier recurrence.

Metastasis to virtually every organ has been reported. The most common sites are the bone (~65%), lungs (~60%), liver (~55%), and brain (~20%). Chest wall cutaneous or soft tissue recurrence is found in ~15–20% of patients. Bone is the first site of metastasis in 40–50% of patients; liver metastases are uncommon in the absence of disease elsewhere. Though the overall prognosis of patients with invasive ductal and invasive lobular carcinomas is similar, differences in the pattern of recurrence bear mention. Lobular carcinoma is less likely to involve the lungs, liver, and brain but more likely to involve bone than ductal carcinomas. Lobular carcinomas have a greater propensity to spread along organ linings resulting in leptomeningeal metastases, pleural and pericardial effusions, and ascites. Diffuse infiltration of the stomach with delayed gastric emptying and impaired absorption similar to primary gastric cancer (*linitis plastica*) is also more common with lobular carcinoma.

Natural history

Breast cancer has a more varied course than most other solid tumor malignancies. Some patients develop evidence of systemic disease shortly after (or concurrently with) diagnosis, while others may not experience symptoms of recurrent disease for more than 20 years. Metastatic breast cancer is generally incurable with a median survival of 18–24 months, however, a large range exists. Some long-term survivors (albeit with disease) can be expected even in the absence of effective treatment. Middlesex Hospital followed 250 patients with advanced breast cancer seen between 1805 and 1933; no patient received any form of therapy. The median survival from the onset of symptoms of breast cancer (generally a palpable breast mass) was 2.7 years. Eighteen percent of patients survived 5 years; 4% survived 10 years or more.

What do we mean by "generally incurable?" Is long-term *disease-free* survival ever an attainable goal for patients with metastatic breast cancer? Investigators at M.D. Anderson Cancer Center reviewed the long-term follow-up of 1581 patients treated on consecutive doxorubicin and alkylating agent-containing front-line treatment protocols between 1973 and 1982. Two hundred and sixty-three (16.6%) patients achieved a complete response (CR); 49 (3.1%) patients remained in CR for 5 years or more. There was a substantial drop in the risk of progression approximately 3 years from initiation of therapy, but recurrences more than 5 years after treatment were reported.

Can we predict which patients are likely to be long-term survivors who therefore might benefit from aggressive initial therapy? Yes, but to a limited degree. In the M.D. Anderson Cancer Center series the long-term CR group had more pre-menopausal patients, a younger median age, a lower tumor burden, and better performance status than the overall CR and total patient populations. Perhaps more importantly, we can predict who will not be a long-term survivor. No patient with an ECOG performance status of 2 – that is, someone ambulatory and capable of self-care, out of bed more than half the day but not able to perform even sedentary work – was a long-term survivor.

Certain clinical and pathologic factors may predict the rate of progression of metastatic breast cancer. Longer survival is more likely in patients with a long disease-free interval, nonvisceral disease and fewer sites of recurrence. The site of recurrence is also important. Longer survival is expected in patients with cutaneous or soft tissue recurrences than in patients with extensive hepatic or lymphangitic pulmonary metastases. Biologic factors important in the prognosis of patients with early stage breast cancer remain important in patients with metastatic disease. Poorly differentiated tumors progress more rapidly. Patients with estrogen receptor positive (ER+) tumors can be expected to enjoy a longer survival; survival is shorter in patients with tumors that overexpress or amplify the human epidermal growth factor receptor-2 (HER-2). Despite the varied natural history, this chapter will focus on generalities and an approach to treatment rather than specific treatment regimens.

Therapeutic approaches

The importance of histologic (or cytologic) confirmation of suspected metastatic breast cancer cannot be overstated. Benign lesions or second nonmammary primary tumors can be easily mistaken for metastatic disease, particularly in patients with solitary lesions. In one autopsy study, 11% of breast cancer patients developed second primary malignancies, often of the genitourinary or gastrointestinal systems, a mean of 7 years from the initial breast cancer diagnosis. A second primary tumor must be considered even in patients previously treated for overt metastatic breast cancer. In a study of patients treated at the M.D. Anderson Cancer Center, seven of 49 patients remaining in complete remission for more than 5 years after anthracycline-based therapy developed a second, nonbreast, malignancy.

Before considering specific therapeutic options, the goal of therapy must be clear. Though a small fraction of patients with overt metastatic disease obtain long-term remissions, most have a median survival of 18–24 months. Should all patients be treated aggressively, with curative intent, in the knowledge that only a few will be saved? Should treatment focus on palliation at the potential expense of the few who may derive long-term benefit from aggressive therapy? Although these goals are not mutually exclusive, there are no simple answers. Nor can (or should) the physicians make this decision independent of the patient. A patient's desire to attend a child's wedding on a given day is quite real and important to her and should be respected – regardless of the adjustments to the chemotherapy schedule that may be required.

An often overlooked, but crucial, component of the treatment of women with metastatic breast cancer is the role of supportive services. Social workers may arrange home care, disability payments, and compassionate use drug discounts. Clinical psychologists may bolster coping skills to decrease the effects of depression and anxiety. Legal assistance may be required to provide for children who are minors. Spiritual counselors may provide hope when drugs fail. Only in an open, multidisciplinary environment and with frank discussion of the nature of the disease and goals of therapy can optimal treatment be delivered.

Though the varied clinical course of patients with overt metastatic breast cancer does not lend itself well to simple treatment algorithms, a general approach can be outlined (Figure 18.1 and Table 18.1). Two distinct therapeutic options are available:

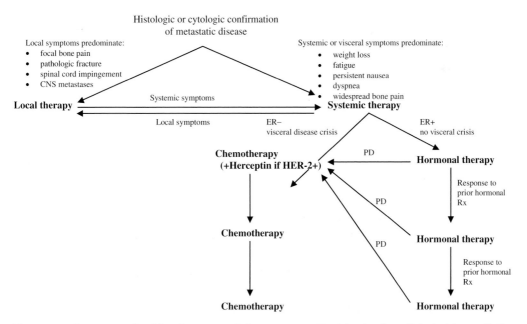

Figure 18.1 Treatment algorithm for metastatic breast cancer. Participation in a clinical trial or palliative care only should be considered at each decision point.

Table 18.1. Approach to the patient with suspected overt metastatic disease

Confirm diagnosis – biopsy if any doubt

↓

Careful history and physical – assess symptoms and tempo of disease

↓

Laboratory and radiographic evaluation – determine extent of disease

↓

Review biologic characteristics of primary tumor

↓

Review previous systemic therapy

↓

Assess patient's general medical and social condition

↓

Determine goals of treatment

local therapies such as surgery, radiation, hyperthermia, or photodynamic therapy and systemic therapies such as hormonal manipulations, cytotoxic chemotherapy, or specific antibodies.

Local therapies, by definition, are limited to the specific part of the body treated (i.e., radiation field, area of tumor resected) and do not affect areas of disease outside the target field. Considering metastatic breast cancer as a systemic disease may lead us to discount the importance of local therapy – to the detriment of our patients. Prioritizing local and systemic treatment requires an honest assessment of the consequences of uncontrolled local disease (pain, pathologic fracture, spinal cord compression) and the virulence of the systemic disease (true visceral crisis versus the mere presence of visceral disease). Local therapies can provide excellent palliation of symptoms with improvement typically faster than that obtained with even the most effective systemic therapy. For instance, a patient with a solitary painful bone metastasis causing impending fracture and asymptomatic pulmonary nodules might best be treated with surgery and radiation to the bone lesion, followed by systemic therapy. Alternatively, a patient with the same bone lesion and rapidly progressive lymphangitic pulmonary metastases might best be treated with analgesics, limited weight bearing, and cytotoxic chemotherapy.

The choice of systemic treatment is based on dual considerations – the probability of response and the toxicity of the therapy. With truly rare exceptions, hormonal therapy offers better palliation than chemotherapy in patients with ER+ tumors. That is, the probability of response is similar with substantially fewer side effects with hormonal therapy. The "most aggressive" therapy is not always the most appropriate or optimal. Hence most patients with ER+ tumors should be offered initial hormonal therapy with cytotoxic treatment held in reserve for when the disease becomes hormone refractory – perhaps years from the initial diagnosis of metastatic disease. Initial chemotherapy may be considered for selected patients with ER+ tumors and rapidly progressive visceral disease; the mere presence of visceral disease does not mandate cytotoxic therapy. Obtaining a response to hormonal therapy requires a longer period of treatment (~2–3 months) than obtaining a response with chemotherapy (~3–6 weeks). If the pace of the disease would not allow a 2–3 month trial of hormonal therapy should that therapy be proven ineffective, initial chemotherapy should be offered.

Tamoxifen has been the mainstay of hormonal therapy for over 25 years and is effective in both pre- and postmenopausal women. Tamoxifen blocks the effects of estrogen thereby decreasing growth and triggering programmed cell death (apoptosis) of estrogen-sensitive breast cancers. Common side effects are hot flashes and vaginal discharge. More serious side effects including thromboembolic events, endometrial cancer, and severe depression are thankfully rare.

Aromatase converts adrenal steroids to estrogen and accounts for most of the circulating estrogen in postmenopausal women. Recently, specific aromatase inhibitors (anastrozole, letrozole or exemestane) have supplanted tamoxifen as the first choice of hormonal therapy in postmenopausal women. As aromatase accounts for only about 10% of the circulating estrogen in premenopausal women, the aromatase inhibitors are not effective in women with functioning ovaries. Many patients can be treated for prolonged periods with the sequential use of different hormonal agents. As a general rule, the response rate and duration of response decreases by about half with each successive hormonal therapy. Other hormonal therapy agents including megesterol acetate, LHRH agonists and androgens are used less frequently but remain excellent options for some patients.

There is no clearly established "first-line" chemotherapy regimen (Table 18.2). Instead, the choice of chemotherapy must take into account the expected toxicity, the patient's opinion about the severity/importance of those toxicities, interaction with comorbid conditions, and the patient's prior therapy. For instance, you may avoid taxanes in a patient with diabetic neuropathy or anthracyclines in a patient with an underlying cardiomyopathy. The use of combination cytotoxic regimens compared with the use of sequential single agents produces modestly higher response rates and slightly prolongs duration of response, but does not increase overall survival or improve quality of life. For most patients, the increased toxicity and more complicated treatment schedules often associated with combination cytotoxic therapy are difficult to justify.

Table 18.2. Single agent activity of commonly used drugs

Agent	Previously treated	Previously untreated	Comments
	Overall response rate (%)		
Antitumor antibiotics			
Doxorubicin	30–78	14–38	Cardiac toxicity – cumulative dose limited to $\sim$450 mg/m^2
Epirubicin	7–67	7–43	Cardiac toxicity – cumulative dose limited to $\sim$900 mg/m^2
Mitoxantrone	23–35	22	Less cardiac toxicity but overall lower response rate
Mitomycin-C	–	18–23	More prolonged myelosuppression
Antimetabolites			
5-Fluorouracil	5–65	–	Commonly used in combinations
Methotrexate	11–66	29	
Capecitabine	–	20	Oral, limited alopecia and myelosuppression
Gemcitabine	14–46	17–25	Limited alopecia
Microtubule inhibitors			
Vinorelbine	0–41	15–36	Central line often required
Paclitaxel	25–61	23–53	Peripheral neuropathy, weekly or once every 3 weeks
Docetaxel	47–67	18–53	Fluid retention with chronic therapy
Alkylating agents			
Cyclophosphamide	10–62	33–40	Commonly used in combinations
Thiotepa	10–42	–	Used primarily in high-dose regimens
Platinum compounds			Potential synergy with Herceptin
Cisplatin	47	0–21	Renal toxicity
Carboplatinum	20–50	0–8	

Hormonal and cytotoxic agents have distinctly different mechanisms of action, providing a rationale for combined chemohormonal therapy in patients with ER+ disease. The addition of a hormonal agent to chemotherapy has been investigated in numerous clinical trials. Unfortunately many of these trials were conducted before routine steroid receptor analysis and thus included many ER (−) or unknown patients. Nonetheless, similar to the results with combination chemotherapy, combined chemohormonal therapy often increases response rates and time to progression but has no consistent impact on overall survival. The concurrent use of hormonal and cytotoxic agents presents the oncologist with a therapeutic quandary – namely, which agent is responsible for the patient's response and therefore should be continued? Prolonging an ineffective therapy, whose ineffectiveness is masked by response to another agent, exposes the patient to unnecessary toxicity and expense.

The optimal duration of chemotherapy for patients with overt metastatic disease represents a balance between potential benefit and ongoing toxicity. Though some chemotherapy agents can not be administered indefinitely (e.g., anthracyclines), many drugs useful in the treatment of breast cancer are not limited by cumulative toxicity. In the clinical trials reported, continuous therapy generally prolonged the duration of remission, but the effect on survival and quality of life were less consistent. Unfortunately the available clinical trial data do not allow firm conclusions nor does an understanding of tumor biology guide duration of therapy with traditional cytotoxics. While continuous treatment prolongs the duration of remission, it is not without toxicity and has a minimal effect at best on overall survival. Rather than making definitive recommendations for or against maintenance therapy, the skilled clinician is guided by patient preference and opinion regarding the balance of potential benefit and extended toxicity.

Knowledge of the basic biology of breast cancer has expanded exponentially over the last three decades with little direct impact on therapy until recently. HER-2 is a growth-factor receptor in the epidermal growth-factor receptor family. HER-2 is overexpressed (or amplified) in approximately 25% of breast cancers and results in a greater risk of recurrence and shortened overall survival. A phase II trial of 222 women with HER-2 overexpressing metastatic breast cancer found a response rate of 15% with six confirmed complete responses using a recombinant humanized monoclonal antibody (Herceptin, Genentech, South San Francisco) directed against HER-2. A randomized phase III trial evaluated the safety and efficacy of adding Herceptin to first-line chemotherapy with either paclitaxel or the combination of doxorubicin plus cyclophosphamide. Overall response rate and time to progression significantly improved with the addition of Herceptin to chemotherapy compared with chemotherapy alone. Perhaps more importantly, the addition of Herceptin prolonged overall survival. Though HER-2 overexpressing breast cancer is typically ER−, combinations of Herceptin and hormonal therapy in patients with dual ER+/HER-2+ disease are currently under investigation. Given the proven survival advantage, Herceptin-based therapy should now be considered standard for all patients with HER-2 overexpressing metastatic breast cancer.

Finally, the option of not continuing systemic therapy should be considered at each point a new treatment is required – whether due to disease progression or unacceptable toxicity with the prior therapy. Rather than a sudden shift in the goals of treatment (from cure to palliation), this recognizes the reality that chemotherapy may no longer accomplish the goal of helping the patient "live longer and better."

Patients, their families and physicians may not reach this conclusion at the same point in the course of the disease. Continuing an open and honest dialogue regarding the patient's symptoms, hopes, and fears can facilitate both an optimal treatment plan and an appropriate referral to a hospice or palliative care program.

Site specific issues

Bone

Metastatic disease involving the bone causes significant morbidity for patients. Bone lesions are commonly painful and may result in pathologic fractures or hypercalcemia. Though nuclear medicine bone scans are more sensitive at detecting bone involvement, plain x-rays are needed to assess the degree of bone destruction and the risk of pathologic fracture in weight-bearing areas. If destruction of more than one-third of the bone cortex is identified, an orthopedic consultation for surgical stabilization should be considered. Abbreviated courses of radiation therapy (generally 10 fractions) provides prompt pain relief for localized bone lesions. Though the use of radionuclides such as strontium or samarium has been suggested for patients with widespread bone metastases, these treatments often result in significant long-term myelosuppression (particularly thrombocytopenia) and should be used in only rare circumstances. Patients with lytic bone lesions benefit from regular treatment with the bisphosphonates to slow the progression of further bone destruction, decrease pain, and limit the incidence of pathologic fracture.

Pleural effusions

Pleural effusions cause gradually increasing dyspnea and a persistent cough resulting in a major decrement in quality of life. Cytology typically identifies malignant cells in the effusion, but cytologic examination of the fluid is unnecessary in patients already known to have malignant disease. A therapeutic thoracentesis provides prompt symptomatic relief but repeated thoracenteses often result in a loculated effusion that is much more difficult to manage. An early referral for pleurodesis provides more consistent long-term symptomatic control.

Liver

Symptoms of hepatic involvement are often subtle and difficult to control: increased fatigue, generalized malaise, persistent nausea. Right upper quadrant pain is uncommon and suggests rapidly expanding liver metastases. Painless jaundice may represent a local area of biliary obstruction that may be amenable to stenting but more often portends diffuse liver involvement and a short expected survival.

Brain

CNS imaging is not routinely performed in asymptomatic patients with advanced breast cancer, thus the incidence and clinical relevance of occult CNS metastases remains unknown. Symptomatic CNS involvement affects approximately 20% of patients at some point during the course of the disease. Frequent symptoms include focal loss of neurologic symptoms, seizure, persistent headache, and intractable nausea. Prompt improvement or complete resolution of symptoms with the initiation of high-dose steroids is expected. Surgical resection of isolated CNS lesions is a reasonable option, particularly if the systemic disease remains under control or is not immediately life-threatening. Radiation therapy, either as a single agent or after resection, prevents recurrence of CNS symptoms in most patients.

Cutaneous

Though 20–25% of patients may experience local chest wall recurrence at some point, significant morbidity from local disease is less common. Death from infection or other complications of local recurrence is rare. In addition to local pain, patients with extensive skin involvement (*en cuirasse*) may develop a restrictive pulmonary deficit. Radiation remains the mainstay of treatment. Photodynamic therapy (systemic administration of a light-sensitizing agent followed by focal laser therapy) induces a local response in over half of treated patients but can not be applied to large, diffuse areas. Consultation with a burns specialist can be helpful in managing local wound complications.

Choroid

A decrease in vision in the absence of parenchymal CNS disease should prompt careful ophthalmologic evaluation to search for choroid metastases. Radiation results in stabilization of vision in most patients, though significant improvement in visual acuity is uncommon.

Future directions

There has never been a more exciting time in breast oncology. Years of painstaking basic laboratory investigation have expanded our knowledge of breast cancer biology and allowed the first rationally designed, targeted therapies to enter the clinic. Interference with growth factors and arrest of the angiogenic cascade offers real promise of more effective, less toxic, individualized treatment. Certainly other unique, biologically based therapies (anti-angiogenics, vaccines, tyrosine kinase inhibitors, gene therapy) will follow. Though the excitement and potential are real, progress will undoubtedly be slow and fraught with surprise.

Until that potential is fully realized, we must remember that the last 40 years of basic research and clinical investigation have clearly improved the treatment of patients with metastatic breast cancer. Treatment options have increased substantially, allowing patients to play a more active role in treatment decisions. Clearly survival is prolonged and quality of life preserved with the careful use of hormonal and cytotoxic agents, but the words of Francis Peabody still ring true, "The secret of the care of the patient is in caring for the patient."

REFERENCES

Sentinel articles

Bloom H, Richardson W, Harrier E. Natural history of untreated breast cancer (1805–1933). *Br Med J* 1962;2:213.

Cobleigh M, Cogel C, Tripathy N et al. Efficacy and safety of Herceptin (humanized anti-Her2 antibody) as a single agent in 222 women with Her2 overexpression who relapsed following chemotherapy for metastatic breast cancer. *Proc Am Soc Clin Oncol* 1998;17:97.

Falkson G, Gelman RS, Pandya KJ et al. Eastern Cooperative Oncology Group randomized trials of observation versus maintenance therapy for patients with metastatic breast cancer in complete remission following induction treatment. *J Clin Oncol* 1998;16:1669–76.

Geels P, Eisenhauer E, Bezjak A et al. Palliative effect of chemotherapy: objective tumor response is associated with symptom improvement in patients with metastatic breast cancer. *J Clin Oncol* 2000;18:2395–405.

Greenberg PA, Hortobagyi GN, Smith TL et al. Long-term follow-up of patients with complete remission following combination chemotherapy for metastatic breast cancer. *J Clin Oncol* 1996;14:2197–205.

Hakamies-Blomqvist L, Luoma M, Sjostrom J et al. Quality of life in patients with metastatic breast cancer receiving either docetaxel or sequential methotrexate and 5-fluorouracil. A multicenter randomised phase III trial by the Scandinavian breast group. *Eur J Cancer* 2000;36:1411–17.

Hortobagyi GN, Theriault RL, Porter L et al. Efficacy of pamidronate in reducing skeletal complications in patients with breast cancer and lytic bone metastases. Protocol 19 Aredia Breast Cancer Study Group [see comments]. *N Engl J Med* 1996;335:1785–91.

Slamon DJ, Leyland-Jones B, Shak S et al. Use of chemotherapy plus a monoclonal antibody against HER2 for metastatic breast cancer that overexpresses HER2. *N Engl J Med* 2001;344:783–92.

Swenerton KD, Legha SS, Smith T et al. Prognostic factors in metastatic breast cancer treated with combination chemotherapy. *Cancer Res* 1979;39:1552–62.

Selected review

Hortobagyi GN. Treatment of breast cancer. *N Engl J Med* 1998;339:974–84.

Internet sites

http://cancer.gov/cancer_information/cancer_type/breast
National Cancer Institute site with comprehensive breast cancer information. Includes ability to search for NCI-sponsored clinical trials.

http://komen.org

    One of the largest single breast cancer advocacy groups. Site includes information and on-line support groups.

http://NABCO.org

    National Alliance of Breast Cancer Organizations. One of the most powerful advocacy groups with extensive support and information capabilities on-line.

http://breastcancer.org

    Site also sponsors regional educational events and monthly on-line chats with breast cancer experts.

19

Colorectal cancer

Charles D. Blanke

Oregon Health & Science University, Portland

Introduction

Cancers of the rectum and colon (CRC) collectively make large bowel malignancy the third-most frequently diagnosed non-skin neoplasm in Americans. Since males do not commonly expire from breast cancer, and females never die from prostate malignancies, CRC is the second biggest cancer killer of Americans. The risk for developing CRC dramatically increases with age up until the 80s, and the lifetime chance of developing large bowel cancer is about 6%.

Worldwide, incidence rates vary more than 10-fold between low- and high-risk areas. Mortality has been decreasing in many countries, including the US, though it has recently increased in China and Japan. It seems likely that environmental exposures (and not some kind of genetic protection) account for much of the difference in incidence rates, since offspring of migrants from low-risk countries have incidence rates approaching those of native residents of the high-risk areas.

About 15% of patients will present with metastatic disease. Of those with localized tumors undergoing potentially curative surgery, one-third to one-half will recur, depending on stage. Thus, approximately half of all patients with CRC will eventually be diagnosed with metastatic disease.

Anatomy and histology

The large bowel is divided between colon and rectum, though prognostic and treatment differences for cancers arising from each are more striking for early-stage disease. Resected tumors are usually considered to have arisen from the colon if they are located above the peritoneal reflection, and to be rectal in origin if they arose at or below this anatomic landmark *or* the lower edge of the tumor was within 12 cm of the anal verge, as measured on rigid proctoscopy. The venous drainage of the colon and upper rectum is through the portal system, while the distant rectum has both systemic and portal drainage. Practically, this means it is very unusual for colon tumors to spread to the lungs or more distantly without the patient having concomitant liver metastases, but that situation is seen fairly commonly with distal rectal cancers (see below).

Adenocarcinomas make up almost 95% of large bowel cancers, and the remainder of this review will be specific to that cell type. Carcinoids, other neuroendocrine cancers, sarcomas, gastrointestinal stromal tumors, and melanomas are also seen, but management of those neoplasms differs dramatically.

Patterns of spread

Cancer of the rectum and colon can spread through the vascular and lymphatic systems, and/or detach from the primary and directly seed the abdomen. The liver is by far the most common site of non-nodal metastases and is the solitary site of spread in roughly 40% of patients. The lungs are the second most common site of hematogenous spread. Metastases to bone and brain are certainly seen, but much less frequently.

Symptoms

Patients with advanced CRC may have symptoms related directly to the location of metastatic spread or generic constitutional cancer symptoms or problems from an intact primary tumor. The vast majority of symptoms from any of these are very nonspecific. Distant metastases can cause site-specific pain (e.g., right upper quadrant discomfort from liver metastases) and other problems related directly to the organ in which they reside (e.g., cough from lung spread and jaundice, fever, and modest liver insufficiency from hepatic involvement; frank liver failure is uncommon). Patients with advanced disease often suffer from constitutional symptoms including weight loss, cancer cachexia, and profound fatigue. Malignant ascites can cause feelings of fullness and/or frank pain, as well as early satiety. Ascitic fluid can become infected by gut bacteria, leading to fever and nausea/vomiting. Patients with advanced disease are also commonly depressed and may express feelings of hopelessness. Intact primary tumors can bleed and cause symptoms of anemia, lead to altered bowel habits (particularly related to partial or complete obstruction), or perforate, potentially causing peritonitis.

Treatment of advanced CRC

Except for differences in patterns of spread (detailed above), metastatic cancers of the colon and rectum act in similar biologic fashion and are usually lumped together under most treatment guidelines. Though surgery alone can successfully treat early-stage large bowel tumors more than 90% of the time, in general, patients with metastatic CRC are incurable, with an overall 5-year survival approximating 6%. However, a distinct subset of patients, those with single or double-organ confined, limited volume disease, may still be cured with aggressive surgery and complete resection. Others with single-organ confined, nonresectable disease may still benefit from other locally directed modalities (see below). Therefore, one must always consider whether a patient is potentially curable with aggressive treatment before relegating him or her to palliative, noncurative systemic chemotherapy.

Standard therapy for patients with extensive metastatic CRC (if performance status allows) is indeed systemic chemotherapy. One can legitimately ask if chemotherapy actually makes any difference, in the absence of curative potential. That is, can it prolong life, extend symptom-free survival, or vanquish those symptoms already present? Unlike the situation with many solid tumors (e.g., melanoma), there is scientific evidence that chemotherapy prolongs survival in metastatic CRC. A Viennese trial randomized patients between a cisplatin/5-fluorouracil regimen and best supportive care, showing a statistically and clinically significant prolongation of life, from 5–11 months, with treatment. Other reviews and scientific models have demonstrated actual shrinkage of tumor is not required for patients to have a survival benefit. Those achieving cessation of tumor growth (i.e., "stable disease") live longer as well. There is even data that second-line therapy benefits patients in terms of improving their overall survival, versus best supportive care.

Though itself potentially toxic, by preventing tumor-related symptoms or diminishing problems already present, modern chemotherapy can actually improve or at least maintain patients' quality of life. In addition, many (though not all patients) can have successful dose reductions, delays, or complete cessation of treatment if toxicity does occur. Thus, the fear that chemotherapy will cause permanent damage to quality of life should not serve as a reason never to try it at all.

Though many patients are sick as a result of their metastatic disease, with aggressive screening programs and modern staging, a significant fraction of advanced disease patients will be found while still having normal performance status. Since chemotherapy will likely cause *some* toxicity and since cancer-related symptoms that are not present cannot be taken away ("you can't palliate the asymptomatic man"), another reasonable question is whether chemotherapy must be given to asymptomatic patients shortly after diagnosis, or whether it can wait until they start to become ill. A Nordic Cancer Study Group randomized trial in asymptomatic patients with advanced disease looked at immediate chemotherapy versus watchful waiting and instigation of therapy after patients became ill. This trial did report that immediate therapy led to a 6-month improvement in how long patients stayed asymptomatic, as well as improving progression-free and overall survival. However, the trial was executed poorly, and many investigators feel it did not decisively answer the question. A more recent trial has suggested that watchful waiting is safe. For now, it seems reasonable to allow completely asymptomatic patients the luxury of observation, if they so desire. If that strategy is adopted, however, the patient must be educated to report to the physician at first symptom development (waiting until one is bedridden will guarantee a chemotherapy failure), and it is also reasonable to periodically scan these patients and treat at rapid or dramatic radiographic progression, even if the patient is still asymptomatic at that point.

Systemic therapy

The recommended chemotherapy for patients with metastatic CRC has included the drug 5-fluorouracil (5-FU) for almost 45 years. 5-FU can interfere with either DNA or RNA synthesis by the neoplastic cells, depending on the route and timing of administration. Despite its widespread use, 5-FU is not an ideal drug. Its oral bioavailability varies dramatically and is wholly unpredictable, requiring its administration in intravenous form. A 10-fold difference in its objective response rate has been noted in the literature, and the true figure is probably a lowly 10–20% or so. A nearly infinite number of schedules and sets of recommended dosages have been published, with the most common two including a once per week administration, and a daily × 5 days in a row (every 4–5 weeks) schedule. The major toxicities of bolus 5-FU include mucositis, diarrhea, dermatitis, and leukopenia. Alopecia and nausea are usually mild with this agent. Unusual toxicities, such as cardiac events (particularly ischemia) can be seen. A small fraction of the population is deficient in dihydropyrimidine dehydrogenase (NADP), the enzyme that catabolizes 5-FU. These patients, when given 5-FU, suffer unusual (e.g., neurotoxicity) and occasionally life-threatening side effects from the drug. Levels of enzyme can be tested, though arranging the process can be difficult. Suspected NADP-deficient patients *must* be tested, however; rechallenging them with drug is an unacceptable option and may kill the patient.

As bolus 5-FU has a short half-life, and since the drug must be present at the time of neoplastic cell division, some investigators choose to give 5-FU by continuous 24-hour per day administration. This is less convenient for the patient, since it requires wearing an ambulatory infusion pump, plus having a central line placed. This route also changes the toxicity profile of the drug, causing almost no myelosuppression but leading to peeling and reddening of the hands and feet (sometimes severe), in a significant fraction of patients.

Other agents, such as the immune modulator interferon, have been added unsuccessfully to 5-FU in attempts to increase its efficacy. Somewhat successful in this setting is the agent leucovorin, a reduced folate cofactor which increases the binding of a 5-FU active metabolite to its target enzyme. The addition of leucovorin clearly improves the response rate (20–45%) over 5-FU alone, but the effect on overall survival is not clear. Individual studies have reported mixed results on the potential survival benefit, and a recent meta-analysis showed *no* improvement on survival, even though the addition of leucovorin doubled the response rate versus single-agent 5-FU. Until recently, the combination of 5-FU with leucovorin clearly represented standard of care therapy for those with advanced CRC.

The most exciting new development in the treatment of CRC is the emergence of the drug CPT-11 (irinotecan). CPT-11 is a topoisomerase I inhibitor and prevents the propagation of tumor DNA or repair of damaged genetic material. CPT-11 was originally developed for second-line use in patients who had failed front-line 5-FU with leucovorin. In that setting, CPT-11 clearly prolongs survival (despite a relatively modest 15% response rate) over best supportive care alone or infusional 5-FU. More recently, a major trial was published in the *New England Journal of Medicine.* This study randomized *untreated* CRC patients between CPT-11 plus 5-FU and leucovorin, CPT-11 alone, or 5-FU/leucovorin alone. The triple therapy arm was clearly superior, leading to a median survival of almost 15 months. Remarkably, the triple combination did not seem more toxic than 5-FU with leucovorin but without CPT-11. The triple regimen clearly now represents the standard of care therapy for patients with untreated metastatic disease.

Despite the statement above, CPT-11 *can* be a toxic drug. It clearly causes more alopecia than 5-FU, and its use has also been associated with late diarrhea, reversible myelosuppression, mild nausea, anorexia, and pulmonary toxicity. Infusion has also been associated with an early-onset cholinergic syndrome (easily treated with, and in subsequent courses prophylaxed against, with atropine), consisting of cramping, diarrhea, and salivation/lacrimation. The severity of the late diarrhea can be markedly reduced with an aggressive program of oral loperamide, instituted at the first loose stool and continued until the patient is diarrhea-free for 12 hours. Use of prophylactic loperamide is not recommended, however.

This is an extraordinarily exciting time to be a colorectal oncologist, because a number of new drugs are in late development. Oxaliplatin is a platinum derivative that has major activity in preclinical models of CRC, and it appears effective, particularly when combined with 5-FU and leucovorin, in de novo and previously treated patients with large bowel cancer. Oxaliplatin was recently approved in the US for second-line treatment of large bowel malignancy. As stated above, 5-FU is not a drug that can be given orally, and continuous infusion by i.v., while more effective than bolus i.v., is inconvenient. A number of 5-FU prodrugs, usually given with competitors of NADP, are entering the market. These drugs mimic infusional 5-FU pharmacokinetics and may be given orally. They appear at least as effective as standard 5-FU in phase III trials, and tend to have similar or better toxicity profiles. Many clinicians now offer elderly or poor performance status patients capecitabine, an oral 5-FU prodrug, as initial therapy for metastatic colorectal cancer.

Ongoing research looks at the use of chemo*preventive* agents in patients with *established* CRC, including the selective COX-2 inhibitors celecoxib and rofecoxib. These are being evaluated in combination with chemotherapy. Agents that block growth of tumor blood vessels are also being tested in treatment of CRC, with or without chemotherapy. These theoretically should be more selective than standard agents and might cause tumor-specific toxicities. Gene therapy approaches, and a host of trials using immune strategies (including tumor-specific mutated ras peptides in vaccine form, modified activated T-cells, bcl-2 antisense oligodeoxy-nucleotides, anti-CEA monoclonal antibodies, and anti-HER-2 receptor antibodies) are in clinical trials.

Prognosis

Untreated patients with metastatic CRC have an average survival of approximately 5 months. Treatment with 5-FU alone can extend that to the 6–10 month range, and standard 5-FU modulation with leucovorin to 10–12 months. The best current therapies using 5-FU, leucovorin, and a third drug such as CPT-11 or oxaliplatin can offer median survival times exceeding 17–20 months.

Special situations – intact primary

One of the reasons computerized tomography of the liver has not been a mandated part of staging newly diagnosed patients found to have large bowel malignancies was the thought that the primary tumor would need to be surgically extirpated, regardless of the presence of metastatic deposits. Classic teaching is that a large proportion of these patients would bleed or obstruct and might need emergency surgery at the worst possible time, e.g., when the patient was neutropenic from chemotherapy. However, the percentage of patients with metastatic disease and intact primary who do ultimately progress locally to the point where intervention is needed has never been definitively characterized. It certainly is possible that patients with distant metastases would die from that disease before the primary could cause trouble, and it is also possible that primary chemotherapy or chemoradiotherapy might directly shrink or at least control the growth of the lesion in the large bowel. A Vanderbilt retrospective review of patients with *asymptomatic* intact primaries, in the face of metastatic disease, showed the vast majority can be treated with systemic chemotherapy or chemoradiotherapy to the primary bowel lesion, as the first therapeutic intervention. None of the patients with colonic primaries, and 18% of those with rectal tumors, needed urgent surgery for obstruction. No patient developed clinically significant bleeding from the primary, and no patient died because of the "watch-and-wait" strategy adopted. In general, it is still recommended that patients with *symptomatic* primaries have their large bowel addressed immediately. Obstructing tumors will still likely need surgery, though it is possible nonemergency bleeding can be controlled with radiation therapy alone or stenting and will never require resection.

Hepatic-only metastases

Approximately 40% of patients will have CRC limited to the liver, and they have options besides observation and systemic chemotherapy. These patients should be divided into those with limited-volume, possibly curable disease, and those with extensive hepatic replacement.

There are a number of techniques for ablating small, limited (in number and volume) lesions. Resection is still considered standard of care, but occasionally limited metastases may be found in anatomically unfavorable locations (e.g., near large vessels), or the patient may be medically unfit for extensive surgery. Other surgical modalities used to treat this pattern of disease include radiofrequency ablation, cryosurgery, and percutaneous alcohol injection. They appear to achieve excellent control at the site of the metastases, but do not prevent disease appearance in other parts of the liver. Of course, they have no impact on nonhepatic spread, so the possibility of combining them with intravenous chemotherapy (to control systemic disease) is attractive.

The treatment for patients with extensive hepatic-only metastases, but with disease too widespread for directed therapy (e.g., radiofrequency ablation, surgery, etc.), is very controversial. These patients can receive treatment directly through the hepatic artery, in addition to or instead of systemic therapy. CRC metastases derive their blood supply through the hepatic artery, while normal liver parenchyma is supplied mainly by the portal vein. Thus, this route of delivery may target tumor and relatively spare normal liver and systemic organs. Hepatic artery infusion of fluoropyrimidines is highly effective in inducing neoplasm shrinkage and decreasing symptoms of tumor bulk, and it certainly does prolong survival versus best supportive care. An improvement on results achievable with chemotherapy (especially the modern CPT-11 or oxaliplatin plus 5-FU and leucovorin regimens) has not been shown. In addition, the treatment can be highly toxic, causing universal fever, pain that requires narcotics, and the additional possibilities of hepatic failure or gut ischemia.

Chemoembolization consists of infusing chemotherapeutic drugs through the hepatic artery, given with agents designed to cause physical blockage of blood flow to the tumor with resultant ischemic insult. Chemoembolization does not appear to add to results achievable with typical systemic therapy.

Locally advanced nonmetastatic colon cancer

Ten percent or so of patients have tumors that penetrate the colonic wall and invade nearby organs. When complete resection can be performed via en-bloc resection, up to 50% of those patients can be cured. Unresectable patients should be treated with radiation therapy, with or without radiosensitizing 5-FU. Responding tumors should then be resected, a situation which occurs in up to 75% of cases.

Locally advanced rectal cancer

Patients presenting with unresectable nonmetastatic rectal cancer have historically been treated with radiation therapy. Using this modality, approximately 50% of cases can be converted to resectable status. However, postradiation local progression rates remain high, ranging up to 55%. Recent efforts have emphasized the use of combination chemoradiotherapy, followed by surgery (in cases with significant downstaging), followed by additional chemotherapy. Resectability rates (with negative margins) as high as 97%, with 4-year local failure rates as low as 30%, have been reported.

Treatment of the elderly patient with advanced CRC

Ninety percent of colorectal cancers occur in patients 50 years of age or older, and it is not unusual to see patients in their 80s or 90s. Physicians fear treating patients above 70 with systemic chemotherapy, and these patients are clearly underrepresented in clinical trials. Meta-analyses and prospective database reviews have demonstrated that 70-year-old patients and greater do not have more frequent or severe side effects overall, and that efficacy (measured by response rates and failure-free survival) is the same in older and younger patients. Thus, chemotherapy should not be arbitrarily withheld from an elderly patient with good performance status.

Conclusions

Colorectal oncology is a dynamic subspecialty that has dramatically evolved over the last 5 years. Some patients with metastatic disease can still be cured with locally directed therapies, though they represent a small fraction of the overall population. Several new drugs, with significant preclinical and clinical activity, have been recently approved or are in late clinical trials. These can be given at only a modest toxic cost to the patient, and they have the potential to improve survival. Still, end-of-life issues will become relevant for the vast majority of metastatic CRC patients within 3 years after diagnosis, and the physician caring for these patients should be able to recognize and effectively treat the symptoms of advanced disease, as well as the cancers themselves.

BIBLIOGRAPHY

Sentinel articles

Advanced Colorectal Meta-Analysis Project. Modulation of 5-fluorouracil by leucovorin in patients with advanced colorectal cancer: evidence in terms of response rate. *J Clin Oncol* 1992;10:896–903.

Cunningham D, Pyrhonen S, James R et al. Randomized trial of irinotecan plus supportive care versus supportive care alone after fluorouracil failure of patients with metastatic colorectal cancer. *Lancet* 1998;352:1413–18.

Fong, Y, Cohen AM, Fortner JG et al. Liver resection for colorectal metastases. *J Clin Oncol* 1997;15:938–46.

Saltz LB, Cox JV, Blanke C et al. Irinotecan plus fluorouracil and leucovorin for metastatic colorectal cancer. *N Engl J Med* 2000;343:905–14.

Scheithauer W, Rosen H, Kornek GV et al. Randomized comparison of combination chemotherapy plus supportive care with supportive care alone in patients with metastatic colorectal cancer. *Br Med J* 1993;306:752–5.

Reference articles

Bleiberg H, DeGramont A. Oxaliplatin plus 5-fluorouracil: clinical experience in patients with advanced colorectal cancer. *Semin Oncol* 1998;25(Suppl. 5):32–9.

Sobrero AF, Aschele C, Bertino JR. Fluorouracil in colorectal cancer – a tale of two drugs: implications for biochemical modulation. *J Clin Oncol* 1997;15:368–81.

Internet sites

http://www.adhf.org/

The American Digestive Health Foundation (ADHF) is a cooperative digestive health group effort of the American Gastroenterological Association and the American Society for Gastrointestinal Endoscopy. Its web site has a nice section on CRC, including a patient quiz.

http://www.fascrs.org/ascrs-home.html

American Society of Colon and Rectal Surgeons. This web site includes more than information on colorectal cancer surgery.

http://www.ccalliance.org/

The Colon Cancer Alliance is an organization of CRC survivors, caregivers, people with a genetic predisposition to the disease, and other individuals affected by colorectal cancer. This web site is heavy on advocacy issues.

http://cancer.gov/cancer_information/cancer_type/colon_and_rectal

National Cancer Institute: Colon Cancer Treatment. Information from the NCI on CRC, including clinical trials.

20

Prostate cancer

Christopher Sweeney

Indiana University Cancer Pavilion, Indianapolis

Prostate cancer is the most common male malignancy in the US. In the year 2000 there were approximately 180 400 new cases of prostate cancer with approximately 31 900 deaths.[1] Most patients present with localized disease and treatment choices include surgery, radiation (external beam or brachytherapy), or observation. It is well recognized that a minority of patients will develop metastatic disease after definitive local therapy or present with metastatic disease. Some of these patients will have a very indolent course and not die of prostate cancer, whereas others will have aggressive disease that will metastasize from the prostate gland and be the cause of the patient's death. Progression is often first manifest by an increasing prostate-specific antigen (PSA). The mere presence of an elevated PSA after definitive local therapy does not portend a poor outlook. For example, in one series of 315 patients who underwent a prostatectomy it was noted that the median survival was more than 10 years if the PSA rose 2 years after the surgery, took longer than 10 months to double and the Gleason's score was 7 or less.[2]

However, survival is shorter once patients have visible metastases on radiographic imaging and/or symptomatic lesions. Standard initial therapy for metastatic disease consists of androgen ablation. Dr. Huggins won the Nobel prize in medicine for his discovery that prostatic epithelium will undergo atrophy with withdrawal of androgen stimulation.[3] Hormonal therapy, either by castration (surgical or medical) and/or by administration of anti-androgens or estrogens is able to engender a response in approximately 90% of men with prostate cancer. Castrate levels of serum testosterone were initially accomplished by bilateral orchiectomy or estrogens. In the early 1980s LH-RH agonists became clinically available and had equivalent therapeutic results.[4] Later in the 1980s the concept of total androgen blockade with the addition of an anti-androgen to block extratesticular sources of androgen became popular. The concept of total androgen blockade initially appeared to be validated by a phase III study demonstrating a 7-month survival advantage for leuprolide and flutamide versus leuprolide alone.[5] However, numerous other phase III studies failed to show any substantial benefit for total androgen blockade including a meta-analysis.[6] This meta-analysis included 27 randomized trials with central analysis of the data from 8275 men. More than 50% were older than 70 years and 72% of patients had died by the time of the analysis. Approximately 80% of the deaths were due to prostate cancer. With total androgen blockade the 5-year overall survival was 25.4% compared with 23.6% with androgen suppression alone ($P = 0.11$). When the studies evaluating anti-androgens (nilutamide or flutamide) alone ($n = 6500$, 20 trials) were analyzed there was a slight 5-year overall survival benefit of 27.6% versus 24.7% ($P = 0.005$) for the combination.

Unfortunately, after a median time of about 20 months patients will become refractory to hormonal therapy. No therapy for hormone-refractory prostate cancer has been shown to confer a survival advantage. However, prostate cancer that grows independent of hormonal ablation also has a varied course. For example, if a patient is on an anti-androgen such as flutamide the standard practice is to withdraw this agent and watch for tumor shrinkage. The latter is known as anti-androgen withdrawal phenomenon and occurs in approximately 15% of patients.[7] This phenomenon is observed more often if patients have been on anti-androgens for a prolonged period (more than 18 months). This event is thought to be due to mutations of the androgen receptor. A variety of second-line hormonal therapies are available. These include institution of an anti-androgen if a patient has not previously received this class of agent, suppression of adrenal androgen production with high dose ketoconazole and hydrocortisone or low-dose corticosteroids. The PSA response rate with these manipulations is about 20% with a few patients experiencing a palliative benefit.[8–10] Predictors for survival have also been identified. Newling et al. have shown that the median survival varies depending on markers of progression.[11] For example 50% of patients succumb to their disease by 13 months if found to be progressing by hormonal therapy alone, 10 months if showing a worsening bone scan, 7 months if lymph node metastases are enlarging, and 3 months if lung or liver metastases progress.

Numerous approaches have been found to improve the quality of life of patients with hormone-refractory prostate cancer. These include localized radiotherapy to symptomatic lesions or radiopharmaceutical injections for more diffuse bony pain. An example of the latter is samarium.[12] In a placebo-controlled randomized study of 118 patients, pain relief was seen for 4 months in 43% of patients who received 1.0 mCi/kg. Bone marrow suppression was mild (no grade 4 hematological toxicity), reversible, with nadir thrombocytopenia and neutropenia occurring at 4–5 weeks and returning to normal at week 8. Another commonly used treatment for these patients has become mitoxantrone and low-dose corticosteroid, based on two randomized studies that compared this combination to the corticosteroid alone.[13,14] In both studies, there was a palliative benefit as evidenced by a decrease in pain but no survival benefit for patients who received the mitoxantrone. In the trial by Tannock et al. all patients had symptomatic disease, and mitoxantrone (12 mg/m^2) every 3 weeks with 10 mg of oral prednisone daily resulted in 33% of patients having a serological response (> 50% decline of PSA) compared with 22% with the same dose of prednisone alone. More importantly, 29% halved their narcotic analgesia or their pain for a median of 43 weeks compared with 12% with a median of 18 weeks treated with prednisone alone given as monotherapy. The median survival for both groups was approximately 12 months.

A variety of agents that block the microtubule apparatus have been evaluated as single agents. Estramustine phosphate, a nor-nitrogen mustard carbamate derivative of estradiol–17 beta-phosphate is cytotoxic by interfering with the microtubule apparatus rather than by an estrogen or alkylating effect.[15,16] In the pre-PSA era, several National Prostate Cancer Project (NPCP) phase II trials were performed using estramustine alone. Only five objective responses were noted out of 262 patients treated.[17] Another group of drugs that block the microtubule apparatus are the taxanes. Single agent paclitaxel was found to be devoid of any meaningful activity in a phase II ECOG study.[18] Twenty-three patients with hormone-refractory prostate cancer and bidimensionally measurable disease were treated with paclitaxel by 24-hour continuous infusion at 135–170 mg/m^2 every 21 days for a maximum of six cycles. One patient (4.3%) experienced a partial response lasting 9 months, and four other patients with radiographically stable disease had minor reductions in the serum PSA of 16–24%. Weekly docetaxel has been evaluated in a phase II study in hormone-refractory prostate cancer in 23 patients.[19] It was given at a dose of 36 mg/m^2 for the first 6 weeks of an 8-week cycle. PSA was evaluable in 19 patients and there was a > 50% decline in 47% of patients and there was significant decrease in pain in 33% of patients as measured by the 6-point Present Pain Intensity scale. Of note is the observation that the PSA decline correlated with pain response.

With the emergence of preclinical data demonstrating synergy for combined anti-microtubular therapy[20] (estramustine, vinblastine or taxane), multiple phase II studies demonstrated that this was an efficacious approach.[21–25] Petrylak completed a phase II study of docetaxel at 70 mg/m^2 on day 2 with estramustine at 280 mg orally three times per day from day 1 to day 5. There was a 71% rate of PSA decline greater than 50% in 35 evaluable patients with a 1-year survival of 77%. Significant toxicity was also observed in this study. There were two deaths associated with granulocytopenic fevers, two patients experienced cerebrovascular accidents (including one patient who died) and two patients had a deep venous thrombosis. The thrombotic complications resulted in the last 15 patients being prescribed aspirin and coumadin for prophylaxis. An Intergroup trial is currently accruing patients to a phase III trial comparing docetaxel (60 mg/m^2 every 3 weeks) plus 5 days of oral estramustine, with mitoxantrone plus low-dose corticosteroid. The lower docetaxel dose is to minimize toxicities seen at 70 mg/m^2 and patients are to be escalated from 60 mg/m^2 to 70 mg/m^2 if there are no grade 3 or 4 toxicities in the first cycle. All patients are receiving thromboembolic prophylaxis. A randomized phase II study of 166 patients evaluating paclitaxel (100 mg/m^2 on days 2, 9 and 16 every 28 days) was compared with the same dose of paclitaxel plus estramustine (280 mg oral three times per day for 3 days). The serological response rate (50% decline in PSA for more than 8 weeks) was greater with the combination, 48% versus 28% and the median survival was also numerically greater (16.3 months versus 13.1 months). Although this study was underpowered to draw any firm comparisons, it adds further support to the concept of combined microtubule blockade. However, this slight advantage comes at the cost of an increased incidence of thromboembolic events (six patients in the estramustine group compared with one in the paclitaxel alone group).

The Hoosier Oncology Group in collaboration with the Fox Chase Cancer Network completed a phase III trial comparing vinblastine (4 mg/m^2) weekly × 6 with the same vinblastine dose plus estramustine on days 1 to 42 with cycles repeated every 8 weeks.[26] The combination arm was associated with an increased incidence of nausea and edema, a 25% incidence of PSA decline > 50% for at least three consecutive months, and an improvement in time to progression (2.2 versus 3.7 months; $P < 0.001$). Of note is that there was also a trend toward improved survival as the median survival was increased by 2.7 months in the combination arm (9.2 versus 11.9 months; $P = 0.08$). It should also be noted that vinblastine was inactive as a single agent with only 4% of patients having a PSA decline > 50% for at least 2 consecutive months.

Vinorelbine is a vinca alkaloid, like vinblastine, that has better activity in non-small cell lung cancer compared with vinblastine and vindesine. Moreover it has less neurotoxicity because its effects on the axonal microtubules are limited. Also of significance is that vinorelbine as a single agent has documented activity in hormone-refractory prostate cancer. In a phase II study of 37 evaluable patients, six patients received 30 mg/m^2 weekly and 31 patients received 22 mg/m^2 weekly because of dose delays due to granulocytopenia in the higher dose cohort.[27] Doses were weekly × 8 and then every other week. Fourteen of 37 evaluable patients (39%) had clinical benefit response (improvement in performance status, 25% or greater improvement in pain visual analog scale or > 50% decrease in analgesics, all lasting for a minimum of 12 weeks). Eleven of these 14 patients were able to discontinue all analgesics. Four of these 14 patients had a concomitant > 50% reduction in serum PSA. Therapy was well tolerated with no unanticipated toxicity. Multiple phase II studies of vinorelbine plus estramustine have shown some degree of efficacy but like all regimens containing estramustine has an increased rate of thrombotic complications.[28,29]

The role of bisphosphonates in the treatment of metastatic prostate cancer is an area of ongoing investigation. This class of agent results in decreased skeletal events in patients with bony involvement with breast cancer and myeloma.[30,31] There are numerous phase II studies of bisphosphonates in hormone-refractory prostate cancer.[32,33] Heidenrich et al. has recently reported an illustrative study of the palliative benefit of bisphosphonates. Clodronate was given intravenously daily for 8 days followed by an oral maintenance phase of 1600 mg daily to 85 patients with a mean Karnofsky Performance Score of 45. A palliative response with a significant decrease in mean pain score from 7.9 out of 10 on a visual analog scale (range 6 to 10) to 2.5 (range 0 to 4) ($P < 0.001$) was achieved in 75% of patients with 22% being rendered completely pain-free without further need of analgesics. The mean duration of bisphosphonate action was 9 weeks (range 4 to 22). More recently, bisphosphonates have been evaluated in hormone-responsive prostate cancer. Clodronate or placebo was given orally in a study of 311 patients being treated with hormonal ablation. After a median follow-up of 3 years 41% of the patients treated with clodronate had progressive disease compared with 58% of the placebo group.[34] The primary endpoint of the study was symptomatic progression or death and again the clodronate group fared better with only 59% of the clodronate patients reaching this endpoint versus 70% with placebo ($P = 0.04$).

In conclusion, patients with prostate cancer have a course that may be indolent or progress rapidly. Physicians have to therefore make treatment decisions that take the nature of each individual's disease into consideration. For example, the patient with a slowly rising PSA on hormonal therapy with no symptomatic progression can be observed closely and thus avoid the side effects of chemotherapy. However, cytotoxic chemotherapy provides effective palliation to many patients with symptoms and the risk–benefit analysis is often in favor of instituting chemotherapy at this time. The foregoing discussion clearly details that many issues need to be resolved to define the optimal therapy for patients with prostate cancer.

REFERENCES

1 Greenlee RT, Murray T, Bolden S et al. Cancer statistics, 2000. *CA Cancer J Clin* 2000; 50:7–33.

2 Pound CR, Partin AW, Eisenberger MA et al. Natural history of progression after PSA elevation following radical prostatectomy. *J Am Med Assoc* 1999;281:1591–7.

3 Huggins C, Hodges CV. Studies on prostatic cancer; effect of castration of estrogen and androgen injection on serum phosphates in metastatic carcinoma of the prostate. *Cancer Res* 1941;1:293–7.

4 The Leuprolide Study Group. Leuprolide versus diethylstilbestrol for metastatic prostate cancer. *N Engl J Med* 1984;311:1281–6.

5 Crawford ED, Eisenberger MA, McLeod DG et al. A controlled trial of leuprolide with and without flutamide in prostatic carcinoma [published erratum appears in *N Engl J Med* 1989;321:1420]. *N Engl J Med* 1989;321:419–24.

6 Maximum androgen blockade in advanced prostate cancer: an overview of the randomised trials. Prostate Cancer Trialists' Collaborative Group. *Lancet* 2000;355:1491–8.

7 Scher HI, Kelly WK. Flutamide withdrawal syndrome: its impact on clinical trials in hormone-refractory prostate cancer. *J Clin Oncol* 1993;11:1566–72.

8 Small EJ, Baron AD, Fippin L et al. Ketoconazole retains activity in advanced prostate cancer patients with progression despite flutamide withdrawal. *J Urol* 1997;157:1204–7.

9 Small EJ, Halabi S, Picus J, Dawson N, Chen Y, Vogelzang NJ. A prospective randomized trial of antiandrogen withdrawal alone or antiandrogen withdrawal in combination with high-dose ketoconazole in androgen independent prostate cancer patients. *Proc Am Soc Clin Oncol* 2001;20:174 (abstr).

10 Small EJ, Vogelzang NJ. Second-line hormonal therapy for advanced prostate cancer: a shifting paradigm. *J Clin Oncol* 1997;15:382–8.

11 Newling DW, Denis L, Vermeylen K. Orchiectomy versus goserelin and flutamide in the treatment of newly diagnosed metastatic prostate cancer. Analysis of the criteria of evaluation used in the European Organization for Research and Treatment of Cancer – Genitourinary Group Study 30853. *Cancer* 1993;72:3793–8.

12 Serafini AN, Houston SJ, Resche I et al. Palliation of pain associated with metastatic bone cancer using samarium-153 lexidronam: a double-blind placebo-controlled clinical trial. *J Clin Oncol* 1998;16:1574–81.

13 Tannock IF, Osoba D, Stockler MR et al. Chemotherapy with mitoxantrone plus prednisone or prednisone alone for symptomatic hormone-resistant prostate cancer: a Canadian randomized trial with palliative end points [see comments]. *J Clin Oncol* 1996;14:1756–64.

14 Kantoff PW, Halabi S, Conaway M et al. Hydrocortisone with or without mitoxantrone in men with hormone-refractory prostate cancer: results of the cancer and leukemia group B 9182 study [see comments]. *J Clin Oncol* 1999;17:2506–13.

15 Stearns ME, Tew KD. Estramustine binds MAP-2 to inhibit microtubule assembly in vitro. *J Cell Sci* 1988;89:331–42.

16 Stearns ME, Wang M, Tew KD et al. Estramustine binds a MAP-1-like protein to inhibit microtubule assembly in vitro and disrupt microtubule organization in DU 145 cells. *J Cell Biol* 1988;107:2647–56.

17 Murphy GP, Slack NH, Mittelman A. Use of estramustine phosphate in prostate cancer by the National Prostatic Cancer Project and by Roswell Park Memorial Institute. *Urology* 1984;23:54–63.

18 Roth BJ, Yeap BY, Wilding G et al. Taxol in advanced, hormone-refractory carcinoma of the prostate. A phase II trial of the Eastern Cooperative Oncology Group. *Cancer* 1993; 72:2457–60.

19 Beer TM, Pierce WC, Lowe BA, Henner WD. Phase II Study of weekly docetaxel in hormone refractory prostate cancer. *Proc Am Soc Clin Oncol* 2000;19:348 (abstr).

20 Speicher LA, Barone L, Tew KD. Combined antimicrotubule activity of estramustine and taxol in human prostatic carcinoma cell lines. *Cancer Res* 1992;52:4433–40.

21 Hudes GR, Greenberg R, Krigel RL et al. Phase II study of estramustine and vinblastine, two microtubule inhibitors, in hormone-refractory prostate cancer. *J Clin Oncol* 1992;10:1754–61.

22 Hudes GR, Nathan FE, Khater C et al. Paclitaxel plus estramustine in metastatic hormone-refractory prostate cancer. *Semin Oncol* 1995;22:41–5.

23 Pienta KJ, Redman BG, Bandekar R et al. A phase II trial of oral estramustine and oral etoposide in hormone refractory prostate cancer. *Urology* 1997;50:401–6; discussion 406–7.

24 Carles J, Domenech M, Gelabert-Mas A et al. Phase II study of estramustine and vinorelbine in hormone-refractory prostate carcinoma patients. *Acta Oncol* 1998;37:187–91.

25 Colleoni M, Graiff C, Vicario G et al. Phase II study of estramustine, oral etoposide, and vinorelbine in hormone-refractory prostate cancer. *Am J Clin Oncol* 1997;20:383–6.

26 Hudes G, Einhorn L, Ross E et al. Vinblastine versus vinblastine plus oral estramustine phosphate for patients with hormone-refractory prostate cancer: A Hoosier Oncology Group and Fox Chase Network phase III trial. *J Clin Oncol* 1999;17:3160–6.

27 Fields-Jones S, Koletsky A, Wilding G et al. Improvements in clinical benefit with vinorelbine in the treatment of hormone-refractory prostate cancer: a phase II trial. *Ann Oncol* 1999; 10:1307–10.

28 Smith MR, Kaufman D, Oh W et al. Vinorelbine and estramustine in androgen-independent metastatic prostate cancer. *Cancer* 2000;89:1824–8.

29 Sweeney C, Monaco F, Hanna M et al. Phase II study of weekly vinorelbine (VNR) and estramustine phosphate for hormone refractory prostate cancer. *Proc Am Soc Clin Oncol* 2000;19:335 (abstr).

30 Hortobagyi GN, Theriault RL, Porter L et al. Efficacy of pamidronate in reducing skeletal complications in patients with breast cancer and lytic bone metastases. Protocol 19 Aredia Breast Cancer Study Group. *N Engl J Med* 1996;335:1785–91.

31 Berenson JR, Lichtenstein A, Porter L et al. Long-term pamidronate treatment of advanced multiple myeloma patients reduces skeletal events. Myeloma Aredia Study Group. *J Clin Oncol* 1998;16:593–602.

32 Adami S. Bisphosphonates in prostate carcinoma. *Cancer* 1997;80:1674–9.

33 Heidenreich A, Hofmann R, Engelmann UH. The use of bisphosphonate for the palliative treatment of painful bone metastasis due to hormone refractory prostate cancer. *J Urol* 2001;165:136–40.

34 Dearnaley DP, Sydes MR, MRC Pr05 Collaborators. Preliminary evidence that oral clodronate delays symptomatic progression of bone metastases from prostate cancer: first results of MRC Pr05 trial. *Proc Am Soc Clin Oncol* 2001;20:174 (abstr).

21

Pancreatic and hepatobiliary cancer

Edward H. Lin and James L. Abbruzzese

U.T. M.D. Anderson Cancer Center, Houston

Definitions

Pancreatic and hepatobiliary cancers are named after their respective anatomical organ sites. Pancreatic cancer does not refer to tumors arising from the endocrine pancreas, which are termed islet cell tumors. Biliary tract cancers include gallbladder cancers, and cholangiocarcinomas arising from the intrahepatic, or perihilar, or distal extrahepatic duct. Cancers arising at the bile duct bifurcation are called Klatskin's tumors. Cancers arising from the ampulla of Vater (the common point of entry of the bile and pancreatic ducts into the duodenum) and surrounding ampulla are termed ampullary cancers and periampullary cancers respectively (Figure 21.1).

Epidemiology and etiology

Pancreatic cancer

Pancreatic cancers afflict about 28 000 Americans per year and rank in fifth place in cancer mortality.[1] The fact that the annual mortality rate of pancreatic cancer almost matches its annual incidence rate best illustrates its grave prognosis and lethality. Men, especially black men, are particularly at risk for the disease. The major risk factors for pancreatic cancer are smoking, with a relative risk of 4.0, and exposure to industrial carcinogens such as benzidine and naphthalamine. Poor dietary habits (high fat and low vegetable and fruit consumption), alcohol consumption, chronic pancreatitis, and diabetes are considered secondary risk factors. Patients with certain hereditary conditions, such as familial adenomatous polyposis (FAP) and Lynch syndrome II, BRCA1 and 2 carriers are also predisposed to pancreatic cancer as well as other types of cancers.[2]

Biliary tract cancer

In the US, gallbladder cancer and cholangiocarcinoma account for 7000 and 5000 cases per year, respectively.[1] Presence of gallstones is the single most important

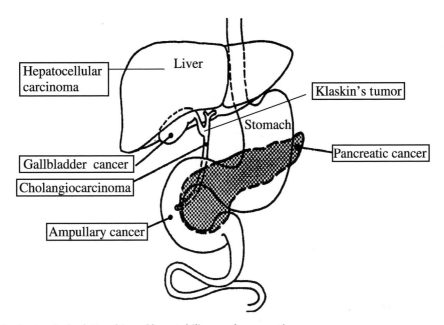

Figure 21.1 Anatomical relationships of hepatobiliary and pancreatic cancer.

risk factor for gallbladder cancers. Larger symptomatic gallstones (> 1 cm) are more carcinogenic than small asymptomatic ones. Other risk factors include gall-bladder polyps, choledochal (bile duct) cysts, *Salmonella typhi* (Typhus) carriers, porcelain gallbladder, pancreas-bile duct fistula, and cholestasis due to excess estrogen. Patients with hereditary Peutz–Jegher's syndrome are also prone to de-velop gallbladder cancer. Gallbladder cancer more commonly afflicts women. In contrast, cholangiocarcinoma more commonly afflicts men, especially among Native Americans, who appear to have a higher incidence of biliary tract cancers than Caucasians. Cholangiocarcinoma is often associated with primary scleros-ing cholangitis with or without ulcerative colitis. Liver fluke infections (*Clonorchis sinenesis* and *Opisthorchis viverini* are found in South-East Asia and the Far East, respectively) predispose to cholangiocarcinoma. Thorotrast, a radio-opaque con-trast agent, is banned due to its association with cholangiocarcinoma. Interestingly, smoking does not appear to be a risk factor for cholangiocarcinoma in contrast to its association with many other types of cancer.[3,4]

Hepatocellular carcinoma

Hepatocellular carcinoma (HCC) is one of the most common cancers in the world, with half a million cases reported worldwide per year. Africa and Asia are the most prevalent continents for HCC, as the incidence of HCC correlates with the regional hepatitis B virus (HBV) epidemics and the exposures to aflatoxin, a potent

Table 21.1. Etiology and epidemiology of pancreatohepatobiliary cancer in the US

	Pancreatic cancer	Cholangiocarcinoma	Gallbladder cancer	Hepatocellular cancer
Incidence/year	28 500	5000	7000	10 000
Male:female ratio	1:1	3:1	1:4	3:1
Ethnic groups most prone	Black	Native American	American Indians	Asians
Risk factors	Smoking	PSC	Gallstones	Hepatitis B, C
	Benzidine	UC	Gallbladder polyp	Alcohol
	High fat diet	Liver flukes		Cirrhosis
	Pancreatitis	Thoratrast		Estrogen
				Aflatoxin
Hereditary risk factors	FAP	NA	Peutz–Jegher syndrome	Wilson's disease
	Lynch syndrome			Tyrosinemia
	BRCA1 and 2 genes			α-AT deficiency

Note: PSC, primary sclerosing cholangitis; UC, ulcerative colitis; FAP, familial adenomatous polyposis; AT, antitrypsin.

carcinogen produced by molds found on poorly stored grains. The incidence of HCC in the US (about 10 000 cases per year) is rising, which is thought to be largely due to hepatitis C (HCV) and, to a smaller extent, to HBV and alcohol. Men are four times more likely to develop HCC than women. Co-infection with both HBV and HCV greatly increases the relative risk of HCC by up to 80-fold. Excess alcohol consumption alone can lead to liver cirrhosis and greatly accelerates the cirrhosis if viral hepatitis is also present. Cirrhosis develops during the first 10 years in 20% of the patients with chronic HCV, with HCC occurring at a rate of 1–4% per year in cirrhotic patients. It is estimated that 2–6% of all patients with chronic HCV (4 million cases in the US) may develop HCC in the next 20 years. Cirrhosis precedes the development of HCC in most cases in the West. This is in contrast to the situation in the Orient, likely due to the much greater frequency of aflatoxin exposure in the Orient. Population-wide hepatitis B vaccination has already produced a trend toward the reduction of HCC incidence in Taiwan. Currently, there are no effective vaccines for hepatitis C. Hereditary metabolic disorders, such as Wilson's disease, that predispose patients to liver cirrhosis also increase their risk for developing HCC.[4–6] Table 21.1 summarizes the etiology and epidemiology of pancreatic and hepatobiliary cancer.

Activation of oncogenes

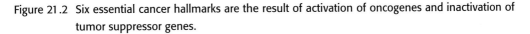

EGFR K-ras	EGFR TGFα	Telomerase	VEGF IL-8	bcl-2	MMP2 MMP9
Self-sufficient growth signal	Insensitivity to antigrowth signals	Limitless replicative potential	Sustained angiogenesis	Evasion of apoptosis	Tissue invasion metastasis
	SMAD4 TGFα		IL-12	p53 Bax	E-Cadherin APC

Inactivation of tumor suppressor genes

Figure 21.2 Six essential cancer hallmarks are the result of activation of oncogenes and inactivation of tumor suppressor genes.

Cancer biology

There are six essential hallmarks of cancer: (1) self-sufficiency in growth; (2) insensitivity to antiproliferative signals; (3) evasion of apoptosis (cell death); (4) limitless replicative potential; (5) sustained angiogenesis (blood vessel formation); and (6) tissue invasion and metastasis. These six cancer hallmarks are due to the gain of many cancer oncogenes and loss of many tumor suppressors; many of these altered cellular proteins are being explored as novel cancer therapeutic targets (Figure 21.2).[7,8]

Clinical presentations

There are often no specific symptoms for patients with pancreatic and hepatobiliary cancer. Commonly encountered complaints are general malaise, nausea, dyspepsia, weight loss, and abdominal pain and clinical depression. The frequent sites of metastasis from these cancers are the regional lymph nodes, liver, adjacent organs, or peritoneal implants also known as abdominal carcinomatosis.

Patients with advanced pancreatic cancer may present with back pain (due to nerve root invasion), ascites, weight loss, or cachexia (failure to thrive). Sudden onset of diabetes, or unexplained uncontrolled diabetes, should raise suspicions for pancreatic cancer. Persistent nausea and vomiting may be due to gastric outlet obstruction caused by the cancer in the head of the pancreas. Distal bile duct obstruction often leads to an enlarged gallbladder that is palpable on exam, a finding known as Courvoisier's sign. Superficial thrombophlebitis is known as Trousseau's syndrome, reflecting the hypercoagulable state present in pancreatic cancer.[2]

Obstructive jaundice is the most common sign for both pancreatic cancer and cholangiocarcinoma. The clay-colored stool reflects the degree of bile duct obstruction. There is a paucity of symptoms for gallbladder cancer, which often eludes early diagnosis. Thus, not uncommonly, the diagnosis of gallbladder cancer is made after laparoscopic or open cholecystectomy. Gallbladder cancer is often associated with a history of gallstones or chronic cholecystitis but the overall incidence of gallbladder cancer among patients with gallstones or cholecystitis is under 1%.[3,4]

Early HCC is generally asymptomatic and is confined to the liver initially. The liver and spleen may be easily palpable. However, pain is unusual even with bulky tumors unless the tumor has invaded adjacent structures. Sudden worsening of portal hypertension is often the result of portal vein involvement by the tumor. Fatal hemorrhage from HCC has been reported. Cirrhosis is graded according to the Child–Pugh classification, based on scores assigned by the assessment of hepatic encephalopathy, albumin, prothrombin time (PT), bilirubin, and ascites. Spider angioma, palmer erythema, and gynecomastia are signs of estrogen excess due to decreased liver metabolism of estrogen. HCC can also be associated with paraneoplastic syndromes such as polycythemia, hypercalcemia, and syndrome of inappropriate anti-diuretic hormones (SIADH).[4]

Diagnosis and staging

Diagnosis

The diagnostic schema for patients with pancreatic and hepatobiliary cancer is shown in Figure 21.3. For obstructive jaundice, ultrasound is initially performed to rule out gallstones and to visualize bile duct dilatation. If jaundice is found to be due to gallstones confirmed by either endoscopic retrograde cholangiopancreatography (ERCP) and/or ultrasound, computed tomography (CT) scan is often not necessary. However, when there is a clinical suspicion of cancer, CT of the target organ should be performed.[3] CT generally provides better resolution than ultrasound in visualizing both intrahepatic and extrahepatic mass. When metastatic disease is present, fine needle aspiration (FNA) or core tissue biopsy under ultrasound or CT guidance often yields a pathological diagnosis. Pathological diagnosis should be established in all patients except possibly those cases with liver mass and AFP (alpha fetal protein, a tumor marker for liver cancer) > 500 ng/ml, which are virtually diagnostic for HCC.[5]

Thin-cut CT with contrast through the target organ should be performed in all potentially resectable pancreatic and biliary tract cancer cases, assessing regional lymph nodes, vascular involvement, and the depth of tumor invasion. ERCP can be used to assess the status of the bile duct and to relieve most cases of biliary duct obstruction. Endoscopic ultrasound (EUS) is increasingly used to assess the portal

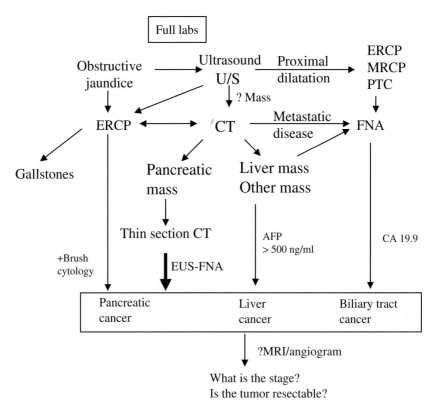

Figure 21.3 Diagnostic work-up for patients with pancreatic and hepatobiliary cancer. ERCP, endoscopic retrograde cholangiopancreatography; MRCP, magnetic resonance cholangiopancreatography; PTC, percutaneous transhepatic cholangiography; CT, computed tomography; FNA, fine needle aspiration; EUS, endoscopic ultrasound; AFP, alpha fetal protein; CA 19.9, a nonspecific serum tumor marker; MRI, magnetic resonance imaging.

vein and regional lymph node involvement in pancreatic cancer and EUS-guided FNA produces quite high diagnostic yields for pancreatic and biliary tract cancer. Percutaneous transhepatic cholangiography (PTC) is a useful adjunct for proximal bile duct obstruction not accessible by ERCP. Magnetic resonance cholangio-pancreatography (MRCP) is noninvasive and can provide quality images of both proximal and distal bile ducts. MRI images also complement CT findings in selected cases.[2–4]

The initial imaging choice for patients with suspected HCC is an abdominal ultrasound. If a mass is present, CT with arterial portography provides the best resolution to distinguish HCC from regenerating cirrhotic nodules. Lipiodol contrast-enhanced CT is often used in Asia and Europe to assess HCC. Magnetic resonance imaging is sometimes used in select HCC cases. Intrahepatic cholangiocarcinoma is often a diagnosis of exclusion, i.e., after HCC and other metastatic cancers to the liver have been ruled out. In this setting, upper and lower endoscopies are routinely performed to rule out metastasis from another gastrointestinal source.[4,5] CA 19.9, a nonspecific serum tumor marker, is often elevated in patients with pancreatic and biliary tract cancer. Laparoscopy or exploratory laparotomy should be reserved for surgical indications only, but not for diagnostic purposes.

Pathology

More than 90% of pancreatic and hepatobiliary cancer cases are adenocarcinomas derived from ductal epithelial cells. Other rare pathologies include squamous cell cancer, giant cell tumor, adenosquamous carcinoma and lymphoma.[2−4] Islet cell tumors have a distinct pathology with an indolent clinical course and are frequently responsive to local and systemic treatment.[9] Two subtypes of HCC, fibrolamellar and hepatoblastoma, are associated with a better prognosis and afflict teenage girls and children, respectively.[4] In addition, many other malignancies metastasize to the liver, thus, accurate pathologic diagnosis is of paramount importance.

TNM cancer staging

Tumor staging is based upon TNM criteria (T = extent of tumor invasion into the organ of involvement, N = nodal metastasis, and M = distant metastasis) established by the American Joint Committee on Cancer (AJCC). Stage I and II are T1 or T2 tumors that are limited to the involved organ without evidence of nodal metastasis (N0). Stage III is characterized by the presence of T3 tumors with regional lymph node metastasis (N1), in contrast to stage IV cancer characterized by T4 tumor with or without distant metastasis (M1).[10] Figure 21.4 illustrates the

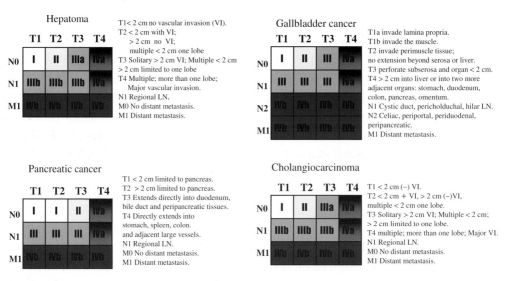

Figure 21.4 Staging of pancreatic and hepatobiliary cancer.

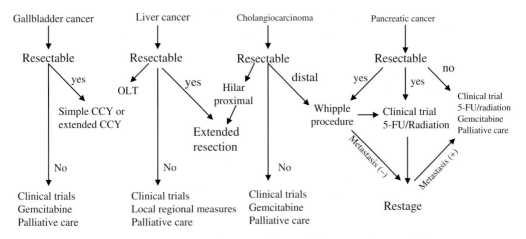

Figure 21.5 Treatment algorithms for pancreatic and hepatobiliary cancer. CCY, cholecystectomy; OLT, orthotopic liver transplantation.

staging of pancreatic and hepatobiliary cancer (stage I white; stage II stippled; stage III light grey; stage IV dark grey).

Management

To date, surgery remains the only curative option for patients with pancreatic and hepatobiliary cancer due to the lack of effective screening and systemic treatment modalities. All patients should be encouraged to participate in appropriately designed clinical trials (Figure 21.5).

Pancreatic cancer

Eighty percent of pancreatic cancer patients present with either locally advanced disease (stage III) or metastatic disease (stage IV). These patients are presumably not candidates for surgery involving a pancreaticoduodenectomy, also known as the Whipple procedure. Thus, only 20% or less of pancreatic cancer cases are surgically resectable. The resection criteria include: (1) no evidence of tumor involvement of the SMA (superior mesenteric artery); (2) no evidence of extrapancreatic disease; and (3) a patent portal vein.[2] In inexperienced hands the Whipple procedure is a very morbid surgical procedure with a postoperative mortality rate of 5–10% or higher. However, at experienced centers the mortality of the Whipple procedure is minimal and morbidity is acceptable. However, the 5-year survival rate of patients who have the Whipple procedure is disappointingly low at 10–20% with many patients still dying of pancreatic cancer 5–7 years after surgery. In contrast, patients with ampullary cancer experience better survival with its 5-year survival rate approaching 35%. The reason for this more optimistic survival is likely due to early disease presentation and the inherent less aggressive biology of ampullary cancers.[2] Thus, preoperative radiation with 5-FU becomes the preferred approach at M.D. Anderson Cancer Center for patients with resectable pancreatic cancer for two reasons: (1) up to 30–50% of patients can be downstaged, facilitating complete surgical resection; and (2) a significant number of patients can be spared this morbid surgical procedure should patients experience rapid disease progression during preoperative chemoradiation.[2,8]

Gallbladder cancer

About 70% of gallbladder cancer patients present in advanced stages. Tis (Tumor in situ) or T1a gallbladder cancers are almost always discovered incidentally after either laparoscopic or open cholecystectomy. These patients are considered cured of their disease with a 5-year survival rate > 90%. Current imaging techniques such as MRI can determine the depth of tumor invasion, a major determinant in resectability. For T1b tumors, extended cholecystectomy with hepatic resection and dissection of regional lymph nodes is recommended. The 5-year survival for patients with T1b tumors approaches 60–80%. Extended cholecystectomy is indicated for patients with T2 cancer as well. For patients with T3–T4 tumors, an extended operation combining hepatic resection with nodal dissection, with or without excision of the common bile duct is sometimes performed, but the results are disappointing. A subset of patients with peripancreatic nodes or invasion into adjacent organs may benefit from a synchronous pancreaticoduodenectomy.[3,4]

Cholangiocarcinoma

Surgical management of cholangiocarcinoma depends on location of the tumor in the bile duct. Distal bile duct lesions have the best resectability rates due to the ability of the surgeon to achieve adequate margins and possibly earlier stage of presentation. This stands in contrast to proximal cholangiocarcinomas that often present late in their natural history of disease. With the following findings patients are generally considered unresectable: (1) lymph node involvement outside the porta hepatis; (2) distant metastases; (3) bilateral tumor extension into secondary hepatic ducts or the hepatic parenchyma; (4) portal vein involvement. Distal cholangiocarcinomas are best treated with the Whipple's procedure. Treatment of perihilar cholangiocarcinomas consists of removal of most of the extrahepatic duct and regional lymph nodes whereas proximal intrahepatic cholangiocarcinomas are approached by extended hepatic dissection.[3,4]

Hepatocellular carcinoma

The frequent association of HCC and cirrhosis poses a serious challenge. This fact is underscored by the observations that at least one-third of HCC patients die of cirrhosis or its complications rather than directly from HCC. Surgically there are eight distinct hepatic arterial/venous/biliary drainage segments, allowing safe liver resection without compromising remnant liver function. The 5-year survival rate for resected stage I or II HCC is about 25–55%, which is comparable to the results achieved by orthotopic liver transplantation (OLT). OLT is indicated for patients with severe cirrhosis that prevents safe liver resection. Best OLT results are achieved in patients with a single HCC mass < 3 cm, within a single lobe of the liver; in contrast, HCC mass > 5 cm is associated with a very high rate of intrahepatic recurrence. Furthermore, shortage of liver donors severely limits the use of OLT in the treatment of HCC.[11]

Although confined to the liver, most HCC cases are not surgically resectable. Many regional treatment options have been developed but these have not been validated by prospective randomized clinical trials. These regional interventions include percutaneous ethanol injection (PEI), RFA (radiofrequency ablation), or HAE (hepatic arterial embolization). PEI is indicated for HCC < 3 cm and is performed under ultrasound by injecting 10–15 ml 100% alcohol directly into the HCC, leading to local tumor necrosis. Although the intrahepatic recurrence rate is high, the 5-year survival rate following PEI approaches 20%. RFA can ablate multiple HCC < 5 cm. This technique involves the insertion of a heat-wave generating probe into the center of the tumor mass, sparing surrounding normal liver tissue. The exact role of RFA in the management of HCC is under investigation. Cryoablation, a technique performed in a similar manner as RFA using liquid nitrogen, has largely lost favor due to its high complication rate. Hepatic arterial embolization (HAE) takes advantage of the fact that HCC derives its blood supply by the hepatic artery, whereas normal liver cells derives their major blood supply through the portal veins. HAE is performed under fluoroscopy guidance by releasing tiny gelform particles that embolize the feeding tumor arterioles, causing tumor necrosis. However, prospective randomized studies have failed to demonstrate survival benefits comparing HAE versus chemotherapy plus HAE versus best supportive care.[5,12]

Palliative measures

Chemotherapy

The current standard for patients with locally advanced pancreatic cancer (unresectable) consists of 5-fluorouracil (5-FU) with concurrent radiation (Figure 21.5). A modest survival benefit was achieved with chemoradiation as compared with radiation alone. Gemcitabine is the only approved chemotherapy agent for advanced pancreatic cancer based on its benefits in improving quality of life, pain control, a modest response rate of < 10% and a gain in median survival of 6 weeks when compared with 5-FU and best supportive care.[3] Gemcitabine has also been used in the palliative therapy of other biliary tract cancers and HCC, producing a 10–20%

response rate in phase II nonrandomized clinical studies. Other chemotherapy agents for palliative therapy include 5-FU, capecitabine (an oral 5-FU prodrug) or camptozar (CPT-11). These agents also produce 10–20% response rates in these malignancies. To date, combination chemotherapies have largely failed to demonstrate superior survival as compared with single agent chemotherapy in pancreatic and hepatobiliary tract cancer.[2–5] Molecular targeted therapy to specific tumor target(s) holds both great promise and great challenges to the development of future cancer therapies.

Management of the symptom complex associated with pancreatic and hepatobiliary cancer

Symptomatic management constitutes a major component of care for patients with pancreatic and hepatobiliary tract cancer. Obstructive jaundice often requires initial biliary stent placement and subsequent replacement under ERCP. In selected cases external or internal biliary bypass is also used to relieve jaundice. Small bowel obstruction due to extensive abdominal carcinomatosis should be managed initially nonsurgically with nasogastric tube suction and bowel rest, with or without permanent gastric tube placement. Unless there is a surgical indication, gastric outlet obstruction may be relieved with a duodenal stent or venting gastrostomy. Total parenteral nutrition (TPN) is applied to these patients sparingly since TPN is quite expensive and does not improve survival in these terminally ill patients. Medical comorbidities also significantly impact treatment tolerance and survival.[13]

Pain and clinical depression in this population of patients are very common and are often undertreated. Pain medications should be aggressively titrated according to the WHO pain assessment ladder with the choices of pain medication ranging from oral nonsteroidal drugs (NSAIDS) to low and high potency narcotics. To reduce the frequency of narcotic intolerance, short-acting narcotics are used for breakthrough pain along with long-acting narcotics. New onset of pain should prompt clinical evaluation for possible progression of disease. Celiac block (injection of alcohol into the splanchnic nerves) is reserved for patients with refractory pain that fails to respond to conventional management.[13] Clinical depression should be aggressively treated with antidepressants and a timely referral for psychiatric counseling should be emphasized.[14]

Performance status is the single most useful predictive prognostic marker in the management of patients with pancreatic or hepatobiliary cancers. Performance status is measured according by either ECOG (Eastern Cooperative Group) scales or Karnofsky scores (KPS) (see Table 2.2). Patients with ECOG performance status > 2 or patients who have become refractory or intolerant to treatment should be managed using supportive measures alone. The physical, emotional, and social needs of these terminally ill patients are best met by a local hospice service through a team consisting of physicians, nurses, pain experts, social workers, and chaplains.[15]

REFERENCES

1 Greenlee RT, Murray T, Bolden S, Wingo PA. *Cancer Statistics* 2000;50:7–33.

2 Evans DB, Abbruzzese JL, Rich TR. Cancer of the pancreas. In *Cancer Principles and Practice of Oncology*, 5th edn, ed. VT DeVita, S Hellman, SA Rosenberg, pp. 1054–87. Philadelphia: Lippincott-Raven, 1997.

3 De Groen PC, Gores GJ, LaRusso NF et al. Biliary tract cancers. *N Engl J Med* 1999;341: 1368–78.

4 Flickinger BI, Lotze MT. Hepatobiliary cancers. In *Cancer Principles and Practice of Oncology*, 5th edn, ed. VT DeVita, S Hellman, SA Rosenberg, pp. 1087–1106. Philadelphia: Lippincott-Raven, 1997.

5 Nakakura EK, Choti MA. Management of hepatocellular carcinoma. *Oncology* 2000;14: 1085–98.

6 Shafer DF, Sorrell MF. Hepatocellular carcinoma. *Lancet* 1999;353:1253–7.

7 Hanahan D, Weinberg RA. The hallmarks of cancer. *Cell* 2000;100:57–70.

8 Wolff RA, Chiao P, Lenzi R et al. Current approaches and future strategies for pancreatic carcinoma. *Invest New Drugs* 2000;18:45–50.

9 Moertel CG, Johnson M, McKusick MA et al. The management of patients with advanced carcinoid tumors and islet cell carcinomas. *Ann Intern Med* 1994;120:302–9.

10 Fleming ID, Cooper JS, Henson DE et al (ed.). *AJCC Cancer Staging Handbook*, 5th edn. Philadelphia: Lippincott-Raven, 1998.

11 Mor E, Kaspa RT, Sheiner, Schwartz M. Treatment of hepatocellular carcinoma associated with cirrhosis in the era of liver transplantation. *Ann Intern Med* 1998;129:643–53.

12 Venook A. Regional strategies for managing hepatocellular carcinoma. *Oncology* 2000;14: 347–54.

13 Levy MH. Pharmacologic treatment of cancer pain. *N Engl J Med* 1996;335:1124–30.

14 Passik SD, Breitbart WS. Depression in patients with pancreatic carcinoma: diagnostic and treatment issues. *Cancer* 1996;78:615–26.

15 Lillemoe KD, Pitt HA. Palliation. *Cancer* 1996;78:605–14.

22

Anal cancer

Rob Glynne-Jones

Mount Vernon Hospital Centre for Cancer Treatment, Northwood

Incidence

Epidermoid cancer of the anus includes the anal canal and perianal skin, i.e., tumors within a radius of approximately 5 cm from the anal orifice. It is a relatively rare disease. In the US, approximately 2000 new cases are registered annually. It comprises about 3% of all colorectal malignancies. There are two peak incidences; one at 40–50 years and another at 70–80 years. Industrialized countries appear to show an age adjusted incidence of < 1 per 100 000. Cancers of the anal canal are approximately three times more common in females than in males. In contrast, carcinomas in the area of the anal margin are slightly more common in males. There is a slight female preponderance overall. A viral etiology has been suggested since 50% of cancers show evidence of human papilloma virus type 16 and 18, similar to carcinoma of the cervix.[1] For this reason receptive homosexual intercourse is accepted as a risk factor and the incidence of anal intraepithelial neoplasia (AIN) is also higher in homosexual activity. Even before the AIDS epidemic an excess risk of 40–50 times was observed in the homosexual population for anal cancer.[2] Immunosuppression is a further important risk factor, and anal cancer is not uncommon in renal and cardiac transplant recipients. Other recognized risk factors include previous pelvic radiotherapy and cigarette smoking.

Carcinoma of the anus usually runs an indolent course with a low rate of distant metastases. This disease often presents at an early localized stage when it is amenable to curative nonsurgical treatment. Historically, cure rates were observed with surgical procedures such as abdomino-perineal excision of the rectum which produced cure rates overall in the region of 50%.[3] More recent randomized studies have shown 5-year survival in the range of 55–70% with chemoradiation.[4–6]

Even small lesions can present with marked pain and rectal bleeding and are often misdiagnosed. The real challenge in managing anal cancer is to provide a treatment which will cure the majority of patients without compromising anal/rectal function.

Pathology

Macroscopically the tumor arises close to the anal margin either in the skin or anal canal. Early appearances are often of a warty nodule or infiltrating ulceration. Microscopic appearances demonstrate more than 90% as squamous cell carcinomas, basiloid or cloacagenic carcinomas. Less than 5% appear to represent adeno-carcinoma arising in the mucous glands of the anus and are usually mucus secreting. Tumors of the anal canal are often poorly differentiated squamous cell carcinomas. In contrast, tumors of the anal margin are more like skin cancers and are often well-differentiated squamous cell carcinomas.

Primary extent

The primary tumor usually grows in an annular fashion extending through the wall of the anal canal and eventually involves the underlying sphincter muscles. There may be invasion of the perianal skin which is occasionally extensive and deeply in-filtrating. In women, the tumor seems to frequently extend anteriorly to invade the recto-vaginal septum and the perineal body. The cancer can spread both circumfer-entially and longitudinally up the anal canal to involve the lower part of the rectum or externally out into the perianal skin with deeper involvement of the muscles. The levator muscles of the sphincters are involved at a relatively early stage which can spread further into the ischiorectal fossa, vagina, or even urethra if left unchecked.

Lymph node spread

The inguinal lymph nodes may be involved in up to 30% of cases overall with anal margin tumors, but much less frequently in cancers of the anal canal. Early tumors (T1, T2) have an even lower rate of approximately 12%. Inguinal lymphadenopathy is usually unilateral and occasionally bilateral but not contralateral to the tumor. The pelvic nodes almost always will also be involved, particularly with increasing tumour stage and in the context of poorly differentiated carcinomas which extend superiorly into the rectum or anteriorly in women. When the rectum is directly involved, the cancer may spread via the inferior mesenteric lymph nodes. The overall incidence of pelvic lymph node metastases is in the region of 25–35%.

Bloodborne metastases are fortunately quite rare at presentation. Only < 5% of patients have spread confirmed in the liver and even fewer in the lungs.

Presenting symptoms

Common symptoms which bring the cancer to light include a discharge from the rectum, itching, pain, bleeding, and a feeling of incomplete emptying of the bowels (tenesmus) and constipation.

There is often little to see unless the cancer extends outside onto the anal margin and perianal skin and so examination of the rectum is essential. The doctor should always palpate for inguinal lymph nodes particularly at the very medial end of the inguinal ligament where an involved gland the size of a marble can be easily missed.

Differential diagnosis

The diagnosis is usually obvious although Crohn's disease, solitary ulcer syndrome, and painless syphilitic ulcer in a homosexual can be confused with an early cancer. It may also be very difficult to distinguish between a warty looking well-differentiated squamous carcinoma and proliferative genital warts.

Investigation and staging

Advanced cancers in the ano-rectum are often very painful for the patient and therefore do not allow an easy digital rectal examination. For this reason, it is often helpful to perform an examination under anesthetic which will both clarify the extent of the local lesion and also define pararectal lymph nodes. To some extent, modern quality magnetic resonance imaging (MRI) can demonstrate both the local extent of the tumor and the presence of suspiciously enlarged lymph nodes in both the perirectal and pelvic areas. Traditionally CT scans have been performed to define metastatic spread, periaortic and pelvic lymph node enlargement – although computerized tomography (CT) scans nearly always underestimate the local extent of the tumor. The UICC 1990 staging system is conventionally used (Table 22.1).

Blood tests which are usually performed include a full blood count, urea and electrolytes and creatinine for renal function to ensure safe delivery of the nephrotoxic drugs *cis*-platinum or mitomycin-c; and liver function tests. HIV status should be explored for younger patients with recognized risk factors. Serum squamous cell carcinoma antigen is routinely used in our unit. This test has a 44% sensitivity and 92% specificity and appears to relate to lymph node involvement. It also correlates with tumor T stage.[7] Elevated squamous carcinoma levels should therefore prompt a careful clinical examination and a review of CT scans for evidence of groin or pelvic lymphadenopathy.

Treatment

Small tumors in the anal margin can be treated by wide local excision alone, but curative surgery may compromise sphincter function for small tumors in the anal canal. There is also a surgical role for placing a diverting colostomy in patients either with recto-vaginal fistula, obstruction, or fecal incontinence. More extensive surgery is usually reserved for salvage when the local disease relapses.

Table 22.1. TNM staging. The UICC 1990 staging system is used
(Note: nodal N stage differs in anal margin and anal canal)

Tx	Primary tumor cannot be assessed
Tis	Carcinoma in situ
T1	Tumor 2 cm or less
T2	Tumor > 2–5 cm
T3	Tumor > 5 cm
T4	Tumor invades other organ (vagina, urethra, bladder, sacrum) – anal canal
	Tumor invades deeper structures (skeletal muscle or cartilage) – anal margin
N	Regional nodes are perirectal, internal iliac and inguinal
Nx	Regional nodes cannot be assessed
N0	No regional node metastases
N1	Metastasis in perirectal nodes
N2	Metastasis in unilateral internal iliac and/or inguinal nodes
N3	Metastasis in perirectal and/or bilateral internal iliac or inguinal nodes
M0	No metastasis
M1	Metastasis present

It is usually accepted that the standard of care for patients with squamous cell carcinoma of the anal canal and margin is primary chemoradiotherapy since it produces better local control and survival than radiotherapy alone or surgery alone. The present authors believe there is a role for preoperative chemoradiation and anteroposterior excision of the rectum for patients with large T4 tumors which have destroyed the levator muscles and hence the sphincters.

Chemotherapy

The standard chemotherapy regimen requires inpatient stay and is given during the first and fifth week of radiotherapy using:

Cisplatin	20 mg/m^2 in 1 litre N saline with appropriate hydration, days 1–5, 29–33
5-FU	750 mg/m^2 in 1 litre N saline over 24 hours, days 1–5, 29–33
or	
Mitomycin C	12 mg/m^2 bolus, day 1 only (max 20 mg)
5-FU	750 mg/m^2 in 1 litre N saline over 24 hours, days 1–5, 29–33.

For patients who are elderly and there is concern as to an increased risk of neutropenic sepsis, use:

Mitomycin C	8 mg/m^2 bolus, day 1 only (max 10 mg)
5-FU	750 mg/m^2 in 1 litre N saline over 24 hours, days 1–4, 29–32.

Prophylactic antibiotics

Ciproflaxacin 250 mg twice daily is given on the commencement of chemotherapy and continues until any areas of moist desquamation following chemoradiotherapy are no longer moist.

Evidence base

The initial studies of Nigro et al.[8,9] demonstrated high rates of local control with the use of approximately 30 Gy of irradiation with concurrent mitomycin C (MMC) and 5-fluorouracil (5-FU). Cummings et al.[10] reported a series of 190 patients treated with radiotherapy or chemoradiotherapy using seven sequential regimens and concluded retrospectively improved local control with chemoradiotherapy and with the addition of MMC to 5-FU.

Only three randomized trials have been performed. The UKCCCR[4] and the EORTC trial[5] compared chemoradiotherapy with radiotherapy alone. The RTOG trial[6] compared mitomycin C versus no mitomycin C in combination with chemoradiotherapy (using 5-FU plus radiotherapy). These three trials confirm that chemoradiotherapy using 5-FU and MMC in combination with radiotherapy is the standard of care. There is still uncertainty concerning the benefit of a boost dose of radiotherapy following chemoradiotherapy where the total dose of radiotherapy is 45–50 Gy.

Prognosis

Overall 5-year survival is about 70%. Patients with cancers in the anal margin do rather better than those with anal canal tumors. It is possible that this reflects the fact that anal canal tumors are poorly differentiated and often clinically understaged. The prognosis is defined by the size of the primary tumor and the presence of lymph node metastases. For cancers of 4 cm or less the overall survival may reach 80–90%.

Historically, Papillon reviewed 5-year survival rates following AP excision of the rectum alone and showed that they varied from 32% to 61%. However, it is not always clear whether radiotherapy has been used either pre- or postoperatively in surgical series of anteroposterior excision of the rectum. The results of series from specialist units who have employed radiotherapy alone have demonstrated local control in the region of 60–80% with 5-year survival of 46–66%.

The management of squamous cell carcinoma of the anal canal and margin has changed dramatically, particularly over the last 15–20 years. There are many unanswered questions but the majority of patients appear to be curable with preservation of reasonable anal function. It is, therefore, appropriate to treat all but the very elderly, very frail and patients with "paper money" skin in the perianal area with chemoradiation unless renal function precludes the use of mitomycin or cisplatin. However, there is another group of patients who have unstable angina for whom the use of 5-FU is considered too dangerous.

Care for the dying patient

Failure to respond to or relapse after primary chemoradiation can sometimes be salvaged by surgical procedures. However, the results of long-term control after salvage surgery are poor. Local recurrence is complicated by pain, bleeding, and discharge. Recurrent disease within the pelvis is similar to the situation experienced by patients with recurrent rectal cancer i.e., pelvic pain extending into the buttocks and often in a sciatic distribution if the recurrence is predominantly presacral and irritating the lumbar sacral plexus. Bilateral ureteric obstruction is often encountered.

A defunctioning colostomy can be very helpful to alleviate symptoms from uncontrolled local disease. Bilateral ureteric stents may often be appropriate particularly if the patient is otherwise fit for further chemotherapy. A small number of patients develop liver or lung metastases and palliative chemotherapy can be considered.

For patients who are dying adequate pain control and stool softeners will be essential components of terminal care. Neuropathic pain may pose particular problems but may respond to amitriptyline, anti-epileptics such as sodium valproate or tegretol, flecainide or gabapentin. Rectal discharge is often an extremely difficult symptom to palliate but occasionally may be relieved by octreotide.

Box 22.1 Summary – anal cancer

- Anal cancer is a rare tumor which should be treated in specialist units.
- Primary chemoradiation is the standard of care.
- HIV status should be sought for patients with risk factors.
- MRI can accurately delineate local extent of tumor.
- Surgical salvage rarely offers long-term control and again should be performed in specialist units experienced in operating in heavily irradiated tissue.
- Adequate pain relief and stool softeners are essential components of terminal care.

REFERENCES

1 Frisch M, Glimelius B, Adriaan JC et al. Sexually transmitted infection as a cause of anal cancer. *N Engl J Med* 1997;337:1350–8.
2 Daling JR, Weiss NS, Hislop TG et al. Sexual practices, sexually transmitted diseases and the incidence of anal cancer. *N Engl J Med* 1987;317: 973.

3 Hardcastle JD, Bussey HJR. Results of surgical treatment of squamous cell carcinoma of anal canal and anal margin seen at St Mark's Hospital, 1928–1966. *Proc R Soc Med* 1968;61:629.

4 The UKCCCR Anal Cancer Trial Working Party. Epidermoid anal cancer: results from the UKCCCR randomised trial of radiotherapy alone versus radiotherapy, 5-fluorouracil and mitomycin C. *Lancet* 1996;348:1049–54.

5 Bartelink H, Roelofson F, Eschwege F et al. Concomitant radiotherapy and chemotherapy is superior to radiotherapy alone in the treatment of locally advanced anal cancer: results of a phase III randomized trial of the European Organisation for Research and Treatment of Cancer Radiotherapy and Gastrointestinal Groups. *J Clin Oncol* 1997;15:2040–9.

6 Flam M, John M, Pajak TF et al. Role of mitomycin in combination with fluorouracil and radiation, and of salvage chemoradiation in the definitive nonsurgical treatment of epidermoid carcinoma of the anal canal: results of a phase III randomised intergroup study. *J Clin Oncol* 1996;14:2527–39.

7 Osborne M, Glynne-Jones R, Makris A. Chemoradiation followed by immediate boost in squamous cell carcinoma of the anus. *Br J Cancer* 2000;83 (Suppl 1, P71):46.

8 Nigro ND, Vaitkevicius VK, Consindine B Jr. Combined therapy for cancer of the anal canal: a preliminary report. *Dis Col Rectum* 1974;17:354.

9 Nigro ND, Seydel H, Consindine B Jr. Combined preoperative radiation and chemotherapy for squamous cell cancer of the anal canal. *Cancer* 1983;51:1826.

10 Cummings B, Keane T, Thomas G, Harwood A, Rider W. Results and toxicity of the treatment of anal canal carcinoma by radiation therapy or radiation and chemotherapy. *Cancer* 1984;54:2026.

23

Esophageal and gastric cancer

Stephen A. Bernard

University of North Carolina School of Medicine, Chapel Hill

Esophageal cancer

In the US, esophageal and gastric cancer are often locally advanced or metastatic at presentation. Management of these patients requires palliation of problems with the ability of the patient to take in food and liquids.

Natural history of esophageal cancer

The esophagus begins at the cricopharyngeal muscle (15 cm from the teeth) and ends at the gastroesophageal junction (40 cm from the teeth). Cancer most frequently occurs in the middle third of the esophagus. The second most frequent location is in the lower third of the esophagus.

Esophageal cancer is uncommon in the US. The disease is most often seen in a region that extends from southwest China to Iran, often called the esophageal cancer belt, and in Africa and South America. In the US, an increase in the frequency in cases of adenocarcinoma of the esophagus has been observed over the last 5–10 years. While squamous carcinoma of the esophagus is most often associated with injury due to cigarettes, alcohol, and lye, adenocarcinoma is associated with Barrett's esophagus, a dysplastic condition of the distal esophagus, which may be initiated by reflux.

In the US the disease is frequently locally advanced at the time of diagnosis. Most patients with esophageal cancer present with difficulty in swallowing (dysphagia). The normal esophagus is elastic and distensible. For dysphagia to be present, approximately 75% of the wall circumference must be involved with tumor. Other symptoms that are commonly seen are weight loss, and pain with swallowing. Less commonly, the local disease is large enough so that pressure is exerted on the recurrent laryngeal nerve and hoarseness results. This symptom would be more likely seen in tumors arising in the middle third of the esophagus. Tumors arising in this part of the esophagus can also erode the bronchus or trachea producing a fistula that manifests itself as coughing when eating. In cervical lesions, or very advanced mid-esophageal lesions, patients may not even be able to swallow saliva. Aspiration can result when a large mass is present that prevents food or secretions from passing.

Therapy, either surgery, radiation, or chemotherapy, usually alters the natural history of the disease. Patients who are severely debilitated at the time they are first seen may receive treatment that is symptom-based and not receive active treatment of their disease. Typically, these individuals die of inanition, and aspiration.

Patterns of spread and recurrence

In contrast to the stomach, the esophagus lacks a serosa or covering over its outer wall. Consequently, penetration through the wall is more easily accomplished and spread along the extensive lymphatic network occurs readily. This network, which begins in the wall, drains to multiple nodes within the mediastinum. These anatomic features partly account for the advanced stage of the disease at presentation and the difficulty in removal of all disease surgically.

Once it has penetrated through the muscle layers, the disease spreads along the wall of the esophagus, and may be seen at several sites along the length of the organ. Nodal involvement can be seen throughout the mediastinum. From these loco-regional sites, spread is to the lung or to distant nodes (gastrohepatic or celiac) below the diaphragm in the case of distal esophageal cancer. The neoplasm may also spread to the liver. Other sites such as bone or central nervous system are infrequently involved. After curative surgery, the disease is still most likely to recur in the mediastinum or nodal groups in the upper abdomen.

Prognosis

The prognosis for this disease is based on the extent of wall invasion, and the involvement of regional nodes. Individuals with nodal involvement in the abdomen or outside the chest, or those with organ involvement such as the liver are considered to have metastatic disease. Life expectancy with disease that is resectable in a patient who is medically fit is in the range of 1–2 years with 10–15% of those individuals surviving to 5 years in the more recent surgical literature. Many patients will have loco-regional disease that is marginally resectable (locally advanced) or their underlying medical condition precludes general anesthesia and surgery. These individuals are often treated with chemoradiotherapy. The limited number of studies comparing a nonsurgical approach to one with surgery have shown similar results for those with locally advanced disease. These patients may survive on average 1–2 years with a small percentage living longer. The pattern of recurrence may be distant in the liver or abdominal nodes or lung. The dominant symptoms following surgery include pulmonary difficulties and problems with swallowing. Long term, patients may have trouble with stricture. For individuals treated with chemoradiotherapy, the initial symptoms are those of pain with swallowing during the treatment; fatigue; vomiting; and symptoms related to bone marrow suppression. Long-term symptoms can include difficulty swallowing related to stricture formation.

For patients with metastatic disease at presentation, prognosis is generally in the range of months. Other features such as medical comorbidities, overall status, and nutritional status also play a role in life expectancy.

Therapeutic approaches

Therapy for local or loco-regional disease is generally surgical if possible. As noted above, for patients who appear to have resectable disease, there is much interest in the addition of chemoradiotherapy prior to surgery. Studies to date have not confirmed an advantage to this approach.

The esophagus has as its main function the passage of food to the stomach. When this function cannot occur, nutrition becomes the central issue in patient management. Surgical treatment provides the quickest solution to the problem. In individuals who cannot undergo surgery, other techniques have been developed to allow an increase in the ability to swallow. Where definitive surgery cannot be done, operative techniques to bypass the obstruction have been developed; however, with the advent of newer approaches to relieve the obstruction these procedures are less often used.

Radiotherapy, given for palliation of swallowing, can be effective. Frequently, external beam radiotherapy is combined with chemotherapy as a radiation enhancer. Use of brachytherapy can reduce small lesions; however, the disease is often outside the organ, and external beam may provide a longer period of symptom control. Laser therapy with photodynamic agents at institutions that have expertise in this area, can also be used to relieve esophageal obstruction.

Stents, either plastic or metal, have been redesigned. These devices can be inserted endoscopically, and can provide good palliation of the inability to swallow and allow for nutrition and hydration. The newer designs remain in place much longer and are less prone to migration into the larynx or distally into the stomach.

Chemotherapy is seldom used alone for local disease that is not amenable to surgery or radiotherapy. Several agents have modest activity in this disease, and drug combinations have been used increasing the likelihood of an initial tumor response, but none of these regimens has been shown to effectively palliate an enlarged mass to allow swallowing. The side effects of many of these agents, especially vomiting, and anorexia also argue against their use for this indication.

Chemotherapy has been used for treatment of metastatic disease. The drug regimens generally have a 10–40% likelihood of producing an immediate response, which lasts for 3–6 months. Balancing these short-term benefits against the morbidity of the drugs requires an open discussion by the physician with the patient and family.

Site-specific rehabilitation issues

Rehabilitation of the patient with esophageal cancer requires little retraining. Two major types of surgical approach exist. One involves a transhiatal approach, which does not require a chest incision. The other requires both a chest and abdominal incision. For individuals who have removal of the esophagus and upper stomach, there will be loss of the lower esophageal sphincter. Reflux is common and may be treated by the use of measures to reduce acid, such as proton pump inhibitors, or H_2 blockers. Individuals receiving chemoradiotherapy as the initial therapy may require several weeks to note an improvement in soreness and difficulty with swallowing. Failure to improve after this therapy, or worsening on therapy, may be due to edema of the wall, especially in high cervical lesions where there is little room for expansion.

Site-specific palliative care issues

Symptoms, arising from the disease, have been discussed above. The decision as to the aggressiveness of palliative therapy must take into account the underlying nutritional status of these patients as well as the presence of comorbidities, such as alcoholism. With the rise of adenocarcinoma in the US, patients are not always as nutritionally depleted as the person with squamous cell cancer whose disease is often a consequence of heavy alcohol and cigarette use. Decision making needs to take all of these issues into account.

For the individual with a significant weight loss, who also has severe lung disease, operative mortality may be extremely high and chemoradiotherapy may be considered. Alternatively, stenting may provide palliation for several months, without exposure to the morbidities of chemotherapy or radiotherapy. Enteral nutrition may be difficult if there has been prior surgery with a pull-up of the stomach into the thorax. Placement of an enteral tube may require an open jejunostomy. The medical fitness of the individual to tolerate such a procedure must be considered.

Management of a fistula may not give relief of symptoms. Although individuals with a fistula may be able to tolerate radiotherapy, the conventional teaching is that the fistula will worsen, with a rapid downhill course. On occasion, a stent can be placed to palliate the chronic aspiration and recurrent episodes of pneumonia, which are the usual causes of death. There are recent reports of the successful resolution of small fistulae with radiotherapy.

Management of the inability to swallow secretions is often difficult. In the past, a fistula was created in the floor of the mouth to drain saliva to an ostomy bag.

This technique is emotionally distressing for the individual, their family, and the healthcare team. The use of anticholinergics may decrease salivary flow. External beam radiation to the major salivary glands may also be considered, but requires several weeks of treatment.

Once there is extensive local disease, life expectancy is very short. The individual may experience pain and recurrent episodes of aspiration. Providing nutritional support is dependent on the general status of the patient. While parenteral nutrition may also alter the state of hydration, it will not prevent the recurrent episodes of aspiration or erosion of the tumor into other structures and is not often given.

In summary, problems with nutrition and hydration dominate the discussion of both early and advanced esophageal cancer. Several techniques are available, ranging from surgery to stents, to allow the individual to be able to eat and drink for much of the remainder of their life.

Gastric cancer

Just as with esophageal cancer, the ability to eat and drink again plays a major role in decision making. Disseminated disease often requires symptom management in gastric cancer.

Natural history of gastric cancer

The highest incidence of gastric cancer (adenocarcinoma) is in Asia, South America, and Scandinavia. The disease has been declining in the US since the early 1900s, where the site of origin of the neoplasm has shifted from one that mainly arises from the distal stomach to a disease that is more often seen in the cardia and gastroesophageal junction. Cancers in the proximal area of the stomach and in the gastroesophageal junction are biologically more aggressive, and have often already spread distantly at time of diagnosis. In Asia, gastric cancer tends to grow more slowly, and remain locally confined; whereas, in the US, the disease is most likely to be disseminated. Recently, genetic differences in the cancer that arises in these two populations have been described.

In the distal stomach, symptoms of obstruction occur earlier. There may be gastric outlet obstruction with symptoms of bloating, early satiety, and discomfort. Bleeding is less common at the initial presentation. When the disease arises in the proximal stomach, or gastroesophageal junction, the cancer has often grown out of stomach and along the wall of the distal esophagus, leading to difficulty swallowing as the first symptom. Another way the disease can present is by spreading to the adjacent transverse colon with the development of symptoms of colonic obstruction at time of initial presentation. As with esophageal cancer, as the disease continues to grow, nutrition and hydration become the central issues, as stomach emptying becomes more difficult. With gastric cancer, cachexia can occur if there is systemic spread, but mechanical issues play a role both early and late in the course of the disease.

Patterns of spread and recurrence

Gastric cancer can spread to the regional nodes, but also has a tendency to spread to more distant sites such as bone, or lung. "Drop" metastases to the pelvis can occur producing pelvic pain. There can be dissemination throughout the abdomen and the development of ascites or small bowel obstruction. Of all gastrointestinal malignancies, gastric cancer has the greatest likelihood of producing systemic spread to sites such as bone, which is seldom involved in other cancers of the digestive tract, or bone marrow. Distant nodes in the neck or axilla may be involved. Many patients will have distant disease in either the liver or abdominal cavity (omentum or serosal surface of bowel) at the time they are first seen.

For those who undergo surgery, the disease recurs both locally in the operative bed and distantly in sites such as the liver, lung, or abdominal cavity where the tumor spreads over the serosal surface of bowel. The frequency of local recurrence varies in the literature and may be as high as 50%. Often, patients have both local and distant recurrences.

Therapeutic considerations

Management of newly diagnosed gastric cancer is dependent on the extent of spread. For those with local or loco-regional disease, surgery is the mainstay of therapy. Unlike esophageal cancer, chemoradiotherapy has not been shown to be effective in palliation, except for those with gastroesophageal junction cancers, which are most often adenocarcinoma, and may respond to a combination of chemoradio-therapy that is used for esophageal cancer. In the surgical literature, the operative technique used is determined by the location of the tumor, with the more proximal lesions requiring a more extensive resection of stomach. There is also controversy in the surgical literature about the extent of nodal dissection. Very extensive nodal resections, as have been practiced in Japan, do not appear to be more beneficial in trials done in western Europe.

There is now early information to suggest that the use of chemoradiotherapy after definitive surgery may delay recurrence locally. Patients may have chronic dyspepsia after such therapy.

The use of chemotherapy for the large proportion of patients who present with metastatic disease continues to show only a modest benefit. Most combination regimens produce a reduction in tumor size in 20–40% of individuals treated, with responses continuing for 12–15 months in some series. Although the use of chemotherapy may give relief of pain or fatigue, similar symptoms may be introduced by the treatment.

Management of symptoms arising from the sites of distant spread is related to the organ involved. For example, involvement of the bone marrow may require transfusion.

Prognosis

Since the most common type of gastric cancer is adenocarcinoma, most of this discussion will focus on this histology. Lymphoma and sarcoma can also be seen and are generally considered more responsive to drug therapy, although surgery is often used for sarcoma. Prognosis for adenocarcinoma is based on tumor penetration through the wall and the serosa of the stomach, as well as regional nodal involvement. Increasing nodal involvement worsens the prognosis. Patients with nodal involvement at presentation have a 5-year prognosis of 15–20%. In the US, approximately two-thirds of individuals will have disseminated disease (disease outside of the regional nodes is also considered metastatic) at the time of diagnosis.

Variations in survivorship are closely related to the nutritional and general status of the individual. Those presenting with weight loss of more than 10–20% or who are mainly bedridden, have a much-shortened prognosis in the range of 8–12 weeks. Active chemotherapy for this group of individuals is not likely to be effective in terms of life extension or in palliation of other symptoms, especially gastric outlet symptoms.

Site-specific rehabilitation issues

For limited disease, the major issue after surgery is the inability to achieve adequate nutrition. Surgery for this disease requires either a subtotal gastrectomy or a total gastrectomy; this decision is dictated by the location and extent of the tumor. More radical node dissections have not always been shown to be helpful in improving cure rates, but may increase postoperative problems – wound healing, postoperative pain, and recovery time. Recently, the creation of a pouch from the jejunum has been shown to improve weight gain. For the individual with a total gastrectomy, 6–12 months may be required before there is weight stabilization. The individual must eat several small meals each day, and allow time for increased flexibility of the intestine. Patients who have a subtotal gastrectomy are able to increase their intake more readily. Gastrostomy tube feedings may be required initially to provide adequate calories in the immediate postoperative period.

In individuals with metastatic disease, there may still be a role for limited debulking surgery to allow nutrition to be given, although this issue remains controversial. The time to convalesce has to be balanced against the extent of the disease, and the overall status of the individual.

Site-specific palliative care issues

In individuals who have had removal of the primary tumor, management of the recurrence may involve palliation of liver failure symptoms, and management of painful liver metastases. There may be recurrence locally, with pain in the upper abdomen. The recurrence may produce small bowel obstruction or ascites, if there are serosal implants. The ascites may be managed medically or with paracentesis. Spread to bone can cause painful fractures. While nutrition may play a role, cachexia is more likely to cause loss of weight.

For those who have a recurrence in the local operative bed or who have an intact primary tumor, weight loss and inanition can be due to mechanical issues or tumor cachexia, especially if the disease has spread. These individuals will often have progressive loss of reservoir function and increasingly can take less and less by mouth. There may be sufficient obstruction that there can be constant or intermittent nausea or vomiting or a combination of the two symptoms. The obligatory production of approximately one liter of gastric secretion daily may need to be addressed. If the individual is still medically fit, and has not lost a large amount of weight, surgical bypass may be considered.

A nasogastric tube may provide immediate relief for these individuals. If possible, a gastrostomy tube may be placed to avoid the need for the nasogastric tube on a chronic basis. The anatomy of the stomach may be distorted, or there can be ascites and bowel adhesions, especially if there was any prior attempt at surgery. Placement of such a tube can be by endoscopic or radiologic techniques but these approaches may also not be possible in this group of patients because of the distorted anatomy and adhesions. Although the lifespan of these individuals may only be a few weeks, the worsening vomiting that does not respond well to medical measures can be the most debilitating symptom, both physically and emotionally. Efforts to decrease gastric secretion may be tried with octreotide but may not be entirely successful.

For a subset of individuals with difficulty with gastric emptying, there is not mechanical obstruction, but rather invasion by the tumor of the myenteric plexus, and a subsequent loss of gastric function. The stomach may appear patent on endoscopy or radiologic testing, but there is not effective emptying. While this problem can also be seen after surgery without a recurrence of the cancer, in individuals with recurrence elsewhere, malignancy is usually the cause of functional delay in emptying. These individuals may not benefit from surgical bypass, as there is often concomitant involvement in the small bowel mesentery. A nasogastric tube or gastrostomy may be required. Use of medications to promote peristalsis can be tried, but where there is also a fixed block, painful cramping can occur.

Large bulky lesions can begin to bleed and on occasion, the bleeding is severe enough that some type of palliation is required. Irradiation of the mass can stop the bleeding for a short period of time.

Pain management for those with recurrent gastric cancer may require a balance of analgesic effectiveness against the slowing of gastric emptying or small bowel emptying. In those with far-advanced disease, where gastric emptying is no longer an issue, pain management may be of paramount importance.

Quality-of-life instruments have been compared with the clinical benefit response in upper gastrointestinal malignancies. These newer scales may help evaluate the effects of therapeutic interventions; however, when they were compared with other quality-of-life instruments such as those of the European Organisation for Research and Treatment of Cancer (EORTC), they were found to overestimate the benefit, especially where pain is the predominant symptom.

Summary

Both esophageal and gastric cancer have problems with nutrition as the most significant symptom. This symptom may arise from purely mechanical features, or from loss of function in the case of the stomach. Efforts to improve this symptom typically involve surgery for early stage disease at both sites. Alternative therapy includes chemoradiotherapy for esophageal or gastroesophageal junction cancer. For patients with recurrent disease or who cannot have either of these types of treatment, stenting may be done in the esophagus. In the stomach, some type of drainage or venting may be required to palliate the symptoms of gastric outlet obstruction. Principles of management must also take into account the need to deal with salivary secretions in the case of esophageal cancer, and gastric secretions in the case of gastric cancer.

BIBLIOGRAPHY

Barton R, Kirkbride P. Special techniques in palliative radiation oncology. *J Palliat Med* 2000;3: 75–83.

Blot WJ, McLaughlin JK. The changing epidemiology of esophageal cancer. *Semin Oncol* 1999; 26(Suppl. 15):2–8.

Coia LR, Minsky BD, Berkey BA et al. Outcome of patients receiving radiation for cancer of the esophagus: results of the 1992–1994 Patterns of Care Study [see comments]. *J Clin Oncol* 2000; 18:455–62.

Hansson LE, Engstrand L, Nyren O et al. *Helicobacter pylori* infection: independent risk indicator of gastric adenocarcinoma [see comments]. *Gastroenterology* 1993;105:1098–103.

Hoffman K, Glimelius B. Evaluation of clinical benefit of chemotherapy in patients with upper gastrointestinal cancer. *Acta Oncol* 1998;37:651–9.

Hundahl SA, Phillips JL, Menck HR. The National Cancer Data Base Report on poor survival of U.S. gastric carcinoma patients treated with gastrectomy: Fifth Edition American Joint

Committee on Cancer staging, proximal disease, and the "different disease" hypothesis. *Cancer* 2000;88:921–32.

Liedman B. Symptoms after total gastrectomy on food intake, body composition, bone metabolism, and quality of life in gastric cancer patients – is reconstruction with a reservoir worthwhile? *Nutrition* 1999;15:677–82.

McLarty AJ, Deschamps C, Trastek VF et al. Esophageal resection for cancer of the esophagus: long-term function and quality of life. *Ann Thorac Surg* 1997;73:1568–72.

Schmitt C, Brazer SR (ed.) *Clinical Aspects of Esophageal Cancer*. 1st edition. Series: *Gastrointestinal Cancers: Biology, Diagnosis, and Therapy*, ed. A Rustgi, pp. 91–114. Philadelphia: Lippincott-Raven, 1995.

Shiraishi N, Inomata M, Osawa N et al. Early and late recurrence after gastrectomy for gastric carcinoma. Univariate and multivariate analyses. *Cancer* 2000;89:255–61.

Svedlund J, Sullivan M, Liedman B et al. Long-term consequences of gastrectomy for patients' quality of life: the impact of reconstructive techniques. *Am J Gastroent* 1999;94:438–45.

Wils J. The treatment of advanced gastric cancer. *Semin Oncol* 1996;23:397–406.

Walsh TN, Noonan N, Hollywood P et al. A comparison of multimodality therapy and surgery for esophageal carcinoma. *N Engl Med J* 1996;335:462–7.

Internet site

http://www.cancer.gov
Overview of both gastric cancer and esophageal cancer. Review is broken up by stage.

24

Head and neck cancer

Merrill S. Kies and Roy S. Herbst

U.T. M.D. Anderson Cancer Center, Houston

Introduction

Head and neck cancers constitute a broad spectrum of disease processes with varying histology, natural history, and treatment outcomes. In this chapter we discuss squamous cell cancers of the oral cavity, pharynx, and larynx constituting about 80% of head and neck malignancies. The annual incidence of such cancers is approximately 45 000 cases per year in the US.[1] This is the fifth most common cancer in the world today. Median age at presentation is 60 years and two-thirds of patients are men. There is a strong association with alcohol and/or tobacco use,[2–4] and most patients present with local or regionally advanced disease.

There exists a dose–response relationship between exposure to tobacco and cancers of the head and neck. Smoking is the preferred method of tobacco use in the United States, and is most strongly associated with malignancies of the floor of mouth, oropharynx, and larynx.[3,4] Other practices, for example chewing tobacco or dipping snuff, tend to be associated with malignancies of the buccal mucosa.[5,6] Alcohol use is an independent risk factor and there appear to be synergistic carcinogenic effects for persons who both smoke and drink,[3,7,8] especially for cancers of the larynx. There is an inverse relationship between the consumption of fruits and vegetables and head and neck squamous cell cancers. Viral exposures have also been implicated in the causation of some uncommon head and neck malignancies. In the Orient, there is a clear etiologic relationship between Epstein–Barr virus and nasopharyngeal carcinoma.[9] In the US, exposure to the human papilloma virus, which has pronounced tropism for epithelial cells, has been associated with oropharyngeal cancers.[10] Wood-dust exposure, asbestos, nickel, and marijuana have also been associated with the etiology of squamous head and neck malignancies.

As smoking cigarettes may have a "field cancerization" effect we have come to appreciate that patients with head and neck cancer are often at risk of developing metachronous second primary tumors especially of the head and neck, esophagus, lung, and bladder.[3,11,12] Nonrandom chromosomal deletions have been defined affecting 3, 8, 9, 17 and 18, with mutations of p53 and p16 commonly observed.[13,14] Overexpression of epithelial growth factor receptor (EGFR) has also been established[15] and this may represent a therapeutic target in the future.

Clinical presentation and staging

The clinical presentation varies with the primary site. Oral cavity malignancies tend to present as a sore or ulcer which is readily identified by patients although often there still is a delay in coming to a physician for evaluation. There is much variability with respect to stage and tumor cell differentiation at diagnosis. The best prognosis in this subgroup of patients is with lip primaries which are obvious and tend to prompt a medical evaluation. Oropharyngeal tumors, on the other hand, are not so readily noticeable. Related symptoms such as sore throat, dysphagia, or otalgia tend to occur late so patients with cancers of the peritonsillar area, base of tongue, as well as hypopharynx, typically have advanced disease at diagnosis. T3/T4 primary tumors and cervical lymph node metastases are present for many if not most patients in this subgroup. Primary tumors in the larynx, however, may present earlier. Often these tumors are associated with hoarseness or shortness of breath. True glottic tumors tend to be well differentiated, and even with early stage disease hoarseness is frequent, encouraging a physician evaluation.

Staging procedures are given in Table 24.1. The emphasis is on the clinical examination, routine blood work and imaging studies of the head and neck. As a generalization, squamous cell carcinoma of the head and neck is localized even if advanced at diagnosis. Patterns of loco-regional dissemination follow lymph node drainage pathways and respect anatomic barriers. Thus, there has been emphasis on local treatment modalities, surgery, and radiotherapy. The majority of patients who succumb to this illness do so because of complications related to local disease progression or recurrence. A minority of patients, 20–30%, will develop systemic metastases usually affecting lung or bone. However, as the efficacy of loco-regional treatment improves there will be an increasing need for effective systemic therapy, at least for a percentage of patients with advanced disease.

Table 24.1. Staging procedures for head and neck cancer

Physical evaluation, complete blood count, chemistry, chest x-ray
Laryngoscopy, nasopharyngoscopy
Panendoscopy?
Head/neck computed tomography/magnetic resonance imaging
Chest computed tomography, bone scans as needed

Table 24.2. Staging of head and neck cancer

T stage
Oral cavity, oropharynx – size dependent
Hypopharynx, larynx, nasopharynx – subsite dependent

N stage
N1   One node $\leq$ 3 cm ipsilateral
N2a One node > 3 cm
   b Multiple ipsilateral
   c Bilateral/contralateral
N3   One node > 6 cm

Groups
I   T1N0M0
II   T2N0M0
III T3N0MO, T1–3N1
IV   T4, N2–3, M1

Table 24.2 offers an outline of staging considerations in head and neck cancer. T stage in the oral cavity and oropharynx is size dependent with T1 lesions less than 2 cm, T2 lesions ranging from 2–4 cm in greatest dimension and T4 disease typically reflective of deeply invasive primary tumors. Stage designations in the hypopharynx, larynx, and nasopharynx are subsite dependent. For further details please consult the AJCC Staging Manual.[16] Nodal stage is listed with the same designations used for oral cavity, oropharynx, hypopharynx, and larynx.

Therapy

A minority of patients, about one-third, present with stage I or II disease.[12] The usual treatment approach for such patients is surgical resection or radiotherapy, the choice largely depending on the precise site of presentation, expertise within the institution, and patients' wishes. For example, most patients with early stage cancers of the lip will undergo surgery. This is a rapid and effective approach, cost effective, and overall results are quite favorable. For early stage laryngeal cancer, on the other hand, radiotherapy has become the standard of care. This too is a highly effective treatment modality for most patients, and with normal or near-normal voice retained. Surgical resection is also available as a salvage procedure for those patients who have disease recurrence. Overall, 60–80% of patients with stages I and II squamous cancers of the head and neck obtain a curative outcome after appropriate local treatment. For this group the prevention of second primary tumors and attention to general medical problems, often related to chronic alcohol and tobacco abuse, have become the focus of current medical treatment and research efforts. Early reports by Hong and colleagues[17] have indicated the potential role of retinoids in prevention of second primary cancers of the upper aerodigestive tract. This has led to major randomized trials[11] and results are eagerly awaited.

The majority of patients with head and neck cancer present with stage III or IV disease.[12] Therapy for these patients has traditionally consisted of surgical resection with postoperative radiation. Patients considered to have unresectable disease related to site (for example nasopharynx) or tumors of massive size have historically been treated with radiotherapy alone. Unfortunately treatment goals in this setting are usually palliative. Although surgery combined with radiotherapy is often effective in loco-regional control, there can be devastating effects on personal appearance and critical functions such as speech and swallowing. Long-term survival rates are generally low ranging from 20–40%.[12,18] As a consequence, intensive efforts are underway to develop more efficacious combined modality treatment programs integrating chemotherapy.[19] Objectives are to improve local and regional disease control, and enhance survival. Ancillary therapeutic goals are to reduce the need for extensive surgery and to maintain critical functions especially voice and swallowing. These notions underlie current approaches to "organ preservation." Rehabilitative therapy focusing on speech and swallowing, attention to dentition, and nutritional support have all become routine therapeutic considerations. Longitudinal assessment of life-quality measures also are now increasingly included in outcome analyses of head and neck cancer treatment programs.

Combined chemotherapy and radiation

Induction chemotherapy, frequently with a cisplatin and 5-FU-based program has been used in sequence with radiotherapy given as a definitive local treatment. Chemotherapy is highly active in this setting, inducing disease remission in 80–90% of previously untreated patients with locally advanced disease. However, randomized trials have failed to demonstrate a clear impact on local tumor control or overall survival.[20] The approach does allow for preservation of the larynx in selected patients with stages III and IV disease.[21,22] The induction treatment format also provides a useful instrument to evaluate a novel drug or regimen. Current efforts are directed toward identifying more active systemic therapy and in determining the best format for integration of chemotherapy with powerful local treatment modalities, surgery, and radiotherapy.

The simultaneous or alternating administration of chemotherapy and radiation is conceptually attractive with application of the principle of "spatial cooperation." The use of chemotherapy provides the potential for better regional and distant tumor control if a systemically effective dose of active agents can be given. Moreover, the concomitant administration of chemotherapy and radiation may markedly enhance the cytotoxicity of radiotherapy resulting in better local antitumor effects. Preclinical studies have elucidated mechanisms of interaction between chemotherapy and radiation. This includes cell–cell synchronization, treatment of hypoxic cell tumor populations, increased cytotoxicity for tumor cells in S-phase, and interference with tumor stem-cell repopulation between radiation treatment fractions. Loco-regional control may be improved in part because most chemotherapy agents have independent activity. Of course, there is potential for increased local and systemic toxicity.

The use of concomitant combination of chemotherapy and radiation has been under intense study for some years.[18,19] There has been clear demonstration of a marked enhancement of tumor responsiveness over treatment schedules with radiation alone and this has led to improved survival. There also has been a substantial increase in related toxicities, especially dermatitis and mucositis. As a consequence, despite some initial anxiety, innovative treatment programs have emerged with radiotherapy administered in split-course or cycling schedules. These trials have shown high complete response rates, feasibility, and the promise of advancing survival with organ preservation.

Under the auspices of the Chicago Oral Cancer Center, we conducted a phase II trial investigating a cisplatin-based induction program followed by a concomitant chemotherapy and radiation regimen consisting of infusional 5-FU, hydroxyurea and radiation (FHX) in patients with stage IV disease.[23] The FHX regimen was given on days 1–5 every 14 days, in effect an alternate-week schedule. Organ preservation principles were maintained with only a minority of patients undergoing limited surgery. Loco-regional control was achieved in 75% of patients with distant control in 90%. Five-year survival exceeded 60%. This experience led to subsequent studies in which cisplatin was added to the FHX regimen (C-FH2X).[24] The radiotherapy was intensified to twice-daily administration, and the induction chemotherapy was deleted. Loco-regional control improved to 92%. This finding adds further evidence that innovative radiotherapy schedules in the presence of concomitant chemotherapy may increase regional control of disease, without surgery, and are feasible. Subsequent Chicago trials have maintained the alternate-week concomitant chemotherapy and hyperfractionated radiation regimen with substitution of paclitaxel for cisplatin.[25,26] An ancillary observation has been that the functional status of patients treated in these trials is acceptable. Organ preservation does not necessarily correlate with preserved function, but a 2-year analysis indicates that 75% of surviving patients had adequate speech and swallowing performance. With respect to this latter issue, long-term follow-up data are awaited.

In recent years, randomized studies have been performed demonstrating the efficacy of chemotherapy and radiation over radiotherapy alone (Table 24.3).[18] Brizel et al.[27] have compared a hyperfractionated radiotherapy arm taken to a total

Table 24.3. Selected randomized concomitant chemotherapy and radiation trials

Study	Patients	Experimental arm	Outcome
Brizel et al.[27]	"Advanced" multisite ($n = 122$)	RT 1.25 Gy bid to 70 Gy with cisplatin and 5-FU given during weeks 1 and 6. Two adjuvant cycles cisplatin/5-FU followed	LRC improved 70% vs. 44% (P = 0.01) and 55% 3-y survival vs. 34% (P = 0.07)
Wendt et al.[28]	Unresectable multisite ($n = 298$)	Split course, accelerated RT 70.2 Gy with cisplatin and leucovorin infusions × 4 days given weeks 1, 4 and 7	LRC was 36% vs. 17% @ 3 year favoring the experimental arm (P < 0.004). OS was 48% vs. 24% (P < 0.004)
Calais et al.[29]	Stage III/IV oropharynx ($n = 226$)	RT every day to 70 Gy – carboplatin and 5-FU starting on days 1, 22, 43	LRC improved in the experimental arm (66% vs. 47%) and OS was 51% vs. 31% (P = 0.02) @ 3 year
Jeremic et al.[30]	Stage III/IV, multisite ($n = 130$)	Hfx RT to 77 Gy – cisplatin 6 mg every day	Improved LRC 50% vs. 36% (P = 0.04); distant control 86% vs. 57% (P = 0.001); and OS 46% vs. 25% @ 5 year

Note: RT, radiotherapy; LRC, loco-regional control; Hfx, hyperfractionated; OS, overall survival.

dose 75 Gy with the same radiation schedule taken to 70 Gy with concomitant cisplatin and 5-FU. The concomitant treatment was followed by two cycles of adjuvant chemotherapy. There was a statistically significant improvement in local disease control and a strong trend toward improved overall survival. Wendt et al.[28] reported a statistically significant 3-year survival advantage after the concomitant use of cisplatin, 5-FU, and leucovorin given in a split-course accelerated radiation format compared with the same radiation schedule given as a single therapeutic modality. Calais et al.[29] compared a more standard once-daily fractionated radiation schedule with the same radiotherapy and concomitant carboplatin and 5-FU. A statistically significant advantage was demonstrated in loco-regional tumor control and overall survival at 3 years. Finally, Jeremic et al.[30] investigated the value of adding cisplatin given to a hyperfractionated radiation therapy program versus the same radiation schedule given alone in patients with locally advanced squamous cell cancers of the head and neck. In this recent report, loco-regional control, distant disease control, and overall survival were statistically improved at 5 years. It is noteworthy that the clearest benefit in three of these four studies was an improvement in local regional control, which then translated into a survival advantage. As a generalization, acute toxicity was increased, especially mucositis and hematological effects, but there was no obvious escalation of long-term sequelae. In aggregate, overall 3-year survival exceeded 50% in these experimental programs, underscoring the important therapeutic efficacy of concomitant chemotherapy and radiation in advanced head and neck cancers.

Quality of care

Despite advances in cancer therapeutics and the attention given to rehabilitation and organ preservation, many patients eventually have local or regional tumor recurrence and the objectives of therapy then become palliative. Recurrent squamous cancer most often occurs in the setting of extensive prior surgery and radiotherapy. A minority of patients are candidates for effective salvage surgical resection or radiotherapy, but many patients are highly debilitated and may have intractable pain, compromised airway, swallowing dysfunction with a tendency to aspiration and complicating pneumonia, or oropharyngeal necrosis or possibly fistula formation. For these patients, the emphasis of care is on symptom control and is most effectively delivered by a multidisciplinary team with cooperation among medical and surgical oncologists. Active anticancer treatment is seldom effective and can most often be considered investigational in the setting. Median survival is 5–7 months.

The principles of palliative care applicable for patients with recurrent disease vary according to the specific problem that a patient may have. Most importantly, patients require that care providers are available. Problems with necrotic tissue that needs debridement, frequent local infection, or airway compromise quickly leads to panic in patients and family if compassionate and confident caregivers cannot be reached. This is a particular issue in head and neck cancer because many nurses and physicians are themselves often uncomfortable with cancers that may threaten the airway or integrity of the carotid artery. Family education and preparation must be considered. Palliative goals should be defined. And there should be "hands on" demonstration of dressing changes, tracheostomy tube manipulation, or whatever is the appropriate specific maneuver for the individual patient. Most family members respond well to this if the caregiver has expertise, patience, and time available.

Many patients are more comfortable with a tracheotomy tube in place and decisions regarding the advisability of this procedure depend upon the status of the airway and prospects for extended survival. Many also benefit from placement of a gastrostomy feeding tube. This access is important not only for maintaining hydration and nutritional status but also for administration of medications. With a limited life expectancy, the addition of tranquilizers such as lorazepam or analgesics such as morphine sulfate can be effective for patients trying to cope with progressive disease. These medications can be used freely, educating patient and family that goals of comfort and relief of anxiety and air hunger are achievable although usually with some sedation. Principles of pain management will tend to be similar in cancer patients with recurrent disease affecting other body systems,

Table 24.4. New agents in clinical trials

Novel retinoids
Cyclo-oxygenase inhibitors
Anti-angiogenic agents
p53 modulation
Signal transduction inhibitors

and should be emphasized (see Chapter 42 for a more detailed discussion). Don't forget the stool softeners.

Future directions

Surgery and radiotherapy are effective treatment modalities for many head and neck cancer patients, and combined modality treatment programs appear to have had an additional significant impact on local disease control and overall survival in patients with advanced disease. Associated toxicity is considerable. Current research efforts focus on the identification of novel agents (Table 24.4) that may be integrated with traditional therapeutic strategies in the attempt to enhance efficacy and diminish toxicity. Clinical trials evaluating efficacy are ongoing. Certainly the care of the head and neck cancer patient is best offered in institutions with experienced multidisciplinary treatment teams and it is imperative that long-term outcome studies be performed to assess quality of life and general medical performance as well as disease control. For patients who have disease recurrence, modern palliative care methods can be well adapted to this setting with the best results obtaining from the cooperation of head and neck cancer specialists and palliative care professionals.

REFERENCES

1 Greenlee RT, Hill-Harmon MB, Murray T et al. Cancer Statistics, 2001. *CA Cancer J Clin* 2001;51:15–36.

2 Blot WJ, McLaughlin JK, Winn DM et al. Smoking and drinking in relation to oral and pharyngeal cancer. *Cancer Res* 1988;48:3282–7.

3 Spitz MR, Zoltan T. Molecular epidemiology and genetic predisposition for head and neck cancer. In *Head and Neck Cancer: A Multidisciplinary Approach*, ed. LB Harrison, RB Sessions, WK Hong, pp. 11–22. Philadelphia: Lippincott-Raven, 1999.

4 Rothman KJ, Cann CI, Flanders D et al. Epidemiology of laryngeal cancer. *Epidemiol Rev* 1980;2:195–209.

5 US Department of Health and Human Services, NIH. *The health consequences of using smokeless tobacco: A Report of the Advisory Committee to the Surgeon General*, No. 86-2874. Washington, DC: NIH, 1986.

6 Winn DM, Blot WJ, Shy CM et al. Snuff dipping and oral cancer among women in the southern United States. *N Engl J Med* 1981;304:745–9.

7 Wynder EL, Bross IJ, Feldman RM. A study of etiological factors in cancer of the mouth. *Cancer* 1957;10:1300.

8 Saracci R. The interactions of tobacco smoking and other agents in cancer etiology. *Epidemiol Rev* 1987;9:175–93.

9 Hsu JL, Glaser SL. Epstein–Barr virus-association malignancies: epidemiologic patterns and etiologic implications. *Crit Rev Oncol Hematol* 2000;34:27–53.

10 Gillison ML, Koch WM, Capone RB et al. Evidence for a causal association between human papillomavirus and a subset of head and neck cancers. *J Natl Cancer Inst* 2000;92:709–20.

11 Khuri FR, Lippman SM, Spitz MR et al. Molecular epidemiology and retinoid chemoprevention of head and neck cancer. *J Natl Cancer Inst* 1997;89:199–211.

12 Vokes EE, Weichselbaum RR, Lippman SM et al. Head and neck cancer. *N Engl J Med* 1993;328:184–94.

13 Mao L, El-Naggar AK et al. Molecular changes in the multistage pathogenesis of head and neck cancer. In *Molecular Pathology of Early Cancer*, ed. S Srivastava, pp. 189–206. Amsterdam: IOS Press, 1999.

14 Mao L. Can molecular assessment improve classification of head and neck premalignancy? *Clin Cancer Res* 2000;6:321.

15 Mendelshon J. Blockade of receptor for growth factors: an anticancer therapy – the fourth annual Joseph H. Burchenal American Association for Cancer Research Clinical Research Award Lecture. *Clin Cancer Res* 2000;6:747–53.

16 Fleming ID, Cooper JS, Henson DE (ed.) Head and neck sites. In *AJCC Cancer Staging Manual* pp. 21–46. Philidelphia: Lippincott-Raven, 1997.

17 Hong WK, Lippman, SM, Itri LM et al. Prevention of second primary tumor with isotretinoin in squamous-cell carcinoma of the head and neck. *N Engl J Med* 1990;323:798.

18 Vokes EE, Daniel JH, Kies MS. The use of concurrent chemotherapy and radiotherapy for locoregionally advanced head and neck cancer. *Semin Oncol* 2000;27:34–38.

19 Kies MS, Bennett CL, Vokes EE. Locally advanced head and neck cancer. *Curr Treat Options Oncol* 2001;2:7–13.

20 Bourhis J, Pignon JP. Meta-analyses in head and neck squamous cell carcinoma: what is the role of chemotherapy? *Hematol Oncol Clin N Am* 1999;13:769–76.

21 The Department of Veterans Affairs Laryngeal Cancer Study Group. Induction chemotherapy plus radiation in patients with advanced laryngeal cancer. *N Engl J Med* 1991;324:1685–90.

22 Lefebvre JL, Chevalier D, Luboinski B et al. Larynx preservation in pyriform sinus cancer: preliminary results of a European organization for research and treatment of cancer phase III trial – EORTC head and neck cancer cooperative group. *J Natl Cancer Inst* 1996;88:890–9.

23 Kies MS, Haraf DJ, Athanasiadis I et al. Induction chemotherapy followed by concurrent chemoradiation for advanced head and neck cancer: improved disease control and survival. *J Clin Oncol* 1998;16:2715–21.

24 Vokes E, Kies M, Haraf D et al. Concomitant chemoradiotherapy as primary therapy for locoregionally advanced head and neck cancer. *J Clin Oncol* 2000;18:1652–61.

25 Kies MS. Combined therapy for squamous head and neck cancer. *Lung Cancer* 1999;25:228–9.

26 Kies MS, Daniel JH, Rosen F et al. Concomitant infusional paclitaxel and fluorouracil, oral hydroxyurea, and hyperfractionated radiation for locally advanced squamous head and neck cancer. *J Clin Oncol* 2001;19:1961–9.

27 Brizel DM, Albers ME, Fisher SR et al. Hyperfractionated irradiation with or without concurrent chemotherapy for locally advanced head and neck cancer. *N Engl J Med* 1998;338:1798–804.

28 Wendt TG, Grabenbauer GG, Rodel CM et al. Simultaneous radiochemotherapy versus radiotherapy alone in advanced head and neck cancer: a randomized multicenter study. *J Clin Oncol* 1998;16:1318–24.

29 Calais G, Alfonsi M, Bardet E et al. Randomized trial of radiation therapy versus concomitant chemotherapy and radiation therapy for advanced-stage oropharynx carcinoma. *J Natl Cancer Inst* 1999;91:2081–6.

30 Jeremic B, Shibamoto Y, Milicic B et al. Hyperfractionated radiation therapy with or without concurrent low-dose daily cisplatin in locally advanced squamous cell carcinoma of the head and neck: a prospective randomized trial. *J Clin Oncol* 2000;18:1458–64.

25

Kidney cancer

Lori Wood

QEII Health Sciences Centre, Halifax

Introduction

Kidney cancer, or renal cell carcinoma (RCC), is the tenth most common malignancy and the thirteenth leading cause of cancer death in the US. In 2001, there were predicted to be 30 800 new cases and 12 100 deaths due to kidney cancer, with an annual incidence that continues to increase.[1] RCC is 2–3 times more common in men and tends to occur between the ages of 50–70 but can occur at any age. Smoking, obesity, diuretic use, and chronic renal dialysis have all been identified as risk factors. A small number of cases have a genetic basis with the most recognized association being the von Hippel–Lindau syndrome, an autosomal dominant disease which often causes multifocal, bilateral tumors. This chapter will review the presentation, prognosis, management, and outcome of patients with RCC.

Presentation

The presentation of RCC is variable; it may present as an incidental finding, with local or systemic symptoms, or with symptoms from metastatic disease. With radiographic investigations for other indications more frequent, an increasing number of asymptomatic kidney tumors are identified. Local symptoms may include hematuria, flank pain, or back pain. Systemic symptoms may include fatigue, weight loss, or anorexia. RCC, even if only localized disease is present, may also produce paraneoplastic syndromes such as erythrocytosis, hypercalcemia, elevated liver function tests, and fever. Symptoms specific to metastatic disease such as bone pain, cough, shortness of breath, or neurological symptoms may occur. RCC can invade the renal vein, inferior vena cava, or hepatic vein resulting in lower extremity edema, ascites, and hepatomegaly.

Approximately 30% of patients present with metastatic disease, 25% with locally advanced disease, and 45% with localized disease.[2] Of patients initially undergoing potentially curative resection, up to 50% may recur. The most common sites of metastatic disease include the lungs (50–75%) followed by lymph nodes (30%), bone (20%), liver (20%), and central nervous system (10%). However, it is important to remember that RCC can metastasize to virtually any site in the body.

Pathology

Tissue diagnosis confirms the clinical and radiological diagnosis of renal cell carcinoma. The majority of RCC will be clear cell RCC and less commonly papillary, granular, or sarcomatoid RCC. However, 10–15% of all kidney tumors will be of different histologies that may have significant therapeutic and prognostic implications. These include: benign lesions, transitional cell carcinomas of the renal pelvis, lymphomas, sarcomas, small cell cancers, oncoctyomas, adult Wilm's tumors, or metastatic lesions. Thus, tissue confirmation is essential.

Staging

The most commonly used staging system is based on the TNM system depending on the tumor size and local extension (T stage), lymph node involvement (N stage) or the presence of metastases (M stage).[3] Stage is the best predictor of prognosis.

Management

Many therapeutic modalities have been studied in RCC including surgery, angioinfarction, chemotherapy, hormonal therapy, and immunotherapy. To date, no chemotherapeutic or hormonal agents have resulted in significant tumor responses or improved survival.[2] If the disease is localized to the kidney or regional lymph nodes, surgery is the primary treatment with a curative goal. If the disease has spread, the goals of therapy may include reduction of symptoms from local or metastatic disease, maintaining or improving quality of life, and potentially prolonging survival.

Localized disease

Primary therapy for localized disease is a radical nephrectomy, or removal of the kidney including Gerota's fascia, the ureter, renal vein, and adrenal gland. Occasionally, a partial nephrectomy can technically and safely be performed. Extended lymphadenectomy has not been shown to improve outcome and is not routinely done. To date, there are no convincing data to support postsurgical radiotherapy or systemic therapy.

Advanced disease
Surgery

The role of nephrectomy in advanced disease has been controversial. It can provide symptomatic relief from pain and hematuria, but transarterial angioinfarction (blocking the arterial supply to the tumor) may similarly be effective and associated with less morbidity. Retrospective studies suggest that prior nephrectomy may be an independent prognostic factor for survival and/or response to immunotherapy. Two recent clinical trials in which high performance status patients with metastatic RCC were randomized to nephrectomy followed by immunotherapy or immunotherapy alone have been performed.[4,5] Overall survival was modestly improved in patients who received surgery in both studies; thus, it appears appropriate to recommend nephrectomy as an option for selected patients.

Surgical resection of isolated metastatic lesions such as lung or brain metastases can be performed in selected patients. The effect of surgery on survival in these patients is not well established; however, there are several reports of good long-term survival after surgical resection of isolated metastatic disease. Patients who may benefit most are those with only one metastatic lesion and a long interval from the initial diagnosis of localized RCC to the development of metastatic disease.

Immunotherapy

To date, immunotherapy approaches have shown the most promise for metastatic RCC.[6,7] These agents mediate their antitumor effect through the activation of host immune mechanisms. Interferon alpha and interleukin-2 (IL-2) have been the most extensively studied agents. Response rates in several phase II trials of interferon alpha have ranged from 0–30%, with an average of approximately 15% of patients having tumor shrinkage. A statistically significant survival advantage was seen in two out of four phase III clinical trials.[8,9] In the largest and most recent of these, the median survival improved from 6 months to 8.5 months with an improvement in 1-year survival of 12% (43% 1-year survival with interferon versus 31% in the control group).[8] It should be noted, however, that the quality of life of patients on interferon was worse than those in the control group; and thus, the clinical significance of the improvement in median survival with interferon should be assessed alongside its toxicities. These toxicities include flu-like symptoms, fever, nausea, depression, loss of appetite, and fatigue. The optimal dose and schedule of interferon alpha is not known, but doses of 5–20 million units daily or three times a week given subcutaneously are currently used.

IL-2 has also been studied extensively in the phase II setting. IL-2 is approved in the US and many parts of Europe based on reproducible results showing a 15% response rate and very durable responses in about 5% of patients (median duration of objective responses of 54 months).[6,7] Like interferon, the optimal dose, schedule, and method of administration are not known. Significant toxicities may include flu-like symptoms, fever, chills, nausea, depression, loss of appetite, and renal and cardiac dysfunction. A sepsis-like syndrome with vascular leak requiring intensive care can occur. To date, there are no data to indicate whether IL-2 is superior to interferon in terms of survival or whether the combination of both drugs is superior to either one alone.

There is wide variation within and across countries as to what constitutes "standard therapy" for metastatic RCC. This controversy exists for many reasons, including how physicians and patients interpret a "significant response" or what they consider "acceptable toxicity." There are also several unique features of RCC that make interpretation of treatment data difficult. One particular feature is that the disease can have a markedly variable and unpredictable course. Some patients have rapidly progressive disease and die in a few weeks to months and yet others will live with stable or slowly progressing metastatic disease for years. In fact, in some cases, metastatic disease has been known to spontaneously regress or disappear. Therefore, caution must be taken when using response rates to interpret phase II treatment data as up to a 7% response rate has been reported in the no-treatment arm of randomized clinical trials.[10] It is also important to recognize that responses may take longer to occur with immunotherapy than what is traditionally observed with chemotherapy; and thus, one must ensure an adequate duration of treatment. In addition, the standard criteria for response may not be ideal in RCC. Traditionally, chemotherapy was judged to be effective depending on its ability to shrink a tumor. However, immunotherapy may produce an antitumor effect by producing prolonged stabilization of disease, as opposed to tumor shrinkage; and thus, time to progression and survival are probably better endpoints than response rates.

For these reasons, many physicians feel supportive care is the standard of care for patients with metastatic RCC. This may especially be appropriate for ill patients with multi-organ involvement or asymptomatic patients with stable or slowly progressing disease. However, this should be an option for all patients.

Symptom management in RCC

Patients with metastatic RCC require a comprehensive and multidisciplinary approach to symptom management with input from all members of the healthcare team. Common symptoms to address include pain, nausea, weight loss, anorexia, and fatigue. The psychosocial stress of the diagnosis, symptoms, and management on both the patients and their families also needs to be addressed.

Radiotherapy may be beneficial for those with painful bony metastases or neurological symptoms from brain or spinal cord involvement. Transarterial embolization may be used to control symptoms in patients with inoperable primary or metastatic tumors. RCC are often highly vascular and blocking the large blood vessels to these tumors may alleviate pain, transiently prevent progression of disease in those sites, and it may help control hematuria from the primary tumor. The procedure is performed by interventional radiologists, usually requiring a short stay in hospital.

Surgery may also be useful, specifically to repair pathological fractures or alleviate spinal cord compression.

Prognosis

The outlook for patients with surgically resected localized RCC can be quite favorable with 5-year survival rates $> 80\%$.[2] Prognosis is significantly worse if there is lymph node involvement or extracapsular spread. Patients with metastatic disease at presentation have a median survival of 1 year and a 5-year survival rate of 0–20%. However, it is critical to remember the highly variable course of this disease and the difficulty in predicting the outcome in any one patient.

Future directions

Renal cell carcinoma is an area of active clinical and basic science research. Novel approaches being explored include modifications of immunotherapy including inducing a graft versus tumor response with allogeneic bone marrow transplantation, dendritic cell therapy, angiogenesis targeting, and gene therapy. All patients should be encouraged to participate in clinical trials evaluating new therapies.

Box 25.1 Summary – kidney cancer
- Common malignancy with a highly variable presentation and clinical course.
- Localized disease accounts for approximately half of the cases and should be managed with surgical resection.
- Treatment for metastatic disease may include surgery, radiotherapy, angioinfarction, immunotherapy, and participation in clinical trials. It will always include the multidisciplinary management of symptoms.
- Natural history of metastatic disease may be indolent in some patients.

REFERENCES

1 Greenlee RT, Hill-Harmon M, Murray T, Thun M. Cancer Statistics, 2001. *CA Cancer J Clin* 2001;51:15–36.

2 Linehan WM, Shipley WU, Parkinson DR. Cancer of the kidney and ureter. In *Cancer: Principles and Practice of Oncology*, ed. VT DeVita Jr., S Hellman, SA Rosenberg, pp. 1271–300. Philadelphia: Lippincott-Raven, 1997.

3 Sobin LH, Wittekind CH (ed.). *TNM Classification of Malignant Tumors*, 5th edn, New York: Wiley–Liss, 1997.

4 Flanigan RC, Blumenstein BA, Salmon S et al. Cytoreduction nephrectomy in metastatic renal cancer: the results of Southwest Oncology Group trial 8949. *Proc Am Soc Clin Oncol* 2000;19:2a (abstr 3).

5 Mickisch GH, Garin A, Madej M et al. Tumor nephrectomy plus interferon alpha is superior to interferon alpha alone in metastatic renal cell carcinoma. *J Urol* 2000;163:176 (abstr, Suppl. 4).

6 Motzer RJ, Russo P. Systemic therapy for renal cell carcinoma. *J Urol* 2000;163:408–17.

7 Figlin RA. Renal cell carcinoma: management of advanced disease. *J Urol* 1999;161:381–7.

8 Medical Research Council Renal Cancer Collaborators. Interferon alpha and survival in metastatic renal carcinoma: early results of a randomized controlled trial. *Lancet* 1999; 353:14–17.

9 Pyrhonen S, Salminen E, Ruutu M et al. Prospective randomized trial of interferon alpha-2a plus vinblastine versus vinblastine alone in patients with advanced renal cell cancer. *J Clin Oncol* 1999;17:2859–67.

10 Gleave, ME, Elhilali M, Fradet Y et al. Interferon gamma-1b compared with placebo in metastatic renal-cell carcinoma. Canadian Urologic Oncology Group. *N Engl J Med* 1998; 338:1265–71.

Internet sites

Kidney Cancer Association
   http://www.kidneycancerassociation.org

26

Bladder cancer

Heather-Jane Au and Scott North

Cross Cancer Institute, Edmonton

Introduction

Bladder cancer occurs in developed and less-developed countries, with 60% of the world cases occurring in more developed countries. The estimated world incidence was 360 000 and mortality 132 000 for the year 2000. Bladder cancer accounts for 2% of cancer deaths worldwide.[1] The incidence of this disease has been increasing over the last several years while the mortality rate has been decreasing. Bladder cancer is the fourth most common cancer in men and the eighth most common cancer in women in the US,[2] with a 3:1 ratio in men versus women worldwide.[1,3]

Transitional cell carcinoma accounts for 90% of bladder cancers diagnosed in developed countries. Known risk factors for the development of transitional cell carcinoma of the bladder include cigarette smoking and occupational exposure to various agents, including aromatic amines used in textile, rubber, and cable industries. Squamous cell carcinoma accounts for 3% of bladder cancers diagnosed in the US compared with 75% in the Middle East and parts of Africa where schistosomiasis is endemic.[3] Other risk factors for squamous cell carcinoma of the bladder may include chronic bladder infections and calculi. Much less common bladder cancer histologies include adenocarcinoma, small cell carcinoma, lymphoma, and melanoma.[4]

Patterns of presentation and progression

In the US, the median age at diagnosis is 65 years. It is rarely diagnosed before the age of 40, and 80–90% of patients present with hematuria, which is often intermittent. Patients over 40 presenting with hematuria should be investigated. Other presenting symptoms may include urinary frequency, urinary infection, flank pain, or urinary obstruction.

Initial work-up includes a complete history, physical examination, and urine for cytology. This is followed by examination under anesthesia to assess for palpable masses and fixation. Endoscopic examination of the urinary tract (cystoscopy) should be completed with appropriate biopsies and/or tumor excision, assessing depth of invasion if disease is identified. Imaging with ultrasound or computed tomography (CT) of the abdomen and pelvis helps to further evaluate depth of invasion, nodal status, and metastases. However, cystoscopic and radiographic assessment of depth of invasion often underestimates the true extent of disease. Other investigations, including magnetic resonance imaging (MRI), intravenous pyelogram, chest x-ray, and radionuclide bone scanning may be warranted depending on prior findings.

Staging of bladder cancer, whether by the Jewett and Strong or TNM system, is based on the depth of tumor invasion into the bladder wall and adjacent organs, lymph node status, and distant metastases. Seventy-five percent of patients with transitional cell carcinoma of the bladder present with superficial disease that is exophytic, confined to the mucosa or submucosa and well differentiated; 20% present with invasive disease, and 5% are metastatic at presentation.[4]

With squamous cell carcinoma of the bladder diagnosed in schistosomiasis-endemic regions, tumours are often large at diagnosis and have a low metastatic rate. However, squamous cell carcinoma of the bladder diagnosed in developed countries tends to have an aggressive course.

Prognosis and treatment

Individuals with bladder cancer may have early stage disease that is confined to the bladder, distant metastatic disease, or the two may coexist. Those with superficial disease are usually curable, though 50–70% will have disease recurrence at the same or different sites within 5 years and 5–20% will progress to more advanced disease.[4] Patients with muscle invasive disease treated with radical cystectomy have a 75% 5-year progression-free survival compared with 20% for those with more deeply invasive disease.[5] Distant metastatic disease is incurable and may involve lung, bone, liver, or brain.

In earlier disease presentations, there are factors in addition to stage that predict for a poorer prognosis. With in situ disease, multiple aneuploid cell lines, nuclear p53 overexpression, Lewis-x blood group antigen expression, and incomplete response to bacillus Calmette–Guerin (BCG) intravesical therapy predict for disease progression. In superficial invasive disease, high grade, large, multiple lesions, and associated in situ disease predict disease recurrence and progression.[5]

Therapeutic options for patients with bladder cancer can be directed at local problems or systemic disease. Depending on the nature of the problem and the comorbidity of the patient, a spectrum of choices exists from conservative to aggressive treatment.

Patients with superficial disease (TNM stage 0–1) are usually managed with transurethral resection and fulguration of bladder lesions. Depending on prognostic findings and previous pattern of recurrence, this may be followed by a course of intravesical therapy. Intravesical BCG therapy has a 70% complete response rate for in situ disease and has been shown to significantly decrease the risk of recurrence and progression. Patients who achieve a complete response have a 20% risk of disease progression at 5 years compared with 95% in those without a complete response.[5] Segmental bladder resection is rarely indicated as the entire urothelium is at risk of disease. Radical cystectomy would only be indicated for extensive or refractory superficial disease.

For the majority of patients with muscle invasion (TNM stage II) a radical cystectomy is indicated. A segmental resection should only be considered in very select cases. In nonsurgical candidates and other select cases, transurethral resection followed by external beam radiation therapy may be employed for local control. If the intent of the radiotherapy is palliative only, concurrent chemotherapy is not used. For patients being treated aggressively, single agent platinum-based chemotherapy may be given concurrently as a radiation sensitizer.

For patients with more deeply invasive disease involving perivesical tissue with or without adjacent organs (TNM stage III), radical cystectomy is again the standard. External beam radiation therapy with or without chemotherapy and salvage cystectomy if residual disease is present can be considered.

Locally advanced unresectable disease extending to the abdominal or pelvic sidewalls, node positive, or metastatic disease (TNM stage IV) usually warrant systemic control of disease with chemotherapy. In these scenarios the goals of treatment include palliating symptoms, improving life expectancy, and improving quality of life.

Standard first-line chemotherapy is usually cisplatin-based. There are two commonly used regimens: cisplatin, methotrexate, doxorubicin and vinblastine (MVAC) or cisplatin, methotrexate, and vinblastine (CMV). The response rate with MVAC is 60%.[6] Patients most likely to benefit are those with good performance status, lack of visceral metastases, and no comorbidities. Median overall survival is 1 year as compared with 6 months with best supportive care.[6–8] Approximately 20% of patients with lymph node metastases and 10% with visceral metastases can expect long-term survival. Average time to progression ranges from 7 to 9 months.

Second-line chemotherapy with single agent gemcitabine or paclitaxel yields response rates of 30–40%.[9] Recently, a phase III trial comparing the combination of gemcitabine/cisplatin to MVAC showed equivalency with respect to response rate and overall survival.[10] However, the gemcitabine/cisplatin combination was significantly less toxic, giving oncologists another useful combination for palliative first-line chemotherapy in this patient population. This regimen is rapidly replacing other more toxic regimens as first-line therapy for metastatic bladder cancer. For patients responding to chemotherapy, a maximum of six cycles is recommended as there has been no demonstrated advantage to continuing beyond this.

Although systemic combination chemotherapy has been shown to improve survival and quality of life, it may be too toxic for some patients. Those with a poor performance status, multiple comorbidities, visceral or bony metastases are less likely to benefit. These patients may be best cared for with supportive measures only. It should be noted that renal insufficiency secondary to obstruction from tumor need not preclude the use of chemotherapy. Ureteric stenting or palliative surgical urinary diversion may reverse renal failure, allowing chemotherapy to be administered.

Caring for the dying patient

Despite therapies with significant activity for bladder cancer, patients with metastatic disease will succumb to their illness. Complications can occur either locally in the pelvis or systemically.

For patients who have had a radical cystectomy, local complications may occur with recurrence in lymph nodes or soft tissue. This can cause pelvic pain syndromes from sacral plexus involvement, obstipation if the rectum is compromised, and lower limb edema from lymph node enlargement. Many of these symptoms can be palliated with external beam radiotherapy.

For patients who have not had local surgery, transurethral resection and fulguration are useful for palliation of bleeding and pain. If these relatively simple measures fail to control the disease, external beam radiotherapy may be employed. Occasionally a palliative cystectomy may be required especially if the patient becomes a "bladder cripple" plagued by pain, bleeding, spasms, and incontinence.

Systemic disease is usually the major cause of problems for endstage patients. Opioids should be used for pain control as clinically indicated. Other means of pain control for bone metastases include radiation therapy and bisphosphonates. Early orthopedic intervention for lytic metastases at risk of pathologic fracture should be pursued. Centrally located pulmonary metastases may cause wheezing, shortness of breath or hemoptysis and can also be effectively alleviated with radiation therapy and/or opioids.

Many patients suffer from anorexia and cachexia. Dietary supplements and megestrol acetate may be helpful in slowing weight loss and stimulating appetite. Some patients may suffer from night sweats and fevers that may benefit from NSAIDs. In refractory cases, thalidomide has been shown to reduce distressing sweats. Although not a common complication, hypercalcemia can develop and usually indicates that the patient's life expectancy is a few weeks to months. Hypercalcemia can be treated with fluids, bisphosphonates, and diuretics as clinically indicated.

In summary, for all patients with distant metastatic disease, judicious use of opioids, radiotherapy, and other supportive care strategies should be employed. Those with an adequate performance status should be considered for systemic combination chemotherapy as it has been shown to improve survival and quality of life.

Conclusion

Bladder cancer often presents with superficial neoplasia. However, the entire urothelium is at risk of disease and the typical course is one of recurrence at the same or different sites with or without progression of disease. For this reason, endoscopic surveillance is an important factor in the management of early-stage patients. Ongoing research is being done to determine whether prognostic markers such as p53 overexpression can be used to direct therapy in early-stage disease. This may allow lower-risk patients with invasive disease to undergo bladder-conserving surgery. Further research is evaluating the role of adjuvant or neo-adjuvant chemotherapy. Clinical trials of chemotherapy are continuing in early stage and advanced stage disease, including studies of paclitaxel and gemcitabine alone or in combination.

Box 26.1 Summary – bladder cancer

- The most common form of bladder cancer in the Western world is transitional cell carcinoma (TCC) and the most common etiologic agent is cigarette smoking.
- Most TCC of the bladder is superficial and can be removed with transurethral resection but virtually all patients will have recurrences, 20% of which will progress to a higher stage.
- For muscle invasive disease, radical cystectomy with or without adjuvant chemotherapy is the treatment of choice. Bladder preservation protocols using radiation therapy and concurrent chemotherapy can be considered.
- For metastatic disease, cisplatin-based regimens have a 50–60% response rate, improve life expectancy, and improve quality of life.
- Patients may develop local complications such as pelvic pain and lymphedema which can be palliated effectively with radiation therapy.
- Median life expectancy for patients with metastatic bladder cancer is 1 year.

REFERENCES

1 World Health Organization. Cancer, http://www.who.int/ncd/cancer.

2 Metts MC, Metts JC, Milito SJ, Thomas CR Jr. Bladder cancer: a review of diagnosis and management. *J Natl Med Assoc* 2000;92:285–94.

3 Johansson SL, Cohen SM. Epidemiology and etiology of bladder cancer. *Semin Surg Oncol* 1997;13:291–8.

4 Scher HI, Shipley WU, Herr HW. Cancer of the bladder. In *Cancer: Principles and Practice of Oncology*, 5th edn, ed. VT DeVita Jr., S Hellman, SA Rosenberg, pp. 1300–22. Philadelphia: JB Lippincott, 1997.

5 National Institutes of Health. Cancernet, http://cancernet.nci.nih.gov/pdqfull.html.

6 Sternberg CN, Yagoda A, Scher HI et al. Methotrexate, vinblastine, doxorubicin, and cisplatin for advanced TCC of the urothelium. *Cancer* 1989;64:2448–58.

7 Harker WG, Meyers FJ, Freiha FS et al. Cisplatin, methotrexate and vinblastine (CMV) an effective chemotherapy regimen for metastatic TCC of the urinary tract, a Northern California Oncology Group Study. *J Clin Oncol* 1985;3:1463–70.

8 Loehrer PJ, Einhorn LH, Elson PJ et al. A randomized comparison of cisplatin alone or in combination with methotrexate, vinblastine, and doxorubicin in patients with metastatic urothelial carcinoma: a cooperative group study. *J Clin Oncol*, 1972;10:1066–73.

9 Pollera CF, Ceribelli A, Crecco M et al. Weekly gemcitabine in advanced bladder cancer: a preliminary report from a phase I study. *Ann Oncol* 1994;5:182–4.

10 Von de Maase H, Hansen SW, Roberts JT et al. Gemcitabine and cisplatin versus methotrexate, vinblastine, doxorubicin, and cisplatin in advanced or metastatic bladder cancer: results of a large, randomized, multinational, multicenter, phase III study. *J Clin Oncol* 2000;17:3068–77.

27

Ovarian cancer

Diane C. Bodurka

U.T. M.D. Anderson Cancer Center, Houston

Natural history

Ovarian cancer is the leading cause of death in women with gynecologic cancers. Often called the "Silent Killer" because there are no obvious symptoms until the disease is in its later stages, more than 23 400 new cases and 13 900 deaths were predicted from this disease in the US in 2001. One in 70 women in the US develop this disease, and 1 in 100 women die from ovarian cancer. Most women have a 1.8% lifetime risk of developing this cancer.

Ovarian cancer occurs most frequently in women aged 40–70, and the greatest number of cases is found in women between 50 and 59 years of age. Eight percent of the cases occur in women less than 35 years of age. A higher incidence is seen in Caucasian women, and this disease is more common in industrialized countries.

Approximately 20% of ovarian cancers are germ cell tumors and sex-cord stromal tumors; these cancers develop in the cells that form the eggs (germ cells) or in the cells that produce the female hormones and form the structure of the ovaries (sex-cord stromal cells). The remaining 80% are epithelial ovarian carcinomas, which begin in the cells that cover the surfaces of the ovaries. These cancers will be the subject of this chapter.

The exact etiology of ovarian cancer is unknown, although events related to incessant ovulatory function have been consistently reported in the literature. Factors associated with decreased risk include parity, use of oral contraceptives, history of breast-feeding, tubal ligation and previous hysterectomy. Suspected risk factors include age, early menarche, late menopause, infertility, use of fertility drugs, and talc use.

Family history is an important risk factor for developing ovarian cancer. Although 90% of ovarian cancer cases are sporadic, an estimated 5–10% of cases occur in women with family histories of breast and/or ovarian cancers. Specifically, women who have mutations in either the BRCA1 or BRCA2 genes are at particularly increased risk of developing ovarian cancer.

If detected early, the survival rate is 95%. However, only about 25% of all ovarian cancers are found in the early stages. Seventy-five percent of women present with advanced disease. The interval from onset of disease to diagnosis is often delayed, since this disease is difficult to detect and often has symptoms that can be confused with other health conditions. The signs and symptoms of ovarian cancer include: abdominal swelling or fullness, digestive problems such as gas, bloating, stomach pain, indigestion, or early satiety, or changes in bowel or bladder habits. Other symptoms may include bleeding between periods or after menopause, pelvic pain, pain during intercourse, a feeling of pressure in the pelvis, leg swelling or pain.

Pattern of spread

Most patients with ovarian cancer will have a palpable adnexal mass. Diagnostic evaluation focuses on whether the adnexal mass requires surgical attention. Thorough evaluation includes taking a history and performing a physical examination including pelvic and rectal examinations, as well as a transvaginal and/or abdominal ultrasound. Other tests may include a chest radiograph, screening mammogram, barium enema, or computed tomography (CT) scan. Such tests may be helpful in identifying other possible primary tumor sites that could result in metastases to the ovaries, as well as to evaluate the possible etiology of obstruction, bleeding, or pain. The serum marker CA-125 (a cell surface glycoprotein) should also be evaluated. Although CA-125 levels are elevated (greater than 35 U/ml) in more than 80% of patients with advanced disease, the CA-125 level is abnormal in only half of women with early stage disease. It is important to note that none of these tests by themselves, including the CA-125 and transvaginal ultrasound, can completely determine the presence of ovarian cancer.

Ovarian cancer is a surgically staged disease (Table 27.1). Staging involves an exploratory laparotomy with thorough evaluation of all areas at risk. It is important that the staging procedure is both accurate and comprehensive since the patient's treatment plan and prognosis will be based upon the results of the clinical, surgical, histologic, and pathologic findings at the time of surgery. Studies have demonstrated a significantly improved prognosis in patients whose tumors have been optimally debulked with the largest piece of residual disease 1 cm or less at the conclusion of surgery. For this reason, it is recommended that a gynecologic oncologist, who has specific training in this field, perform the surgery.

Ovarian cancer may metastasize via the lymphatics or hematogenously. This disease has a particular propensity to spread transcoelomically, and most often is found coating the surfaces of the peritoneum, bowel serosa, liver, and the diaphragm. It

Table 27.1. International Federation of Gynecology and Obstetrics (FIGO) staging system for ovarian cancer

---

Stage I: Growth limited to ovaries

1A   Growth limited to one ovary; no tumor on the external surface, capsule intact

1B   Growth limited to both ovaries; no ascites; no tumor on the external surfaces, capsule(s) intact

1C   Tumor either stage 1A or stage 1B but with tumor on the surface of one or both ovaries; or with capsule(s) ruptured; or with ascites present, containing malignant cells or with positive peritoneal washings

Stage II: Growth involving one or both ovaries with pelvic extension

IIA   Extension and/or metastases to the uterus and/or tubes

IIB   Extension to other pelvic tissues

IIC   Tumor either stage IIA or IIB but with tumor on the surface of one or both ovaries; or with capsule(s) ruptured; or with ascites present containing malignant cells or with positive peritoneal washings

Stage III: Tumor involving one or both ovaries with peritoneal implants outside the pelvis and/or positive retroperitoneal inguinal nodes; superficial liver metastases equals stage III; tumor is limited to the true pelvis but with histologically verified malignant extension to small bowel or omentum

IIIA   Tumor grossly limited to the true pelvis with negative nodes with histologically confirmed microscopic seeding of abdominal peritoneal surfaces

IIIB   Tumor of one or both ovaries with histologically confirmed implants of abdominal peritoneal surfaces, none exceeding 2 cm in diameter; nodes negative

IIIC   Abdominal implants greater than 2 cm in diameter and/or positive retroperitoneal or inguinal nodes

Stage IV: Growth involving one or both ovaries with distant metastases; if pleural effusion is present, there must be positive cytologic test results to allot a case to stage IV; parenchymal liver metastases equals stage IV

---

is often very difficult to remove all of the tumor, due to the studding of virtually all intra-abdominal and pelvic surfaces with small tumor implants.

Therapeutic approaches

The treatment and diagnosis of ovarian cancer requires an exploratory laparotomy and staging. Unfortunately, the majority of women with ovarian cancer present with advanced disease (Table 27.2). Recommendations for adjuvant chemotherapy are based on the stage and histology of the disease. Patients who have stage IA or IB disease and borderline, well- or moderately differentiated tumors have a

Table 27.2. Distribution by stage of ovarian cancer patients

Stage	Percent
I	23
II	13
III	48
IV	16
Total	100

very favorable prognosis from surgery alone, with a 5-year survival approximating 95%. Consequently, these patients do not require adjuvant chemotherapy. Since all other patients are at significant risk of recurrence, postoperative chemotherapy is recommended. Clinical trials have demonstrated that a platinum-based agent, in combination with paclitaxel, is the most active regimen for ovarian cancer.

Prognosis and recurrence

Unfortunately, the majority of women who have responded well to chemotherapy will develop recurrent disease. The average time to recurrence is 18 months, and the average survival of women with advanced disease is 24 months. Patients who have platinum-sensitive tumors are usually re-treated with platinum, especially if the patient has remained without disease for 12 months.

The response to platinum is low in patients with platinum-resistant tumors. Selection of an appropriate second-line or "salvage" regimen requires an assessment of the risks and benefits of therapy. The overall response rate to second-line agents is usually in the range of 15–35%. Patients and their physicians must carefully evaluate which salvage treatment regimen can maximize both survival time and the patient's quality of life.

Rehabilitation issues

When a patient undergoes initial treatment for ovarian cancer, her primary goal is cure, with a return to as normal a life as possible once treatment has been completed. Rehabilitation issues vary according to the patient's age, physical status, and pre-existing medical issues. Patients who may have developed deep venous thromboses during treatment require continued anticoagulation. Patients who have decreased mobility may benefit from physical therapy. Often, neurologists are consulted for assistance with management of neuropathies associated with chemotherapy, such as persistent numbness and tingling in the hands and feet or difficulty writing or buttoning clothing. Patients may also feel extremely fatigued, and may not return to what they perceive as a "normal" level of energy for more than a year after treatment.

Palliative care issues

When ovarian cancer persists or recurs, goals change from cure to prolongation of life and palliation of symptoms, again with as normal a life as possible. Limited surgery or radiation may be used to control symptoms from locally progressive disease. Symptom management often focuses upon bowel-related issues, as this type of cancer frequently causes a "functional" rather than "mechanical" bowel obstruction. Tumor implants often coat the bowel surfaces, thereby severely limiting bowel peristalsis. Most patients with ovarian cancer do not experience severe pain. Rather, their symptoms are bowel-related, and often consist of nausea, vomiting, and dehydration. Many women with advanced ovarian cancer are unable to absorb nutrients due to a lack of gastrointestinal function, and succumb due to starvation. The average lifespan of a patient with recurrent ovarian cancer who presents with a bowel obstruction is only 3 months.

If a single site of obstruction is present, it may be possible to surgically bypass this area. If multiple sites of obstruction exist, however, a surgical approach is not technically feasible. Options are then restricted, and often the patient undergoes percutaneous gastrostomy tube placement. The gastrostomy tube is hooked up to a bag the patient is able to conceal under her clothes. When the valve between the gastrostomy tube and the bag is open, the patient is able to take nutrition by mouth. However, the stomach contents drain directly into the bag. The purpose of this tube is to provide symptomatic relief due to persistent nausea and vomiting from a bowel obstruction. If left unclamped, no nutrition is provided.

Patients with ovarian cancer may also have persistent pleural effusions and recurrent ascites. Thoracentesis may be performed to alleviate shortness of breath. Recurrent, symptomatic pleural effusions may be treated with pleurodesis or placement of a Denver catheter.

Paracentesis may be performed to alleviate abdominal distension due to ascites. Frequent paracenteses are discouraged, however, as this may lead to loculated pockets of fluid which are difficult to drain via a single puncture site. A catheter may be placed into the abdomen under fluoroscopic guidance. This is then hooked up to a bag which the patient may empty as needed to drain the fluid.

Ovarian cancer is a devastating disease, due to the inability to cure recurrent cancer. Current efforts are focusing upon early detection and prevention due to the improved prognosis of early-stage disease. It is incumbent upon the attending physician to address end-of-life issues with patients who develop recurrent disease in order to help the patient maximize her quality of life and address important personal issues while she is able to.

Box 27.1 Summary – ovarian cancer

- Patients with ovarian cancer require surgical exploration and staging.
- Surgery is usually followed by chemotherapy consisting of a platinum-based compound and paclitaxel.
- The prognosis for patients with advanced stage disease remains poor.
- Patients and their physicians must carefully evaluate which salvage treatment regimen can maximize both survival time and the patient's quality of life.
- Current efforts are focused on prevention and early detection in order to help improve the survival of women with ovarian cancer.

BIBLIOGRAPHY

Anderson B. Quality of life in progressive ovarian cancer. *Gynecol Oncol* 1994;55:S151–5.

FIGO Cancer Committee. Staging announcement. *Gynecol Oncol* 1986;25:383–95.

Kornblith AB, Thaler H, Wong G et al. Quality of life of women with ovarian cancer. *Gynecol Oncol* 1995;59:231–42.

Patnaik A, Doyle C, Oza A. Palliative therapy in advanced ovarian cancer: balancing patient expectations, quality of life and cost. *Anti-Cancer Drugs 1998*, 1998;9:869–78.

Pettersson F. *International Federation of Gynecology and Obstetrics Report.* Stockholm: FIGO, 1991.

Internet sites

American Cancer Society
    1-800-4-CANCER
    www.cancer.gov
Cancer Information Service
    1-800-ACS-2345
    www.cancer.org
Gynecologic Cancer Foundation
    1-800-444-4441
    www.wen.org
M. D. Anderson Cancer Center
    www.mdanderson.org

28

Gynecologic malignancies: endometrial and cervical carcinoma

William Paul Irvin, Jr.

University of Virginia Health Center, Charlottesville

Introduction

Gynecologic malignancies account for approximately 15% of all new female cancers diagnosed in the US each year. Based upon US population estimates, 80 000 women were diagnosed with gynecologic cancers in 1998. In that same year, an estimated 27 000 women died as a result of these cancers. Worldwide, cervical cancer represents the second leading cause of cancer-related death among women, second only to breast cancer. In certain developing countries of the world, cervical cancer is the leading cause of death among women of reproductive age.

Endometrial cancer

In the US, endometrial cancer is the most common invasive neoplasm of the female genital tract. It is estimated that 36 000 new cases of endometrial cancer will be diagnosed this year, and that approximately 6000 women will die from their disease.

Endometrial cancer is predominantly a disorder of older women, with 75% of all cases arising in the postmenopausal age group (Table 28.1). The average age at diagnosis is 58 years. Only 2–5% of all cases of endometrial cancer are diagnosed in women less than 40 years of age.

Endometrial cancer arises as a result of unopposed estrogenic stimulation of the endometrial lining. A number of constitutional factors have been identified in women who develop endometrial cancer. These include obesity, nulliparity, early menarche, late menopause, diabetes, hypertension, gallbladder disease, unopposed exogenous estrogen therapy, and prior history of pelvic irradiation (Table 28.2). Protective factors that mitigate against the development of endometrial cancer include the use of combination oral contraceptives. Worldwide, the variable incidence

Table 28.1. Frequency of endometrial carcinoma by age group in women with postmenopausal bleeding

Age group	Total cases	Corpus cancer	
		N	%
< 50	34	0	0.0
50–59	161	15	9.3
60–69	92	15	16.3
70–79	43	12	27.9
> 80	5	3	60.0

Table 28.2. Risk ratios estimated for certain factors correlated with endometrial cancer

Factor	Relative risk
Overweight (lb)	1.9–11
20–50	3
> 50	9
Parous vs nulliparous	0.1–0.9
Late menopause (age ≥ years)	1.7–2.4
Diabetes	1.3–2.7
Radiation therapy	8.0
Exogenous estrogen use	1.6–12.0
Oral contraceptive use	
Sequential	0.9–7.3
Combined	0.1–1.0
Hypertension	1.2–2.1

of endometrial cancer is most strongly associated with socioeconomic status and total dietary fat consumption.

The primary presenting symptom of endometrial carcinoma is abnormal uterine bleeding. In fact, greater than 90% of postmenopausal women diagnosed with endometrial cancer will present with vaginal bleeding as their initial complaint. Though the causes of postmenopausal bleeding are numerous, 10–20% of patients presenting with this complaint will in fact be found to have a gynecologic malignancy, usually endometrial cancer (Table 28.3). The 25% of women diagnosed with endometrial cancer who are premenopausal invariably have abnormal uterine bleeding as well, often characterized as menometrorrhagia or oligomenorrhea. Other important presenting symptoms of endometrial carcinoma include a purulent vaginal discharge or pelvic pain. Only 1–5% of the cases of endometrial

Table 28.3. Etiology of postmenopausal bleeding

Etiologic factor	Hawwa et al. (1970) (n = 335; %)	Pacheco and Kempers (1968) (n = 401; %)
Estrogen therapy	27	27
No pathology (atrophic endometrium)	23	20
Cancer	19.5	18
Endometrium	(13)	(16)
Cervix	(4)	(1)
Other	(2.5)	(1)
Atrophic vaginitis	10	9
Endometrial polyps	7	23
Cervical polyps – cervicitis	6.5	14
Endometrial, benign	3	–
Other (myoma, caruncle, trauma, etc.)	4	9

cancer are diagnosed while the patient is asymptomatic, usually resulting from the investigation of an abnormal Pap smear found to have atypical or malignant endometrial cells.

Following the diagnosis of endometrial cancer, a thorough physical examination and chest x-ray are then performed to look for clinical evidence of extrauterine involvement. In over 75% of the patients there will be none. In those patients without evidence of extrauterine spread, operative surgical exploration and staging is indicated. Such staging typically entails a total abdominal hysterectomy, complete bilateral pelvic lymphadenectomy, and in certain instances a para-aortic lymph node sampling. The final pathology report on these surgical specimens provides an accurate "stage" (I–IV) and grade (1, 2, 3) for the patient's disease (Table 28.4), and thus helps prognosticate the likelihood of cure, versus relapse and/or persistence, of the patient's cancer.

If the patient is found to have metastatic cancer within the resected pelvic or para-aortic lymph nodes removed at the time of the patient's surgical "staging" procedure, with no other evidence of extrauterine spread noted, generally the entire pelvis and the para-aortic lymph node chain will be irradiated postoperatively. Such radiation therapy is designed to destroy any residual remaining microscopic cancer within the pelvis, as well as the para-aortic lymph node chain. The 5-year survival rate for this group of patients would be expected to range from 40–80%.

In those patients found to have gross metastatic disease outside of the pelvis at the time of their surgical exploration, or those with liver, lung, bone, or brain metastases diagnosed preoperatively at the time of their initial presentation, systemic cytotoxic chemotherapy is recommended. Adriamycin and cisplatin are the two

Table 28.4. FIGO surgical staging for carcinoma of the corpus uteri (1988)

Stage I	
Stage Ia G123	Tumor limited to endometrium
Stage Ib G123	Invasion to less than one-half the myometrium
Stage Ic G123	Invasion to more than one-half the myometrium
Stage II	
Stage IIa G123	Endocervical glandular involvement only
Stage IIb G123	Cervical stromal invasion
Stage III	
Stage IIIa G123	Tumor invades serosa and/or adnexa, and/or positive peritoneal cytology
Stage IIIb G123	Vaginal metastases
Stage IIIc G123	Metastases to pelvic and/or para-aortic lymph nodes
Stage IV	
Stage IVa G123	Tumor invasion of bladder and/or bowel mucosa
Stage IVb	Distant metastases including intra-abdominal and/or inguinal lymph nodes

most active agents in the management of metastatic endometrial carcinoma, resulting in objective response rates of 30% and complete response rates of 5–10% when used individually. When used in combination, adriamycin/cisplatin-based chemotherapy induces a complete remission in 15% of patients treated. Treatment is continued for 6–12 cycles, provided that the patient continues to respond in terms of measurable tumor regression. The 5-year survival rate for this group of patients would be expected to range from 10–30%.

Approximately 75% of patients who ultimately fail their initial therapy and develop evidence of persistent or recurrent disease will do so within 2–3 years of the completion of their primary therapy. Isolated local or regional recurrences that arise following primary surgical therapy have a much better prognosis than do similar recurrences following primary radiation therapy.

Localized recurrences can be managed with radiation therapy, surgery, or a combination of the two. In particular, large localized lesions should be excised whenever possible. If the area has not been previously treated, the tumor bed can then be irradiated postoperatively. An isolated pelvic recurrence is potentially curable, particularly when it appears more than 1 or 2 years after the completion of primary therapy. Extended or radical surgical resection, including total pelvic exenteration, may be justified in the setting of recurrent disease limited to the pelvis for those patients having previously received radiation therapy. Distant recurrences resulting from hematogenous metastatic tumor spread typically arise in the lungs, liver, bone, or brain. Clearly, such distant recurrences have a much worse prognosis than do the localized central recurrences. The 5-year survival rate for patients with recurrent endometrial cancer, taken as a whole, would be expected to range from 25–50%.

Palliative therapy is directed towards patients with advanced or recurrent endometrial cancer not amenable to cure by surgery and/or radiation therapy. Such therapy is designed to minimize the physical and emotional impact of symptoms associated with the disease process, in order to maximize the quality of remaining life for the patient. Palliative therapy is often multidisciplinary, and may include pelvic radiation therapy or hysterectomy offered to provide local tumor control and prevent bleeding, palliative chemotherapy to decrease tumor-associated pain and discomfort, and/or hormonal therapy designed to increase appetite, maintain tumor dormancy, and improve the patient's overall sense of well-being.

Complications arising from the management of endometrial cancer are dependent upon the treatment modalities employed. Surgical staging carries with it the attendant risks of any surgical procedure, including bleeding, infection, damage to surrounding organs, or risk of re-exploration. The pelvic lymph node dissection can rarely be associated with postoperative lymphocyst formation, in the short term, and with lower extremity lymphadema, in the long term. The latter is a rare event in the surgical management of endometrial cancer.

Radiation therapy, when employed in the management of endometrial cancer, is generally associated with both short-term as well as long-term side effects. In the short term, radiation cystitis, proctitis, sigmoiditis, and enteritis may occur, giving rise to nausea, dysuria, intermittent diarrhea, constipation, hematochozia, and tenesmus. Management involves the use of urinary analgesics, antispasmodics, bulking agents, low residue diets, and steroid suppositories. In the long term, the most significant complication associated with the use of radiation therapy is that of bowel injury. Radiation injury to the bowel, when it occurs, most commonly presents as bowel obstruction. The incidence of significant bowel injury following radiation therapy is approximately 5%; it generally results in the need for repeat surgical exploration with subsequent bowel resection or bypass.

Systemic cytotoxic chemotherapy, when employed in the management of endometrial cancer, can be associated with both short-term as well as long-term side effects. In the short term, cisplatin has the usual side effects of nausea, vomiting, and myelosuppression. In the long term, cisplatin can be associated with nephrotoxicity, ototoxicity, and irreversible peripheral paresthesias. Adriamycin, in the short term, can be associated with myelosuppression, alopecia, stomatitis, nausea, vomiting, hyperpigmentation, and diarrhea. In the long term, the most important and unique side effect associated with adriamycin therapy is cardiotoxicity. This includes the acute toxicities of pericarditis, myocarditis, and electrophysiologic aberrations, as well as a cumulative cardiomyopathy. The former effects appear reversible. The cardiomyopathy, on the other hand, presents as classic congestive heart failure that may be refractory to the usual measures and is typically irreversible.

Cervical cancer

Cervical cancer is a significant female health problem worldwide. Approximately 500 000 new cases of cervical cancer are diagnosed worldwide each year, making cervical cancer the second leading cause of cancer-related death among women throughout the world. In developing countries of the world, where approximately 75–80% of all cases of cervical cancer occur, cervical cancer is the leading cause of cancer-related death among women of reproductive age. In certain developing countries of the world, cervical cancer is the leading cause of death among women of reproductive age.

In the US approximately 16 000 new cases of cervical cancer are diagnosed each year. Among gynecologic cancers, it is surpassed in frequency by both endometrial cancer (36 000 cases/year) as well as ovarian cancer (26 000 cases/year). With the advent of mass population screening utilizing cervical/vaginal cytology, a dramatic and progressive drop in the incidence rate of cervical cancer was observed in this country between 1947 and 1970. Mortality rates have shown a significant decline as well. In 1960, an estimated 8000 women died of cervical cancer in this country, compared with an estimated 6000 deaths in 1999.

Incidence rates for cervical cancer are highest in lower socioeconomic groups, likely accounting for differences in the racial incidence of this malignancy in the US. The probability that a white woman at birth will eventually develop invasive cervical cancer is approximately 0.7 to 1.0%, while the risk for a black, Hispanic, or Native American woman is 1.6%. In addition to race and socioeconomic status, numerous other risk factors for the development of cervical cancer have been recognized, many of which relate to sexual behavior. Among the most consistent and significant is age at first intercourse, particularly when sexual activity is initiated within one year of menarche. The number of sexual partners one has, particularly if greater than four prior to the age of 16, as well as a history of cigarette smoking, herpes simplex infection, or venereal warts have all been associated with an increased risk for the development of cervical cancer (Table 28.5).

Cervical cancer is one of the few solid neoplasms whose development can be almost completely attributed to a viral source. The term "human papillomavirus" (HPV) refers to a family of more than 70 different types of virion, all sharing a predilection for the infection of epithelial surfaces. Twenty-three subtypes of the human papillomavirus have the ability to infect the epithelial surfaces of the lower female genital tract. Of these, subtypes 16, 18, 31, and 45 have the ability to bring about malignant transformation of the cervical epithelium, thereby ultimately

Table 28.5. Cervical carcinoma: relative risks of selected factors

Risk factor	Relative risk
Age at coitarche (years)	
< 16	16
16–19	3
> 19	1
Years from menarche to coitarche	
< 1	26
1–5	7
6–10	3
> 10	1
Total number of sexual partners	
0–1 vs. > 4	3.6
Number of sexual partners before age 20 years	
0 vs. > 1	7
Genital warts	
Never vs. ever	3.2
Smoked > 5 cigarettes/day	
< 1 year vs. > 20 years	4.0

giving rise to the development of cervical carcinoma. HPV-16 is strongly correlated with the development of squamous cell carcinoma of the cervix, accounting for roughly 85% of all cervical cancer. HPV-18 is associated with the development of the less common adenocarcinomas and neuroendocrine tumors of the cervix.

There are four stages of cervical cancer, stages I–IV (Table 28.6). Stage I refers to disease that is limited to the cervix, and carries with it an 85–95% 5-year survival. Stage II refers to disease that has extended beyond the cervix to involve either the proximal aspect of the supporting pelvic ligaments of the cervix, or to the upper two-thirds of the vagina. Stage II disease has a 60–75% 5-year survival. Stage III disease refers to disease that extends beyond the cervix, either completely to the pelvic sidewall, or into the lower one-third of the vagina. Stage III disease has a 30–45% 5-year survival. Stage IV disease refers to disease that has invaded the bladder and/or rectal mucosa, or to distant metastatic disease. The 5-year survival for stage IV disease is <10%.

Though radiation therapy can be used effectively to manage all stages of cervical carcinoma, small-volume stage I disease is generally managed surgically with a radical hysterectomy, complete bilateral pelvic lymphadenectomy, and para-aortic

Table 28.6. FIGO staging of cervical cancer

Stage	Features
0	Carcinoma in situ, intraepithelial carcinoma
I	The carcinoma is strictly confined to the cervix (extension to the corpus should be disregarded)
Ia	Preclinical carcinomas of the cervix, that is, those diagnosed only by microscopy
Ia1	Minimal microscopically evident stromal invasion
Ia2	Lesions detected microscopically that can be measured. The upper limit of the measurement should not show a depth of invasion of more than 5 mm taken from the basis of the epithelium, either surface or glandular, from which it originates. A second dimension, the horizontal spread, must not exceed 7 mm. Larger lesions should be staged as Ib
Ib	Lesions of greater dimensions than stage Ia2 whether seen clinically or not. Preformed space involvement should not alter the staging but should be specifically recorded so as to determine whether it should affect treatment decisions in the future
II	The carcinoma extends beyond the cervix, but has not extended on to the pelvic wall. The carcinoma involves the vagina, but not as far as the lower third
IIa	No obvious parametrial involvement
IIb	Obvious parametrial involvement
III	The carcinoma has extended on to the pelvic wall. On rectal examination there is no cancer-free space between the tumor and the pelvic wall. The tumor involves the lower third of the vagina. All cases with a hydronephrosis or nonfunctioning kidney should be included, unless they are known to be due to other cause
IIIa	No extension on to the pelvic wall, but involvement of the lower third of the vagina
IIIb	Extension on to the pelvic wall or hydronephrosis or nonfunctioning kidney
IV	The carcinoma has extended beyond the true pelvis or has clinically involved the mucosa of the bladder or rectum
IVa	Spread of the growth to adjacent organs
IVb	Spread to distant organs

lymph node sampling. The basic design of the operation is the removal of the uterus, along with the adjacent portions of the vagina, cardinal ligaments, rectal pillars, uterosacral ligaments, and bladder pillars (Figure 28.1). Patients found to have metastatic disease within the resected pelvic or para-aortic lymph nodes following their surgical procedure go on to receive postoperative adjuvant whole pelvic irradiation with concomitant weekly cisplatin chemosensitization. For all other patients with cervical cancer, specifically those patients who present with bulky stage I disease through stage IV disease, the primary therapy employed is

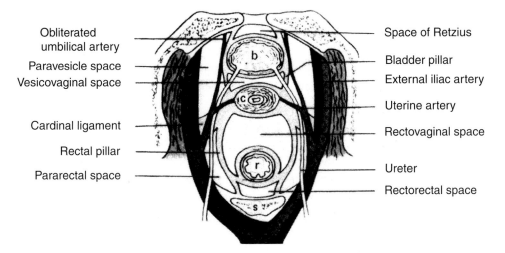

Figure 28.1   The spaces and ligaments of the female pelvis. The primary route of extension for cervical carcinoma is via the cardinal ligaments. The pubovesicle cervical fascia encompasses the bladder (b), cervix (c), and rectum (r), forming protective membranes and spaces that permit the excision required to cure early cervical cancer.

radiation therapy. Whole pelvic irradiation with or without an extended para-aortic field, followed by intravaginal brachytherapy, is administered over a period of 6–8 weeks. Weekly cisplatin chemosensitization is given concomitantly in an effort to increase the lethality of the radiation therapy. A set amount of radiation is prescribed in order to maximize the potential for cure; specifically, 8500 cGy is administered to the central cervical tumor, and 5500 cGy to the pelvis and the pelvic lymph nodes. Though this is a very high radiation dose, such high doses are typically required in order to have a successful chance of destroying the large, often metastatic tumors with which patients initially present.

Despite the fact that carcinoma of the cervix is one of the more curable human malignancies, treatment is unsuccessful in nearly one-half of the cases. Approximately 50% of patients that recur will do so within 1 year of completing their initial therapy, 75% within 2 years, and 95% within 5 years. Thus, the 5-year survival rate for cervical cancer is a reasonably accurate measure of cure. Persistent or recurrent carcinoma of the cervix generally becomes apparent within the pelvic, para-aortic, mediastinal, or supraclavicular lymph nodes. Rarely, however, it can also present as an isolated hepatic, pulmonary, or brain metastasis. Persistent or recurrent carcinoma of the cervix, the consequence of treatment failure, carries with it a 1-year survival rate of 15%, and a 5-year survival rate of less than 5%.

Treatment failure after surgical therapy is generally managed with radiation therapy. However, most treatment failures occur in the more advanced stages of disease, those managed initially with radiation therapy. A central pelvic recurrence following radiation therapy, without evidence of pelvic sidewall extension or extra-pelvic metastases, can be successfully managed with total pelvic exenteration. A total pelvic exenteration involves the en-bloc resection of the uterus, cervix, vagina, bladder, and rectum. Roughly 25–50% of patients with localized central pelvic recurrences following radiation therapy can be cured with such radical surgical resection.

Systemic chemotherapy is generally prescribed for the management of recurrent or disseminated carcinoma of the cervix not amenable to management with surgical resection or radiation therapy. Though numerous chemotherapeutic drug combi-nations have been evaluated in patients with advanced or recurrent carcinoma of the cervix, no randomized or controlled trials conducted to date support the use of any combination of chemotherapeutic agents over cisplatin alone in terms of tumor response.

Several features common to this group of patients often preclude the possibil-ity of a beneficial drug response with palliative chemotherapy. First, nearly all of these patients have had previous radiation therapy, limiting their bone marrow reserve and subsequent tolerance to cytotoxic chemotherapy. The loss of marrow reserve, as well as the loss of pelvic tissue vascularity, prevents the administration of chemotherapy at desired dose intensity. Second, the frequent association of pelvic recurrence with bilateral ureteral obstruction and renal dysfunction significantly limit the treatment of this disease with nephrotoxic or renally excreted chemo-therapeutic agents, such as cisplatin.

The therapeutic side effects for patients diagnosed with cervical cancer are varied and largely depend upon the treatment modalities employed. With primary sur-gical management, the most serious potential side effect results from unavoidable injury to the innervation of the bladder and rectum that occurs during the radical surgical dissection and resection. Such injury can cause life-long problems both with complete bladder emptying, as well as with defecation, in up to 20% of patients that undergo radical surgical management. A certain percentage of these patients will be unable to void spontaneously and will require life-long self-catheterization.

The most serious constellation of complications associated with the manage-ment of cervical cancer are those that follow primary radiation therapy. In the short term, patients managed with radiation therapy can experience problems with radiation cystitis, proctosigmoiditis, and enteritis. As previously mentioned, these complications can result in dysuria, frequency, hematuria, diarrhea, nausea, colicky abdominal pain, pelvic pain, hematochezia, and tenesmus. Symptomatic management involves the use of urinary analgesics, antispasmodics, anti-emetics, bulking agents, low residue diets, and steroid suppositories. In the long term, radia-tion complications can include refractory proctitis, sigmoiditis, rectovaginal fistula, vesicovaginal fistula, small bowel obstruction, or vaginal stenosis. Management of these complications is generally surgical and can involve separately, or in combination, bowel resection, bowel bypass, colostomy formation, urinary diversion, and vaginal reconstruction.

Radiation-induced second cancers are a justifiable concern with patients undergoing primary or adjuvant radiation therapy. Patients treated with radiation therapy for cervical cancer are at increased relative risk (RR) 10 years or more after treatment for bladder (RR 2.8), rectal (RR 1.7), and genital cancers other than those of the uterus or ovary (RR 3.1). These risks increase with age. At 30 years or more following treatment, the cancer RR is 8.5, 4.1, and 4.8 for the respective organs. The risk for uterine and ovarian cancer also increases with age following pelvic irradiation.

Conclusion

Gynecologic cancers continue to represent a significant source of morbidity and suffering for the women of the world. Though we have become more proficient in the management of these disease processes, true breakthroughs in terms of reducing the mortality associated with these cancers must arise from two specific areas. First,

---

Box 28.1 Summary – endometrial and cervical cancer

- Endometrial and cervical cancer are highly curable gynecologic malignancies if detected early and managed appropriately.
- Abnormal vaginal bleeding (menorrhagia, postcoital spotting, or postmenopausal bleeding) is the primary presenting symptom for both endometrial cancer as well as cervical cancer.
- 75% of endometrial cancers occur in postmenopausal women (average age at diagnosis 58). It is the most curable of all gynecologic neoplasms.
- Surgery is the primary therapy for the management of endometrial cancer; occasionally adjuvant radiation therapy is prescribed for those patients felt at high risk for recurrence following surgical "staging."
- Palliative therapy for incurable endometrial cancer can include surgery (to decrease vaginal bleeding or pain), chemotherapy (adriamycin and cisplatin), and/or radiation therapy (to decrease vaginal bleeding, pain, and improve local tumor control).
- The average age for diagnosis for cervical cancer is 40 years of age.
- Radiation therapy can be used to manage all stages of cervical cancer; curative surgical management is limited to early stage disease only (stage I).
- Palliative therapy for incurable cervical cancer can include surgery (to divert fistula formation, to bypass bowel obstruction, to bypass ureteral obstruction), chemotherapy (cisplatin), and/or radiation therapy (to decrease vaginal bleeding and/or pain). Unrealistic patient expectations should be avoided, in that they tend to increase, rather than alleviate, suffering.

we need to stress the significance of early detection. Patients must be made to appreciate the necessity for routine screening tests, such as cervical cytology, and the possibility such tests hold for early detection of potentially lethal disease. Patients need to be educated about the warning signs for these disease processes and the need to seek immediate medical care if such signs arise.

Second, only through the advent of novel biologic and immune therapies will we begin to impact in any significant way on the survival in that unfortunate group of patients who continue to present with advanced or recurrent gynecologic malignancy. Research in gene therapy, vaccine therapy, and other immunotherapies is making huge leaps, and one can but eagerly await the future promise such new therapies may hold for women who continue to struggle with gynecologic malignancies.

BIBLIOGRAPHY

Sentinel articles

Boice JD, Day NE, Andersen A. Second cancers following radiation treatment for cervical cancer: an international collaboration among cancer registries. *J Natl Cancer Inst* 1985;74:955.

Boronow RC, Morrow CP, Creaseman WT. Surgical staging in endometrial cancer: clinicopathologic findings of a prospective study. *Obstet Gynecol* 1984;63:825.

Burke TW, Stringer CA, Morris M. Prospective treatment of advanced or recurrent endometrial carcinoma with cisplatin, doxorubicin, and cyclophosphamide. *Gynecol Oncol* 1991;40:264.

Creaseman WT, Morrow CP, Bundy BN. Surgical pathologic spread patterns of endometrial cancer: a gynecologic oncology group study. *Cancer* 1987;60:2035.

Montana GS, Martz KL, Hanks GE. Patterns and sites of failure in cervix cancer treated in the USA in 1978. *Int J Radiat Oncol Biol Phys* 1991;20:87.

Morris M, Eifel PJ, Lu J et al. Pelvic radiation with concurrent chemotherapy compared with pelvic and para-aortic radiation for high risk cervical cancer. *N Engl J Med* 1999;340:1137–43.

Thigpen T, Brady M, Homesley HD, Soper JT, Bell J. Tamoxifen in the treatment of advanced or recurrent endometrial cancer: a gynecological oncology group study. *J Clin Oncol* 2001;19:364–7.

Review articles

Rose PG. Endometrial carcinoma. *N Engl J Med* 1996;335:640–9.

Stoler M. Human papillomaviruses and cervical neoplasia: a model for carcinogenesis. *Int J Gynecol Pathol* 2000;19:16–28.

Thomas GM. Improved treatment for cervical cancer – concurrent chemotherapy and radiotherapy. *N Engl J Med* 1999;340:1198–9.

Tinga DJ, Beentjes JA, Van de Wiel HB. Detection, prevalence and prognosis of asymptomatic carcinoma of the cervix. *Obstet Gynecol* 1990;76:860.

29

Testicular cancer

David B. Solit[1] and Pamela N. Munster[2]

[1] Memorial Sloan–Kettering Cancer Center, New York
[2] Lee Moffitt Cancer Center, Tampa

Germ cell tumors (GCT) of the testis are the most common cancers of young men 15–35 years of age. Although relatively uncommon overall, their incidence has doubled over the past 40 years. Since the introduction of platinum-based combination regimens, the majority of patients with this disease are now cured.

Natural history

The majority (> 90%) of GCTs arise in the testis. Less common primary sites include the mediastinum, retroperitoneum, and the pineal/suprasellar region. Cryptorchism (the incomplete descent of one or both testes) is a well-defined risk factor for the development of this disease and the surgical correction of this problem (orchiopexy) performed prior to puberty reduces the risk for tumor development. Additional well-defined risk factors include a prior history of GCT and genetic syndromes including Klinefelter's and Down's syndromes.

Germ cell tumors can be divided by histologic type into seminomas (30%) and nonseminomatous germ cell tumors (NSGCT). Nonseminoma tumors may include any combination of the embryonal, endodermal sinus, choriocarcinoma, and teratoma histologies. A seminomatous component may also be present. The serum tumor markers human chorionic gonadotropin (HCG) and alpha-fetoprotein (AFP) are often elevated in patients with either nonseminoma or seminoma, though elevated AFP is found only in patients with NSGCT and confirms the presence of a nonseminomatous component.

Pattern of spread and recurrence

The classic presentation of a testicular GCT is a painless scrotal mass though this finding occurs in only a minority of patients. Rather, the majority present with testicular pain or swelling that may be difficult to distinguish from epididymitis and/or orchitis, and a trial of antibiotics may be warranted in these patients. A testicular ultrasound should be performed in all patients with persistent symptoms or a palpable mass following antibiotics. More advanced disease may present with lower back pain due to retroperitoneal metastasis or gynecomastia resulting from HCG secretion. Initial evaluation should include a testicular ultrasound and serum tumor markers. Over 95% of testicular masses are malignant and testicular biopsy is not recommended prior to orchiectomy. Radical inguinal orchiectomy with high ligation of the spermatic cord is the preferred procedure to confirm the diagnosis. Trans-scrotal orchiectomy or biopsy should not be performed as this approach disrupts the normal vascular and lymphatic drainage of the testis and may promote scrotal skin and lymph node metastasis.

Staging is based upon the level of serum tumor markers and extent of disease. The beta-subunit of HCG (B-HCG), AFP and serum lactate dehydrogenase (LDH) are all incorporated into the American Joint Committee on Cancer staging system and should be obtained. GCTs have a relatively predictable pattern of spread from the testicle to retroperitoneal lymph nodes to visceral sites (only 10% metastasize to distant sites without lymph node involvement). Lymph node metastases follow the pattern of venous drainage with right testicular tumors most commonly metastasizing to the inter-aortocaval lymph nodes and left-sided tumors to the para-aortic lymph nodes. Staging evaluation should therefore include a computed tomography (CT) scan and chest x-ray to evaluate for lymph node and pulmonary spread. Stage I disease includes tumors limited to the testis, stage II disease dissemination to retroperitoneal lymph nodes, and stage III disease, patients with distant spread to supradiaphragmatic nodes or visceral sites.

Therapeutic approaches

Initial treatment for GCT is guided by tumor histology and stage at diagnosis.

Stage I NSGCT

All patients with testicular GCTs should initially be treated by high inguinal orchiectomy. Patients with disease confined to the testis and normal tumor markers following surgery, are managed by either nerve-sparing retroperitoneal lymph node dissection (RPLND) or surveillance. The rationale for RPLND is based upon the predictable pattern of spread seen in patients with this tumor histology (testis to retroperitoneal lymph nodes to distant sites). Surveillance is typically offered to patients with T1 disease (i.e., no lymphatic or vascular invasion and no extension to the tunica, spermatic cord, or scrotum) who are predicted to be compliant with follow-up. Though no randomized study has compared surveillance to RPLND in this population, large retrospective trials suggest equivalent results with cure rates exceeding 95% with either approach. Patients with lymphatic or vascular invasion or local tumor extension have a higher risk of clinically silent stage II disease and typically undergo RPLND.

Stage II NSGCT

Primary RPLND is indicated for patients with lymph node metastases less than 3 cm in size. In patients with low-volume disease (less than 6 nodes involved, all less than 2 cm in diameter) and normal tumor markers following RPLND no further therapy is indicated. Patients with more extensive disease at the time of RPLND benefit from adjuvant chemotherapy. Persistently elevated serum markers following RPLND indicate residual tumor and these patients should be treated with systemic chemotherapy. In patients with pelvic or retroperitoneal lymph nodes greater than 3 cm in diameter and in those with an extragonadal primary site, initial therapy is systemic chemotherapy.

Stage III NSGCT

Independent predictors of survival in patients with disseminated GCT include not only extent of disease and the level of serum tumor markers at diagnosis but also tumor histology and primary tumor site. The International Germ Cell Cancer Collaborative Group has incorporated these pretreatment factors into a prognostic factor-based staging system for patients with disseminated disease. The goal of this and other earlier classification systems was to define a subgroup of patients with "good risk" disease in which less intensive, less toxic regimens could be identified that retain the high cure rate (~90%) achieved with earlier cisplatin-based combination regimens. Novel or more intensive regimens would be directed at poor-risk patients with disseminated disease, who have only a 40–60% cure rate following standard first-line therapy. The results of several multi-institutional randomized trials have identified two regimens, three cycles of BEP chemotherapy (bleomycin, etoposide, cisplatin) or four cycles of EP (etoposide, cisplatin), as standard approaches in the good risk population with each regimen achieving ~90% cure. In the poor risk subgroup, only half achieve a complete response with the standard four cycles of BEP. Therefore, patients with poor-risk disease are encouraged to participate in ongoing clinical trials of newer conventional dose and high-dose combination regimens.

Surgical resection should be considered an integral component of treatment in patients with persistent radiographic disease and normal serum tumor-markers following chemotherapy. Surgery may reveal the presence of necrotic debris, viable tumor or mature teratoma. In patients with histologically confirmed viable tumor, two additional cycles of chemotherapy are indicated. Resection of mature teratoma is necessary as it may grow rapidly precluding later resection or undergo malignant transformation.

Stage I seminoma

Fifteen to twenty percent of patients with stage I seminoma that receive no adjuvant therapy following orchiectomy will recur. Seminomas are exquisitely sensitive to radiation therapy and standard treatment for early-stage patients incorporates prophylactic radiation therapy to the retroperitoneal and ipsilateral pelvic lymph nodes. As the morbidity of radiation therapy in this setting is low, surveillance of patients without radiation therapy is not advisable.

Stage II seminoma

Radiation therapy alone is an option for patients with low-volume disease (defined as all lymph nodes < 5 cm in size). Patients with a greater disease burden should receive good-risk platinum-based combination chemotherapy as defined above for patients with NSGCT (i.e., BEP $\times$ 3 or EP $\times$ 4).

Stage III seminoma

Patients with disseminated disease are treated with systemic chemotherapy (BEP $\times$ 3 or EP $\times$ 4). If residual masses (> 3 cm in size) are present following therapy surgical resection should be considered.

Site-specific rehabilitation issues

Following conventional dose chemotherapy, 20–30% of patients will have persistent long-term side effects though these may not impair quality of life. Infertility is common in patients treated for GCT. RPLND may result in retrograde ejaculation and chemotherapy and radiation therapy are commonly associated with azoospermia or oligospermia. Sperm banking should therefore be considered for all patients with GCT prior to RPLND, chemotherapy, or radiotherapy. No increase in the rate of fetal malformations has been noted in offspring of men treated for GCT.

Patients treated for GCT are also at increased risk for second malignancies; 1–2% will develop a second primary GCT. Secondary leukemias and myelodysplastic syndromes have been associated with both radiotherapy and chemotherapy (particularly etoposide), while excess solid tumor malignancies appear to be confined to patients treated with radiotherapy. Long-term organ toxicities from chemotherapy are primarily attributable to cisplatin and include renal insufficiency, ototoxicity, and neurotoxicity. Carboplatin was evaluated as a less-toxic alternative in this setting but was associated with an unacceptable increase in disease recurrence. Long-term sequelae of bleomycin-induced pulmonary toxicity are rare.

Site-specific palliative care issues

Patients with stage I NSGCT and normal tumor markers following orchiectomy are managed by either RPLND or surveillance. Disease recurrence will occur in approximately 25% of the patients who choose observation alone. The high cure rates (~95%) achieved in this population, are therefore predicated upon careful surveillance to ensure that salvage therapy is initiated early, when the likelihood for cure is greatest. Patients should be monitored closely with serum tumor markers, chest x-ray and abdominopelvic computed tomography (CT) scans repeated every 3 months for the first 2 years. The majority of recurrences will occur within 2 years and the interval between follow-up evaluations can be gradually lengthened thereafter. In patients with more advanced disease treated with systemic chemotherapy, follow-up evaluation should include serum marker measurements and chest x-ray at 1-month intervals for the first year, at 2-month intervals for the second year, with increasing intervals thereafter. As late recurrences and second primary tumors do occur, patients with GCT should receive life-long follow-up.

Between 20–30% of patients with metastatic disease do not achieve a durable complete response following initial cisplatin-based chemotherapy. These patients are treated with salvage regimens that typically entail greater toxicity. The likelihood that conventional dose second-line chemotherapy will result in a durable complete response and cure is influenced by the patients' response to first-line therapy, the location of the primary tumor site, and the extent of disease and level of serum marker elevation at the time of recurrence. Ifosfamide, vinblastine, and paclitaxel have activity as second-line therapy and in appropriately selected populations, favorable response rates as high as 80% have been reported with ifosfamide-based second-line combination regimens. Patients who have had an incomplete response to cisplatin and etoposide with or without bleomycin should be considered for intensive-dose chemotherapy with stem cell support as initial second-line therapy. Fewer than half of patients with relapsed extragonadal nonseminomatous tumors achieve a complete response following conventional or dose-intensive salvage chemotherapy. Novel approaches will be needed for this population and for patients with chemorefractory disease.

BIBLIOGRAPHY

Sentinel articles

Bajorin DF, Sarosdy MF, Pfister DG et al. Randomized trial of etoposide and cisplatin versus etoposide and carboplatin in patients with good-risk germ cell tumors: a multiinstitutional study. *J Clin Oncol* 1993;11:598–606.

Bosl GJ, Geller NL, Bajorin D et al. A randomized trial of etoposide + cisplatin versus vinblastine + bleomycin + cisplatin + cyclophosphamide + dactinomycin in patients with good-prognosis germ cell tumors. *J Clin Oncol* 1988;6:1231–8.

Broun ER, Nichols CR, Kneebone P et al. Long-term outcome of patients with relapsed and refractory germ cell tumors treated with high dose chemotherapy and autologous bone marrow rescue. *Ann Intern Med* 1992;117:124–8.

Einhorn LH, Donohue J. Cis-diaminedichloroplatinum, vinblastine, and bleomycin combination chemotherapy in disseminated testicular cancer. *Ann Intern Med* 1977;87:293–8.

Einhorn LH, Williams SD, Troner M, Birch R, Greco FA. The role of maintenance therapy in disseminated testicular cancer. *N Engl J Med* 1981;305:727–31.

Einhorn LH, Williams SD, Loehrer PJ et al. Evaluation of optimal duration of chemotherapy in favorable-prognosis disseminated germ cell tumors: a Southeastern Cancer Study Group protocol. *J Clin Oncol* 1989;7:387–91.

Herr HW, Sheinfield J, Puc HS et al. Surgery for a post-chemotherapy residual mass in seminoma. *J Urol* 1997;157:860–2.

Horwich A, Sleijfer DT, Fossa SD et al. Randomized trial of bleomycin, etoposide, and cisplatin compared with bleomycin, etoposide and carboplatin in good-prognosis metastatic nonseminomatous germ cell cancer: a multiinstitutional Medical Research Council/European Organization for Research and Treatment of Cancer trial. *J Clin Oncol* 1997;15:1844–52.

International Germ Cell Cancer Collaborative Group. International Germ Cell Consensus Classification: a prognostic factor-based staging system for metastatic germ cell cancers. *J Clin Oncol* 1997;15:594–603.

Loehrer PJ, Johnson D, Elson P, Einhorn LH, Trump D. The importance of bleomycin in favorable prognosis disseminated germ cell tumors: an Eastern Cooperative Oncology Group trial. *J Clin Oncol* 1995;12:470–6.

Loehrer PJ, Gonin R, Nichols CR, Weathers T, Einhorn LH. Vinblastine plus ifosfamide plus cisplatin as initial salvage therapy in recurrent germ cell tumor. *J Clin Oncol* 1998;16:2500–4.

Motzer RJ, Mazumdar M, Sheinfeld J et al. Sequential dose-intensive paclitaxel, ifosfamide, carboplatin, and etoposide salvage therapy for germ cell tumor patients. *J Clin Oncol* 2000;18:1173–80.

Motzer RJ, Sheinfeld J, Mazumdar M et al. Paclitaxel, ifosfamide, and cisplatin second-line therapy for patients with relapsed testicular germ cell cancer. *J Clin Oncol* 2000;18:2413–18.

National Comprehensive Cancer Network. NCCN practice guidelines for testicular cancer. *Oncology* 1998;12:417–62.

Nichols CR, Williams SD, Loehrer PJ et al. Randomized study of cisplatin dose intensity in poor-risk germ cell tumors: a Southeastern Cancer Study Group and Southwest Oncology Group protocol. *J Clin Oncol* 1991;9:1163–72.

Warde P, Gospodarowicz MK, Panzarella T et al. Stage I testicular seminoma: results of adjuvant irradiation and surveillance. *J Clin Oncol* 1995;13:2255–62.

Williams SD, Birch R, Einhorn LH, Irwin L, Greco FA, Loehrer PJ. Treatment of disseminated germ-cell tumors with cisplatin, bleomycin, and either vinblastine or etoposide. *N Engl J Med* 1987;316:1435–40.

Review articles

Bosl GJ. Germ cell tumor clinical trials in North America. *Semin Surg Oncol* 1999;17:257–62.

Bosl GJ, Motzer RJ. Testicular germ-cell cancer. *N Engl J Med* 1997;337:242–53.

Einhorn EH. Testicular cancer: an oncological success story. *Clin Cancer Res* 1997;3:2630–2.

Einhorn LH, Donohue JP. Advanced testicular cancer: update for urologists. *J Urol* 1998;160:1964–9.

Kollmannsberger C, Kuzcyk M, Mayer F, Hartmann JT, Kanz L, Bokemeyer C. Late toxicity following curative treatment of testicular cancer. *Semin Surg Oncol* 1999;17:275–81.

Travis LB, Curtis RE, Storm H et al. Risk of second malignant neoplasms among long-term survivors of testicular cancer. *J Natl Cancer Inst* 1997;89:1429–39.

Internet sites

The Association of Cancer Online resources
www.acor.org/TCRC/

Memorial Sloan–Kettering Cancer Center
http://www.mskcc.org/patients_n_public/about_cancer_and_treatment/cancer_information_by_type/testicular_cancer/index.html

The National Cancer Institute
http://cancer.gov/cancer_information/cancer_type/testicular

People Living with Cancer (ASCO web site)
www.plwc.org

30

Unknown primary site cancer

Renato Lenzi

U.T. M.D. Anderson Cancer Center, Houston

Introduction

Patients with cancer of an unknown primary site present the healthcare professional with many challenges. Managing the problems related to the advanced stage of their condition is difficult and the unresolved diagnosis confronts patients, their families, and their caregivers with an added level of uncertainty. In this chapter, we review the natural history, the diagnostic evaluation, patterns of disease spread, treatment, and palliative care issues related to the management of patients with cancer of an unknown primary site.

Definition and natural history

Cancer of an unknown primary site (CUP) is defined as a pathologically proven malignancy in the absence of a known site of origin after an adequate diagnostic work-up. Cancers with a specific histology that portend a specific treatment, such as lymphomas, melanoma, and sarcomas, are not considered cancers of an unknown primary site, even if the area in the body where they originated cannot be determined.

The incidence of CUP has been estimated at between 0.5% and 7% of all patients with invasive cancer in the US.

Unlike that of most patients who present with an obvious primary tumor, the natural history of patients with CUP does not display an ordinate sequence of events: Progression from the original site to neighboring anatomical structures, regional lymph nodes, and distant metastatic sites is usually not apparent. The diagnosis of CUP is based on the absence of a known site of origin of the cancer and therefore requires a painstaking exclusion of all possible primary sites. This process begins with a careful review of the biopsy material.

Initial morphologic microscopic evaluation (i.e., hematoxylin-eosin staining) will identify most patients with nonepithelial malignancies and will differentiate specific epithelial malignancies that can be diagnosed by morphologic appearance (e.g., well-differentiated hepatocellular carcinoma) from the more common epithelial neoplasms with a non-site-specific morphologic appearance. Usually a diagnosis of adenocarcinoma, carcinoma (including poorly differentiated carcinoma), squamous cell carcinoma, neuroendocrine carcinoma, or a poorly differentiated malignant neoplasm will be made at this stage. Most patients (approximately 60%) will be found to have adenocarcinoma histology. For these patients, further pathologic evaluation is often of limited value. Conversely, patients presenting with poorly differentiated carcinoma or with a poorly differentiated malignant neoplasm require additional studies to further refine the pathologic diagnosis. In those patients, immunohistochemistry, electron microscopy, and genetic and molecular studies may yield a diagnosis of lymphoma, a germ cell tumor, melanoma, or sarcoma. Commonly used immunohistochemical markers include cytokeratins (positive in epithelial cancers), common leukocyte antigen (positive in lymphomas and negative in epithelial cancers), chromogranin and synaptophysin (positive in neuroendocrine tumors), prostate-specific antigen (PSA) (prostate cancer, salivary gland carcinomas), S-100, HMB-45 (melanoma), thyroglobulin (follicular thyroid carcinoma), calcitonin (medullary thyroid carcinoma), β-human chorionic gonadotropin (β-HCG) (choriocarcinoma and germ cell tumors), and alpha-fetoprotein (germ cell tumors and hepatocellular carcinoma). Electron microscopy may be very helpful in selected instances: The presence of cell junctions will rule out lymphomas and leukemias; amelanotic melanoma can be diagnosed if premelanosomes are detected; microvilli projecting into acinar spaces will be diagnostic of an adenocarcinoma; mitochondrial morphology may point to an adrenal cortical carcinoma; large cell lymphomas can often be identified by their ultrastructural characteristics.

Molecular studies of unknown primary tumors have shown altered expression of HER-2-neu, p53, and ras, but at this time the clinical and diagnostic relevance of these findings is unclear. Chromosomal analysis has linked abnormalities of chromosome 12 to germ cell tumors. Comparative genomic hybridization analysis of paraffin-embedded biopsy material that shows a gain of 12p material, identifies the germ cell origin of a morphologically unclassifiable carcinoma. The presence of Epstein–Barr genomic material has been used to diagnose primary nasopharyngeal carcinoma. Advances in our ability to study multiple gene expression may in the future contribute substantially to the molecular identification of the primary site and result in a decrease in the number of patients diagnosed with unknown primary malignancies.

In addition to the pathologic evaluation, the initial diagnostic work-up of patients referred with suspected CUP includes a medical history and a physical examination including breast and pelvic examinations for women and rectal and prostate examinations for men. The initial laboratory evaluation includes a complete blood cell count, a blood chemistry profile, and a PSA test for men. Imaging studies should include a chest radiography, a computed tomographic (CT) scan of abdomen and pelvis, and a mammogram for women. Clues obtained from the history and physical examination and abnormalities detected in these baseline studies should be followed by appropriate additional tests. This "complete" diagnostic work-up will yield a diagnosis of a specific primary cancer in approximately 20% of patients with suspected CUP. The remaining patients will be diagnosed with metastatic cancer of an unknown primary site.

Patterns of metastatic spread at presentation

Several patterns of metastatic spread at presentation have been recognized and are of considerable therapeutic and prognostic significance.

Women with metastatic axillary node carcinoma or adenocarcinoma

These women should be carefully evaluated for a primary breast cancer. Biopsy material needs to be studied for estrogen and progesterone receptors. If no additional sites of disease are identified, the patients should be treated as if they had stage II breast cancer, including local treatment by axillary dissection, mastectomy, or radiation therapy and adjuvant chemotherapy. Women with distant metastatic disease in addition to metastasis in axillary nodes have been shown to have a survival comparable to that of women with stage IV breast cancer, and should be treated accordingly.

Women with peritoneal carcinomatosis

Carcinomatous involvement of the peritoneal cavity in women can be secondary to cancer spread from an ovarian or extraovarian müllerian primary, a gastrointestinal primary (e.g., pancreas, colon, stomach, cholangiocarcinoma), or a breast primary. In many of these women no primary tumor can be demonstrated. Certain features may be suggestive of a müllerian origin of the cancer including serous papillary carcinoma histology, the presence of psammoma bodies, and elevation of CA-125. Metastatic extraperitoneal disease is often absent, although sometimes pleural effusion is noted. Several investigators have reported high rates of response to debulking surgery and platinum-based chemotherapy, with a response rate of 68% and a survival of 15 months in a recent study.

Patients with squamous cell carcinoma metastatic to high and mid-neck nodes

Patients presenting with this pattern of metastatic spread of squamous cell carcinoma are considered to harbor a primary squamous cell carcinoma of the head and neck. Their diagnostic evaluation includes a computed tomographic scan or magnetic resonance imaging of the head and neck and an endoscopic evaluation of the upper aerodigestive tract that includes the head and neck with biopsy of all potentially involved areas. If the primary site is not identified despite such evaluation, patients are treated with surgery followed by radiation therapy. Disease-specific survival rates at 2, 5, and 10 years in a recent retrospective series were 82%, 74%, and 68% respectively. Microsatellite analysis of biopsy material in a small series of patients with this presentation suggests that the primary tumor may arise clonally in mucosal areas that appear histopathologically benign but that harbor neoplastic cells genetically related to the metastatic lesions. Patients with adenocarcinoma involving neck nodes have a poorer prognosis. Patients with squamous cell carcinoma involving lower cervical or supraclavicular nodes also have a poorer prognosis and should be carefully evaluated for primary lung cancer by computerized axial tomographic scan of the chest and by bronchoscopy.

Patients with squamous cell carcinoma metastases to inguinal nodes

These patients usually have regional metastatic spread from a primary tumor in the anus, urethra, cervix, vagina, vulva, penis, or scrotum. It is essential to proceed with meticulous evaluations of the above areas, since some of those primaries are amenable to curative treatment despite the presence of nodal metastases. Treatment most commonly involves surgery and radiation therapy with or without chemotherapy.

Men with mediastinal and/or retroperitoneal involvement

This subgroup of patients is characterized by a pattern of midline chest and/or abdominal involvement, often accompanied by a marked elevation of alpha-fetoprotein and β-HCG levels and age < 50 years. The histology is typically poorly differentiated carcinoma. The importance of this pattern of metastatic disease is that it identifies a subgroup of patients who may have germ cell cancer, which is very responsive to platinum-based chemotherapy. In the absence of the other clinical features described, poorly differentiated carcinoma histology is not associated with prolonged survival.

Prognosis

In a series of 1109 consecutive patients with cancer of an unknown primary site the overall median duration of survival was 11 months. Several factors associated with prognosis have been identified. Favorable prognostic factors include female gender, lymph node involvement (with the exception that the presence of supraclavicular lymph node involvement may represent an unfavorable prognostic factor), and a lower number of metastatic sites (a metastatic site is defined as each organ involved by metastasis regardless of the total number of metastatic lesions). Patients with

CUP as a group have a worse prognosis as the number of metastatic sites increases from one to two to three or more. In that series, the median duration of survival for patients with one site of metastatic disease was 14 months, for patients with two disease sites 11 months, and for those with three or more sites 8 months. Histology also had a bearing on survival: patients with adenocarcinoma had a mean survival duration of 9 months; patients with carcinoma, 12 months; patients with poorly differentiated carcinoma, 13 months; patients with squamous cell carcinoma, 24 months and patients with neuroendocrine carcinoma, 53 months.

Therapeutic approaches

Most patients with cancer of an unknown primary site do not belong to the subgroups previously described in the section on patterns of spread. These patients are treated most frequently with systemic chemotherapy. Radiation therapy is often indicated, commonly for palliation of metastatic lesions in the bone and brain. Surgery is usually reserved for patients with resectable single-site or isolated metastatic lesions (bone, brain, lymph nodes) and may prevent life-threatening or potentially incapacitating complications (bowel obstruction, pathologic fractures of weight-bearing bones). Several chemotherapy regimens have been used for the treatment of patients with CUP, usually including the most active drugs available for the treatment of the most common primary cancers at the time that studies were conducted. Presently, the standard for treatment of CUP is a regimen of paclitaxel, carboplatin, and etoposide. While longer survival has been described among certain patients with poorly differentiated carcinoma – the median survival of complete responders was approximately 3 years in one study – the remarkable response rates achieved with the more recent taxane-based chemotherapy regimens have, unfortunately, not translated into an increased survival expectation for most patients. For example, while a recent study using carboplatin, paclitaxel, and etoposide chemotherapy has shown an overall response rate of 48% with 15% complete responses, the median duration of survival remained only 11 months. No established salvage treatment has been identified as the standard to be given in the event of lack of response or progression after the initial chemotherapy regimen. Gemcitabine has recently been studied in previously treated patients, with an observed response rate of approximately 10% and a favorable impact on quality of life.

Rehabilitation issues

A successful approach to the rehabilitation of patients with CUP needs to recognize the great heterogeneity of these patients' needs. The most diverse subgroup of patients are probably those with isolated metastatic lesions, which includes patients with isolated axillary node involvement, patients with brain lesions, and patients with neck node involvement. The rehabilitation needs of these patients are similar to the needs of patients with primary breast, brain, and head and neck cancers. Patients presenting with metastatic bone disease of the spine, pelvis, or extremities will require specific care to address difficulties with function including weight bearing and ambulation, and to maximize recovery after radiation therapy or surgical treatment. Therapeutic exercises and devices such as braces and walking aids, in combination with pain management, are often necessary to address the needs of these patients. Assessment of neuropsychological impairment and neuro-rehabilitation are frequently needed in patients with metastatic brain disease. Most patients will be treated with combination chemotherapy and will be in need of chemotherapy rehabilitation.

Palliative care issues

Issues related to the palliative care of patients with metastatic cancer of an unknown primary site are also complex, as expected given the wide spectrum of clinical presentations in these patients. Although being diagnosed with any type of cancer has been shown to be associated with increased uncertainty and difficulty in psychosocial adjustment, no systematic investigation of the psychosocial adjustment of or the levels of distress experienced by patients with cancer of an unknown primary site has been published. Typically, all recommendations for the treatment and prognosis of patients with cancer are based on the accurate diagnosis of the primary cancer and on careful staging. Patients with CUP may feel uncomfortable about the physician's inability to make a more precise diagnosis and may have the sense that their work-up has been incomplete. Yet, it is clear from the literature that additional diagnostic tests beyond those that comprise a "complete" set have a very low diagnostic yield in these patients, and most of them will ultimately be treated without the knowledge of the specific site of origin for their metastatic disease. While data from studies focusing on the specific psychosocial adjustment problems of patients with CUP are necessary to devise specific interventions, these patients should be provided with the reassurance that although the primary site is not known, treatment is possible and guidelines and information adequate to rationally develop a therapeutic strategy are available. These patients may suffer from clinically significant anxiety and depression, which often go unrecognized in patients with cancer and need to be appropriately evaluated and treated.

Data on the incidence of pain in this patient population have not been systematically collected, but the incidence is probably significant, given the fact that patients with CUP present at an advanced stage of disease, which in other types of cancer has been shown to correlate with pain incidence. Somatic, visceral, and neuropathic pain are common, as would be expected given the distribution of metastatic lesions. In a review of 1000 consecutive patients with carcinoma of an unknown primary site, the main metastatic sites were lymph nodes, 418 (42%); liver, 331 (33%); bone, 289 (29%); lung, 263 (26%); pleura, 112 (11%); peritoneum, 90 (9%); brain, 64 (6%); adrenal, 60 (6%); skin, 38 (4%); and bone marrow, 34 (3%). The drugs used and the pain-management techniques and procedures involved in the care of these patients encompass the whole spectrum of the available pain-control armamentarium. The choice of the preferred palliative approach should factor in the patient's expected duration of survival, performance status, and comorbidities. If of equivalent efficacy, the less invasive approach should generally be preferred in this patient population. However, while for many patients with metastatic disease progress in the understanding of the pathophysiology and clinical aspects of the metastatic process have resulted in the development of sophisticated and effective conservative treatment strategies, in certain patients preservation or restoration of function are best achieved by an invasive approach, and the presence of metastatic disease should not be regarded as an absolute contraindication to a major surgical procedure.

Conclusion

The management of patients with cancer of an unknown primary site is complex and requires a well-integrated multidisciplinary approach if optimal care is to be delivered. Much is known regarding the preferred diagnostic and treatment approaches to CUP, however this diagnosis still presents a significant management challenge for all the health professionals involved in the care of these patients.

The application of more sophisticated molecular diagnostic techniques will hopefully progressively lower the number of patients who cannot be diagnosed with a specific primary. Additional research on the palliative care needs of patients with carcinoma of an unknown primary site is necessary to better define and quantify those needs and to continue to develop effective therapeutic approaches.

BIBLIOGRAPHY

Sentinel articles

Abbruzzese JL, Abbruzzese MC, Hess KR, Raber MN, Lenzi R, Frost P. Unknown primary carcinoma: natural history and prognostic factors in 657 consecutive patients. *J Clin Oncol* 1994;12:1272–80.

Califano J, Westra WH, Koch W et al. Unknown primary head and neck squamous cell carcinoma: molecular identification of the site of origin. *J Natl Cancer Inst* 1999;91:599–604.

Greco FA, Hainsworth JD. One-hour paclitaxel, carboplatin, and extended-schedule etoposide in the treatment of carcinoma of unknown primary site. *Semin Oncol* 1997;24(Suppl. 19):S19-101–5.

Hainsworth JD, Wright EP, Johnson DH, Davis BW, Greco FA. Poorly differentiated carcinoma of unknown primary site: clinical usefulness of immunoperoxidase staining. *J Clin Oncol* 1991;9:1931–8.

Motzer RJ, Rodriguez E, Reuter VE, Bosl GJ, Mazumdar M, Chaganti RS. Molecular and cytogenetic studies in the diagnosis of patients with poorly differentiated carcinomas of unknown primary site. *J Clin Oncol* 1995;13:274–82.

Richardson RL, Schoumacher RA, Fer MF et al. The unrecognized extragonadal germ cell cancer syndrome. *Ann Intern Med* 1981;94:181–6.

Review articles

Abbruzzese JL, Lenzi R, Raber MN. Carcinoma of unknown primary. In *Clinical Oncology*, ed. MD Abeloff et al. Philadelphia: Churchill Livingstone, 2000.

Greco FA, Hainsworth JD, Cancer of unknown primary site. In *Cancer. Principles and Practice of Oncology*, 6th edn, ed. VT DeVita, SH Hellman, SA Rosenberg. Philadelphia: Lippincott Williams & Wilkins, 2001.

Internet sites

http://www.cancer.gov/cancer_information/cancer_type/carcinoma_of_unknown_primary

31

Mesothelioma

Ralph Zinner

U.T. M.D. Anderson Cancer Center, Houston

Malignant mesothelioma is a deadly disease with a median survival of 6–15 months in affected patients. It is diagnosed in 2000–3000 Americans per year. There is not yet a well-validated effective treatment for any stage of the disease. It is derived from cells lining serosal surfaces including the pleura, pericardium, peritoneum, and rarely the tunica vaginalis, which is embryonically derived from the peritoneum. About 80% of mesotheliomas arise from the pleura, the focus of this chapter.

There are three main pathologic types of malignant mesotheliomas: epithelioid, mixed/biphasic, and sarcomatoid. Patients with the epithelioid type, the most common (50–70%) have the best prognosis.

Mesotheliomas typically occur in people over 40 years of age; the median age at diagnosis is 60. The male:female ratio is 5:1 which reflects the occupational exposure to asbestos, the most important risk factor. Indeed, asbestos exposure is found in 50–80% of patients though the percentage may be higher since even brief exposure may result in mesothelioma and the latency period averages 20–50 years. Considering this long latency and the fact that stiffer regulations to limit asbestos exposure to prevent mesothelioma were instituted only in the early 1970s, the incidence is expected to peak in 2010. Tobacco use is not a risk factor.

Most patients with mesothelioma present with shortness of breath (80%) and/or nonpleuritic chest pain or discomfort (50–60%), often many months in duration. Other symptoms include malaise, coughing, and sweats. Presenting signs include weight loss and fever. Physical examination findings at diagnosis may be unremarkable except for dullness to percussion and decreased breath sounds at the affected hemithorax.

Mesothelioma usually progresses locally. Symptomatic metastases are less common. The tumor often invades local structures, including the lung parenchyma, chest wall, mediastinum, and diaphragm. In late disease, the tumor encases the hemithorax. On exam, there can be decreased chest wall excursion on the affected side. Increasing contraction of the chest wall contributes to shortness of breath.

Dyspnea may appear out of proportion to the radiographic findings which can be explained by shunting of blood through the poorly ventilated lung. In 10–20% of patients, palpable soft tissue masses develop in the chest wall when the tumor extends into the intercostal spaces through a thoracentesis or thoracotomy incision. These can be prevented with local radiation therapy. Less commonly, involvement of the esophagus, vertebrae, nerves, and blood vessels leads to dysphagia, paralysis, numbness, and superior vena cava syndrome, respectively. Obvious ascites may be present and indicates metastatic disease. Any symptomatic distant metastases usually occur late. Hematogenous metastases are most often found postmortem. The most common sites are brain, bone, and liver. Patients most often die of respiratory failure or pneumonia.

Mesothelioma shows a variable and nonspecific radiographic appearance. Often, the only finding at presentation is a large pleural effusion. Subpleural thickening or small pleural masses may be seen on computed tomography (CT) scans. As the disease progresses, these pleural-based masses become more evident and effusions become multiloculated. With further progression, a thick irregular pleural rind develops, encasing the lung and obliterating the pleural space. With more advanced disease a CT scan finding of a frozen thorax with a shift of the mediastinum towards the effusion can be seen. This is in contrast to the behavior of most other effusions. Additionally, in locally advanced disease, there can be mediastinal adenopathy and direct extension of the tumor into local structures such as the pericardium (with pericardial effusion), the chest wall, or the diaphragm. Though CT scanning is the most accurate noninvasive way to stage disease, it is limited in its ability to assess the depth of chest wall invasion or extension through the diaphragm. Magnetic resonance imaging (MRI) is useful for determining chest wall invasion when planning for surgery. Distant metastases are typically late findings. Since most patients present with a pleural effusion, thoracentesis is usually the initial diagnostic procedure. However, it reveals malignancy only 26% of the time. Thoracoscopy is more accurate, showing tumor in 98% of cases. When the pleural space is obliterated by locally advanced tumor, an open pleural biopsy may become necessary to reach a diagnosis. Bronchoscopy does not provide a diagnosis of mesothelioma since results are uniformly normal, although it can be used to rule out a primary lung cancer.

The International Mesothelioma Interest Group (IMIG) tumor, nodes, metastases (TNM) system is the standard staging system. The extent of the primary tumor, the number and types of lymph nodes involved by disease, and the presence of distant metastases are used to determine the stage of disease. This staging system as a predictor of outcome is tentative until prospective clinical study results confirm its accuracy. Other indicators of poor prognosis include nonepithelioid histology, age less than 55, chest pain at diagnosis, poor performance status, weight loss, age greater than 75 years, elevated platelet count, and fewer than 6 months between symptom onset and diagnosis.

There is no standard treatment of mesothelioma. Surgery, radiation therapy, and chemotherapy have been minimally effective in controlling this disease when used as single modalities, though each can be palliative. Since mesothelioma is a relatively rare disease it makes it difficult to demonstrate a survival benefit for any treatment.

Though malignant mesothelioma is most often clinically localized to one hemithorax, surgery rarely removes all visible gross disease. Even when all gross disease is removed, relapse occurs soon, with the 5-year survival rate approaching 0%. Besides the three mentioned above, there are several palliative procedures. For example, large pleural effusions can be relieved by thoracenteses or placement of a permanent drain, though the latter poses a risk of disease growth through the tracts and is therefore not generally recommended. These can be done as outpatient procedures. In pleurodesis, talc or another sclerosing agent can be introduced through a chest tube to induce fibrosis between the parietal and visceral pleurae, causing them to adhere limiting the size of the effusion. This is often an inpatient procedure. Other surgical methods such as pleurectomy and extrapleural pneumonectomy are rarely indicated as single modalities.

Radiation therapy as a single modality can palliate loci of painful invasive disease. However, since mesothelioma diffusely involves the pleura, including the interlobar pleura, to eradicate disease, the entire hemithorax needs to be encompassed in the radiation ports. When the entire lung is irradiated at doses sufficient to eradicate disease, severe fibrosis develops diffusely which results in intolerable shunting.

Chemotherapy is minimally active against mesothelioma; no drug consistently shows response rates greater than 20%. Chemotherapy provides symptomatic relief in some patients. However, combination chemotherapy has not yet proved to be superior to single-agent chemotherapy. Larger studies now under way comparing chemotherapy with best supportive care will clarify whether chemotherapy improves survival. However, at present, supportive care without direct treatment of the cancer is still considered one of the standard options. This is not recommended since there is a need to identify effective treatment through clinical trials in order to improve the outcome for these patients.

Surgery, radiation therapy, and chemotherapy are also being developed as multimodality regimens. Trimodality regimens have shown some promising survival results. The idea behind this approach is that the limitations of any given modality may be overcome by combining them. For example, radiation-induced shunting can be prevented if the lung is removed first using extrapleural pneumonectomy. Likewise, the microscopic disease inevitably remaining after surgery may be sterilized by radiation. On the other hand, chemotherapy given simultaneously with radiation therapy may increase radiation-induced tumor-cell kill by radiosensitizing the tumor tissue. Chemotherapy may also destroy micrometastic disease or at least delay the onset of clinically significant metastatic disease. Triple modality regimens have shown some promise, though the impressive survival seen may in large part result not so much from the treatment but rather from selection of very fit patients who have superior prognoses. No combined modality regimen is known to lead to a long-term cure. Indeed, few patients survive beyond 4 years.

At present, antimesothelioma therapy is largely palliative. Although there is preliminary evidence of some modest survival advantage from triple modality regimens, mesothelioma remains incurable. If currently available therapies can be proven to prolong survival in randomized trials, their use may become standard. However, at best these survival advantages will be quite limited. Therefore, patients should be readily referred for clinical trials to develop better regimens while they can still tolerate therapy. In this postgenomic era in which multiple molecular-targeted therapies are under development, we can look forward with guarded optimism to substantial improvements in the care of these patients.

BIBLIOGRAPHY

Sentinel articles

Bissett D, Macbeth FR, Cram I. The role of palliative radiotherapy in malignant mesothelioma. *Clin Oncol* (*R Coll Radiologists*) 1991;3:315–17.

[This study shows radiation can offer transient relief from chest pain caused by invasion of the chest wall by mesothelioma.]

Butchart EG, Ashcroft T, Barnsley WC et al. Pleuropneumonectomy in the management of diffuse malignant mesothelioma of the pleura: experience with 29 patients. *Thorax* 1976;31:15–24.

[This is an early staging system presently superseded by the TNM staging system below.]

Byrne MJ, Davidson JA, Musk AW et al. Cisplatin and gemcitabine for malignant mesothelioma: a phase II study. *J Clin Oncol* 1999;17:25–30.

[This study showed an excellent response rate and good palliation in responding patients to cisplatin and gemcitabine chemotherapy. These results will need to be confirmed in future trials.]

International Mesothelioma Interest Group. A proposed new international TNM staging system for malignant pleural mesothelioma. *Chest* 1995;108:1122–8.

[Unlike the Butchart staging system, the TNM staging system includes nodal status. It shows nodal status has predictive value in patients treated with surgery. However this system, which was developed through retrospective study, requires validation through prospective studies.]

Middleton GW, Smith IE, O'Brien ME et al. Good symptom relief with palliative MVP (mitomycin-C, vinblastine, and cisplatin) chemotherapy in malignant mesothelioma. *Ann Oncol* 1998;9:269–73.

[This study demonstrates improved symptom control using chemotherapy even in some patients who had no tumor shrinkage seen on radiographs.]

Sugarbaker DJ, Strauss GM, Lynch TJ et al. Node status has prognostic significance in the multi-modality therapy of diffuse, malignant mesothelioma. *J Clin Oncol* 1993;11:1172–8.

Sugarbaker DJ, Flores RM, Jaklitsch MT. Resection margins, extrapleural nodal status, and cell type determine postoperative long-term survival in trimodality therapy of malignant pleural mesothelioma: results in 183 patients. *J Thorac Cardiovasc Surg* 1999;117:54–63.

[Sugarbaker shows good survival using a trimodality regimen consisting of extrapleural pneu-monectomy followed by chemotherapy and radiation therapy. Additionally, information about the predictive value of staging and pathology are described. However, since patients who are able to tolerate this full regimen may have a better prognosis irrespective of therapy type, the contribution of trimodality therapy to outcome will require further study.]

Wagner JC, Sleggs CA, Marchand P. Diffuse pleural mesothelioma and asbestos exposure in the North Western Cape Province. *Br J Ind Med* 1960;17:260–71.

[This is the first study to show a strong link between asbestos exposure and the development of mesothelioma.]

Review articles

Bass P, Schouwink H, Zoetmulder FAN. Malignant pleural mesothelioma. *Ann Oncol* 1998; 9:139–49.

[This is an excellent general review of malignant mesothelioma.]

Kindler HL. *Curr Treat Options Oncol* 2000;1:313–26.

[This is an up-to-date general review with special emphasis on chemotherapy.]

Ong ST, Vogelzang NJ. Chemotherapy in malignant pleural mesothelioma: a review. *J Clin Oncol* 1996;14:1007–17.

[This is a comprehensive review of chemotherapy for malignant mesothelioma.]

Internet sites

Malignant mesothelioma, National Cancer Institute
http://cancer.gov/cancer_information/cancer_type/malignant_mesothelioma
Center Watch (Clinical Trials Listing Service)
http://www.centerwatch.com/patient/studies/CAT192.html

32

Adult soft tissue sarcoma

Alan Sandler and Laura McClure-Barnes

The Vanderbilt Clinic, Vanderbilt University, Nashville

Incidence and demographics

Soft tissue sarcomas are tumors of mesenchymal origin that include muscle, cartilage, endothelium, and supporting structures. They are extremely rare and represent only 1% of all adult malignancies. The incidence is 1.5 per 100 000 population or 8000 new cases per year in the US. The incidence and mortality of soft tissue sarcomas in the US has not changed in the last 10 years. There is a slight male predominance of 1.1:1.0. The majority of adult soft tissue sarcomas occur in patients 50 years or older (51.8%), while 20% occur in patients 40–60 years old and 20% occur in patients less than 40 years old. They can arise anywhere in the body including the viscera, breast, vascular, and genitourinary system. Approximately 50% occur in the extremities, 40% in the trunk and retroperitoneum, and 10% in the head and neck.

Etiology

The etiology of soft tissue sarcoma is unknown. Multiple genetic and environmental factors have been implicated and studied. Specific genetic syndromes that are associated with increased risk of developing soft tissue sarcomas include neurofibromatosis, familial polyposis, Gardner's syndrome and Li–Fraumeni syndrome. Recognized associations exist between sarcoma and radiation exposure. Approximately 5% of newly diagnosed sarcomas are associated with a history of prior radiation. Patients who have undergone previous radiation therapy are at increased risk of developing sarcomas in the field of radiation exposure. The latency period between exposure and development of sarcoma is typically greater than 10 years. Most radiation-associated sarcomas are osteosarcomas but soft tissue sarcomas also occur. Patients with a past history of retinoblastoma or Ewing's sarcoma have a higher risk of developing secondary sarcoma after radiation exposure.

Patients having undergone prior lymphadenectomy with chronic edema are also at increased risk of a sarcoma developing in the affected extremity as well as patients with chronic lymphedema from peripheral vascular disease. This is associated with lymphangiosarcoma. Immunosuppression due to medications or illness such as AIDS, chronic lymphocytic leukemia, or autoimmune diseases is also associated with an increased incidence of soft tissue sarcoma.

Histopathology

Multiple different histological subtypes of soft tissue sarcomas exist due to the wide spectrum of tissue from mesenchymal origin. They are classified according to the mesenchymal tissue they most closely resemble. There are at least 30 different histological subtypes of soft tissue sarcomas. The most common subtype of soft tissue sarcoma is liposarcoma (18%), followed by malignant fibrous histiocytoma, and fibrosarcoma. As tumors become less differentiated, the assignment of a distinct histological subtype becomes more difficult. Comparative studies of pathological review frequently demonstrate poor concordance of histopathological diagnosis. Assignment of a histological subtype is less important with soft tissue sarcomas because mortality and risk of metastasis is based on tumor size and grade. Tumor grade is based on several parameters including the amount of tissue necrosis, vascularity, mitotic activity, and cellularity. They are divided into low, intermediate, or high-grade tumors based on these parameters.

Clinical presentation

Symptoms are based on the location of the tumor. Extremity tumors usually present with a palpable mass. This generally causes patients to present to the physician early. The symptoms are usually related to compression of surrounding structures and may include lymphedema and paresthesias. Only one-third of patients will have pain or swelling at the tumor site. Many patients will give a history of prior trauma to the site but a causal relationship between sarcoma and trauma has not been established.

Retroperitoneal and visceral sarcomas may present with vague symptoms including abdominal pain, early satiety, nausea, and paresthesias. Significant weight loss only occurs in 15% of patients at the time of diagnosis. Due to these nonspecific symptoms, a longer delay occurs before diagnosis and patients present with later stage disease.

Pattern of spread

Soft tissue sarcomas of the extremity spread locally along fascial planes. Fewer than 5% of tumors will invade blood vessels and nerves. Lymph node metastases are rare but may occur in 10% of rhabdomyosarcoma and synovial cell sarcoma subtypes. Distant spread of extremity sarcomas occurs hematogenously with lung being the primary site of metastases. Retroperitoneal sarcomas will spread into the peritoneal cavity and metastasize to the liver. Metastatic disease may also occur hematogenously to bone, subcutaneous tissues, and the central nervous system as disease progresses.

Staging/prognosis

Sarcomas are generally given a stage based on the American Joint Committee on Cancer Staging. The overall stage considers histologic grade, tumor size, regional node involvement, and the presence of distant metastases. The staging criteria will not be reviewed here. The most important prognostic indicators for patients with soft tissue sarcoma are histologic grade and tumor size. Patients with a high-grade tumor or a tumor larger than 5 cm have a poorer overall prognosis. Age older than 60 years is also associated with a poorer prognosis. Inadequate surgical margins, limb-sparing surgery for extremity sarcomas and high histological grade are prognostic factors that increase the risk of local recurrence. The 5-year survival rates based upon stage are as follows: stage I 70–90%; stage II 55–70%; stage III 20–50%; and stage IV 4–20%.

Therapeutic options

Complete surgical excision remains the cornerstone of effective therapy. Adjuvant therapy with radiation and chemotherapy also play a role. Surgical excision for well-differentiated extremity tumors less than 5 cm is generally curative. In patients with narrow or involved surgical margins, radiation therapy is utilized to decrease the risk of local recurrence. Systemic chemotherapy provides no survival advantage in patients with stage I and II disease. High-grade and large (> 5 cm) sarcomas (stage II and III) are treated with a multimodality approach involving a limb-sparing surgical technique with either pre- or postoperative radiation or amputation. This provides better local control of tumor.

Complete resection of retroperitoneal sarcomas is difficult and often impossible. Radiation delivery to the retroperitoneum also causes significant toxicity to the visceral organs causing dose limitations. These difficulties lead to a higher loco-regional failure and overall lower 5-year survival. Sarcomas of the head and neck are also subject to high (50%) loco-regional failures after surgical resection due to difficulty in obtaining adequate surgical margins.

Systemic chemotherapy has been utilized in patients with stage II–III sarcomas in the adjuvant setting. The drugs with the most activity include doxorubicin, ifosfamide, and dacarbazine. Individual trials of chemotherapy in the adjuvant setting have given mixed results, however, meta-analysis has shown an improvement in recurrence-free survival with a trend toward overall survival in patients with extremity sarcomas.

Local recurrence

The treatment of locally recurrent disease is with surgical re-resection if this can be achieved with low morbidity. Adjuvant radiotherapy may be considered in patients who are candidates for re-resection of local recurrence.

Metastasis disease

Even when control of the primary tumor can be achieved, approximately 50% of patients will die of metastatic or locally advanced disease. The median survival at the time of recognized metastatic disease is only 8–12 months but 25% of patients will be alive 2 years after diagnosis of metastatic disease. Patients are often asymptomatic when metastatic disease is found radiographically. Surgical resection may be an option for selected patients with pulmonary recurrence. Patients with isolated pulmonary metastases may be appropriate candidates for surgical resection if adequate control of the primary tumor has been achieved and they have a low number of metastatic lesions. The 5-year survival for patients undergoing metastectomy with up to five pulmonary metastases is 25%. Patients with a long disease-free interval have a better prognosis. There are studies suggesting a limited number of patients may benefit from repeat metastectomy. The subsets of patients with metastatic sarcoma with the highest response rate to anthracycline-based therapy are those with high-grade lesions, younger age, and absence of liver metastases.

BIBLIOGRAPHY

American Joint Committee on Cancer, American College of Surgeons. *AJCC Staging Handbook*. Philadelphia: Lippincott-Raven, 1998.

Brennan MF, Casper ES, Harrison LB. Soft tissue sarcoma. In *Cancer: Principles and Practices of Oncology*, 5th edn, ed. VT Devita Jr., S Hellman, SH Rosenburg, pp. 1738–88. Philadelphia: Lippincott-Raven 1997.

Enzinger FM. *Soft Tissue Tumors*, 2nd edn. Washington, DC: CV Mosby, 1988.

Sarcoma Meta-analysis Collaboration. Adjuvant chemotherapy for localized resectable soft-tissue sarcoma of adults; meta-analysis of individual data. *Lancet* 1997;350:1647–54.

Internet site

http://www.cancer.gov/cancer_information/cancer_type/soft_tissue_sarcoma

33

Osteosarcoma and Ewing's sarcoma

Sharon Soule and David Seitz

Indiana Cancer Pavilion, Indianapolis

Ewing's sarcoma

Background

Ewing's sarcoma is a poorly differentiated tumor derived from a primitive neuro-ectodermal cell. It occurs most commonly within bones, but may also be seen in extraosseus locations. There are approximately 2.1 cases of Ewing's sarcoma per 1 million Caucasian children under 15 years of age in the US. The disease is extremely rare in African–American and Asian children. Seventy percent of all patients with Ewing's sarcoma are under 20 years of age. The peak incidence of Ewing's sarcoma is in females from 11 to 12 years of age and males from 15 to 16 years of age. Seventy percent of patients with localized disease treated with multimodality therapy will be alive 5 years after treatment. In contrast, the 5-year event-free survival for patients with metastatic disease is only 25%.

Diagnosis

The most common presenting symptoms of Ewing's sarcoma are pain and localized swelling at the site of disease. The pain is initially intermittent but later progresses to constant pain that typically wakes the patient at night. Patients may also present with systemic symptoms such as weight loss and fever. The erythrocyte sedimentation rate is commonly elevated. Three percent of patients will be diagnosed because of paraplegia. Ewing's sarcoma is frequently mistaken for osteomyelitis as both diseases cause similar initial symptoms. Patients with such symptoms should therefore be questioned about recent dental procedures, as actinomycosis of the bone can be radiographically and clinically similar to Ewing's sarcoma.

The most common primary sites of Ewing's sarcoma are distal extremity (27%), proximal extremity (25%), pelvis (20%), and chest (20%). Spine and skull primary sites are rare (9%). Physical examination should include close inspection and palpation of the skull to detect primary, but more importantly metastatic lesions.

Ewing's sarcoma lesions originate in the diaphysis of the bone, then extend toward the metaphysis. The radiologic appearance is of a lytic or a mixed sclerotic/lytic lesion with parallel, lamellated new bone formation. This is often described as an "onionskin" appearance on x-ray.

Metastases are present in 30% of patients at the time of diagnosis. When metastases are present, 50% occur in the lungs and 25% occur in other bones, bone marrow, or vertebrae. Central nervous system metastases are extremely rare. Approximately one-third of patients with metastatic disease can be cured with multimodality therapy.

There is no definite staging system for Ewing's sarcoma; disease is usually defined as localized versus metastatic. Staging work-up should include computed tomography (CT) or magnetic resonance imaging (MRI) of the involved lesion, radionuclide bone scan, chest CT, serum sedimentation rate (ESR) and lactate dehydrogenase (LDH), and bone marrow biopsy. Consultation with an orthopedic surgeon with experience in bone tumors prior to diagnosis is imperative as an improper incisional biopsy can significantly complicate subsequent tumor resection.

Prognosis

The most powerful prognostic factor for subsequent disease recurrence is the presence of metastatic disease at diagnosis. Those patients with only lung metastases experience a higher survival rate than do patients with bone metastases. Patients under 15 years of age at diagnosis and those with nonaxial primary sites of disease also have a statistically significant improvement in overall survival. Other poor prognostic factors include tumor diameter greater than 8 cm, tumor volume greater than 100 ml and elevated serum LDH. Pathologic response to chemotherapy is a powerful predictor of overall survival. Patients whose tumor is completely necrotic at the time of surgery have a 95% 5-year survival rate, compared with 68% survival in patients with a microscopic focus of viable tumor at the time of surgery.

Treatment

Treatment for localized Ewing's sarcoma typically involves 9–15 weeks of initial chemotherapy followed by local control measures. After high-dose radiotherapy or surgery, chemotherapy is continued, usually for a total of 48 weeks. Chemotherapy is recommended for all patients, regardless of tumor size, location, or disease stage; only 10% of patients will be cured with surgical resection alone. Chemotherapy regimens usually consist of vincristine, doxorubicin, cytoxan, and/or actinomycin alternating with ifosfamide and etoposide. A randomized study showed a 37% difference in 5-year survival when dactinomycin was added to vincristine, doxorubicin, and cytoxan. Another randomized study done by the CCG/POG cooperative group showed that the addition of etoposide and ifosfamide to the chemotherapy regimen significantly improved event-free and overall survival.

Local control in Ewing's sarcoma may be achieved with either high-dose radiation therapy to the lesion or surgical resection. There have been no randomized trials comparing surgery versus radiation therapy for local control; such a trial would be extremely difficult. Central lesions are treated with radiation therapy alone as resection is often difficult. Most radiotherapy trials in Ewing's sarcoma have delivered 4500–5500 cGy to the tumor, followed by a boost of 1000 cGy to the surrounding tissues. Extremity tumors may be treated with either radiation or surgical resection. The decision of treatment modality is tempered by the observation of second bone tumors in the irradiated field in 10–30% of patients receiving primary radiotherapy 20 years after treatment. The incidence of secondary tumors following radiotherapy is greater in Ewing's sarcoma than in osteosarcoma. Radiation therapy may benefit patients with gross residual tumor or positive margins after surgery.

Patients rendered disease-free after treatment should have a physical examination and chest x-ray every 2–3 months for the first 2 years. When appropriate, an MRI of the involved area every 6 months is recommended. After the first 2 years, the interval of such examinations should be increased.

Patients with metastatic Ewing's sarcoma at the time of diagnosis have a much poorer prognosis than patients with localized disease. However, cure of the disease is still attainable in these patients. Two Pediatric Intergroup Ewing's sarcoma studies included combination chemotherapy with vincristine, adriamycin, cytoxan, and dactinomycin, with or without 5-FU, as well as radiation to the primary tumor and all sites of metastatic disease. Surgical resection of the primary tumor was allowed when possible if all metastatic disease had been eradicated. Thirty percent of patients on these studies were alive at 5 years after treatment. Surgical resection of metastatic pulmonary lesions has not been shown to improve overall survival. However, whole lung radiation of Ewing's sarcoma patients with pulmonary metastases has been shown to improve overall outcome. The addition of ifosfamide and etoposide to the chemotherapy regimen for patients with metastatic disease has not been shown to improve survival, but it is a reasonable treatment option in patients with relapsed disease who did not previously receive these drugs.

The role of high-dose chemotherapy followed by stem cell rescue in metastatic or high-risk Ewing's sarcoma is still unclear. One study involving 20 patients with metastatic disease, centralized tumor location, or high tumor volume received treatment with myeloablative chemoradiotherapy and autologous stem cell rescue in first complete remission. The 3-year overall survival rate was 65% in these patients. Studies involving high-dose chemotherapy for patients with metastatic disease at diagnosis are conflicting with regard to efficacy; two studies showed an impressive event-free survival, while another showed no advantage over standard therapy.

Osteosarcoma

Background

Osteosarcoma is the most common primary malignant bone tumor. It occurs predominantly in children and young adults. It is a relatively rare tumor, with 21 cases diagnosed per million people per year. There are approximately 900 new cases per year in the US. It is also a very treatable disease; approximately 75% of patients are cured. Osteosarcoma occurs more commonly in males than in females, and there is a bimodal age distribution, with peaks at 20 and 60 years of age. Of patients over 40 years of age who are affected, most have a pre-existing condition that increases the risk of disease. These conditions include prior exposure to radium, postmastectomy or lumpectomy radiation therapy, and Paget's disease of the bone.

Eighty-five percent of osteosarcomas originate in the distal femur, proximal tibia, or proximal humerus. Involvement of the axial skeleton is rare. Twenty-five percent of patients have metastatic disease at the time of diagnosis. There are eleven histologic variants of osteosarcoma which have varying clinical courses.

Diagnosis

Osteosarcoma typically presents as a firm soft tissue mass that may be tender to palpation and is fixed to the underlying bone. The skin overlying the lesion is often stretched and shiny with prominent vascular markings. Occasionally patients will present with symptoms related to metastatic lesions such as cough, shortness of breath, or pain at the site of a bony metastasis. The pain is usually initially intermittent and therefore is often dismissed as "growing pains." Radiologic findings vary and may include increased intramedullary radiodensity, an area of radiolucency, a pattern of permeative destruction with poorly defined borders, cortical destruction, or periosteal elevation and extraosseous extension. This may be described as a "sunburst" appearance on x-ray. Serum alkaline phosphatase will be elevated in 45–60% of patients at diagnosis.

Patients with osteosarcoma are staged as either localized or metastatic disease. Imaging should include x-rays of the affected bone, followed by a CT or MRI of the lesion. Patients should also have a chest CT at diagnosis to evaluate for pulmonary metastases. A baseline angiogram may help with future surgical decisions. Imaging of any other symptomatic bones should be obtained as well.

As in Ewing's sarcoma of the bone, biopsy of the affected lesion should be performed only after consultation with an orthopedic surgeon and a pathologist who are experienced in the diagnosis of bone tumors. The incision tract must be removed at the time of surgery to avoid seeding with tumor cells. Therefore, an incorrectly placed incisional biopsy could leave the patient ineligible for limb-salvage surgery or could increase the chance of local tumor recurrence.

Prognosis

Although prognostic factors are not usually utilized to guide therapy, they do provide important information for patients. One variable that has been shown to correlate with survival is the extent of tumor necrosis and tumor size following neoadjuvant chemotherapy. In addition, the expression of P-glycoprotein by the tumor, which is independent of tumor response to chemotherapy, is associated with a significantly decreased rate of event-free survival. Axial tumor locations also correlate with a decreased overall survival rate. Tumor size at diagnosis and patient age do not affect the overall prognosis.

Treatment

Two randomized trials done in the 1980s showed a significant improvement in overall and event-free survival ($< 20\%$ to 66%) for patients who received adjuvant multi-agent chemotherapy compared with those who received no chemotherapy. Chemotherapy should include doxorubicin and cisplatin. Other agents, such as high-dose methotrexate, bleomycin, cyclophosphamide, and actinomycin-D, are frequently added to such regimens, but their utility has not been rigorously proven.

Preoperative chemotherapy is now standard in most patients, although it has not been definitively shown to improve survival. However, the advantages of preoperative chemotherapy include an increased likelihood of limb-sparing surgery as well as important prognostic information regarding postchemotherapy tumor necrosis. This treatment should involve two to six cycles of at least two of the following drugs: doxorubicin, cisplatin, ifosfamide, and high-dose methotrexate with leucovorin rescue. Chemotherapy may be given intravenously or intra-arterially; there are few randomized trials comparing the two methods of administration. Patients with a good pathologic response to preoperative chemotherapy should receive several postoperative courses with the same agents. Patients with a poor response to preoperative chemotherapy should be treated with different drugs.

Surgery should involve an en-bloc dissection with wide margins. There is no difference in overall survival between patients treated with limb-preserving surgery or amputation. Limb preservation should be performed when it is feasible to achieve adequate surgical margins. After preoperative chemotherapy, limb preservation is possible in nearly 85% of patients. There is no improvement in local recurrence rate or survival when radiation therapy is used in osteosarcoma patients, even in those with close or positive surgical margins.

Relapses after therapy commonly occur in the first 2 years following treatment. Patients with metastatic pulmonary lesions should undergo surgical resection, especially if there are five or fewer lesions. Prognosis is better for patients with unilateral pulmonary lesions compared with bilateral disease. Patients who present initially with metastatic disease should have resection at the time of primary tumor resection when possible. Further chemotherapy for patients with unresectable recurrent or metastatic disease is dictated by performance status, prior chemotherapy, and patient wishes. Referral to a specialized center for consideration for a clinical trial is a reasonable option as well.

The majority of patients with incurable Ewing's sarcoma and osteosarcoma will eventually succumb to respiratory failure due to metastatic disease. The sensation of dyspnea may improve with measures such as positioning, oxygen therapy, and relaxation techniques. However, patients with severe dyspnea due to terminal cancer will experience significant relief with narcotic treatment. Narcotics work by several actions: Altered perception of breathlessness, reduced respiratory drive, and reduced oxygen consumption.

REFERENCES

Sentinel articles

Cangir A, Vietti TJ, Gehan EA et al. Ewing's sarcoma metastatic at diagnosis. *Cancer* 1990;66: 887–93.

Eilber F, Giuliano A, Eckardt J, Patterson S, Moseley S, Goodnight J. Adjuvant chemotherapy for osteosarcoma: a randomized prospective trial. *J Clin Oncol* 1987;5:21–6.

Link M, Goorin AM, Miser AW et al. The effect of adjuvant chemotherapy on relapse-free survival in patients with osteosarcoma of the extremity. *N Engl J Med* 1986;314:1600–6.

Link M, Goorin AM, Horowitz M et al. Adjuvant chemotherapy of high-grade osteosarcoma of the extremity: updated results of the Multi-Institutional Osteosarcoma Study. *Clin Orthoped* 1991;270:8–14.

Rosito P, Mancini AF, Rondelli R et al. Italian Cooperative Study for the treatment of children and young adults with localized Ewing's sarcoma of bone: a preliminary report of 6 years of experience. *Cancer* 1999;86:421–8.

Review articles

Grier H. The Ewing family of tumors: Ewing's sarcoma and primitive neuroectodermal tumors. *Pediatr Clin N Am* 1997;44:991–1004.

Jaffe N, Shreyaskumar RP, Benjamin RS. Chemotherapy in osteosarcoma. *Hematol Oncol Clin N Am* 1995;9:825–39.

Picci P, Ferrari S, Bacci G, et al. Treatment recommendations for osteosarcoma and adult soft tissue sarcomas. *Drugs* 1994;47:82–92.

Yasko A, Johnson M. Surgical management of primary bone sarcomas. *Hematol Oncol Clin N Am* 1995;9:719–31.

Internet site

www.cancer.gov

34

Melanoma

Mark Harries[1] and Tim Eisen[2]

[1] The Royal Marsden Hospital, Sutton
[2] University College London, London

Introduction

Melanoma is the eighth most common cancer in the US, accounting for 3% of cancers. In women it is increasing worldwide at a rate exceeding all other cancers except lung cancer. It has now become the leading cause of cancer mortality in the US for women aged 25–29 years.

The outlook for patients with advanced melanoma has traditionally been pessimistic. Indeed, despite recent advances in the understanding of its biology and immunology, patients whose tumor has spread beyond the primary site generally have a poor prognosis. However, as shall be discussed in this chapter, there is considerable palliative benefit to be gained from the appropriate use of surgery, chemotherapy, and radiotherapy. In addition, for the patient with advanced disease, the judicious use of these conventional modalities may lead to worthwhile disease-free survival. Newer treatments such as biochemotherapy and immunotherapy have also been widely tested in this setting and occasionally have resulted in the long-term survival of a small group of patients with advanced disease.

It is clear that patients with advanced melanoma should be managed in a multidisciplinary setting. In few other cancers is the involvement of such a range of specialists and professions as important. Primary care physicians, dermatologists, surgeons, medical oncologists, radiation oncologists, palliative care physicians, and clinical nurse specialists will all often be concerned with a patient at some time during the course of their disease.

Background

Natural history

Melanoma is a malignant tumor of melanocytes. Most lesions arise from the skin, although tumors may also occur on mucosal surfaces or in other sites. Rarely, melanoma may arise within the eye; uveal melanoma is particularly resistant to most treatment modalities. Melanoma most commonly occurs in adults, and in women arises most frequently in the extremities whereas in men it is more frequently found on the trunk or head and neck.

Predisposition

Like other skin cancers, melanoma is most common in white-skinned populations and especially amongst people with the fairest skins (having a so-called Celtic complexion) living in sunny climates. Seventy-five percent of melanomas occur on exposed sites, and the poor ability of skin to tan and exposure to sun have long been recognized as important factors in the development of the disease. More recently, it has been felt that it is the type of sun exposure rather than cumulative exposure that is important, with especially blistering sunburns in childhood predisposing to melanoma in later life. Other risk factors include the presence of greater than 10 dysplastic nevi or 100 common nevi.

Genetic studies in families with a high incidence of melanoma have identified a melanoma predisposing gene, CDKN2A/p16 that is located on chromosome 9. Germ line mutations or deletions in this gene occur in such families, which represent 8–10% of all melanoma cases. In sporadic melanomas, 25–40% of all lesions have mutations or deletions that functionally silence the CDKN2A/p16 gene.

Prognosis

The prognosis of the disease depends principally on the depth of the primary lesion (microstage) and the presence of involved lymph nodes and distant metastases (clinical stage). A number of staging systems exist but they all reflect these two most important parameters. The commonly used American Joint Committee on Cancer staging system has recently been updated to take account of sentinel lymph node biopsy techniques to detect micrometastatic disease (Table 34.1). For the purposes of this chapter, advanced disease is taken as stages III and IV. Stage III melanoma, implying the presence of involved lymph nodes, carries a 5-year survival of 10% (if more than four lymph nodes are involved) to 46% (if one lymph node is involved). For patients with stage IV disease, with distant metastases, the median survival is just 7–8 months. This is in contrast to those patients who have no evidence of regional spread and whose tumors are less than 1.0 mm thick (stage I) who have a 5-year survival of 98%. In addition to stage, the volume of disease and serum lactate dehydrogenase (LDH) are independent prognostic factors.

Pattern of spread and recurrence

Melanoma can spread by local extension through the lymphatics to local and regional lymph nodes and/or by hematogenous routes to distant sites. Any organ may be involved by metastases, but the lungs and liver are common sites. In

Table 34.1. American Joint Committee on Cancer (AJCC) staging of melanoma

(*a*) TNM (Tumor, node, metastases)

Primary tumor (pT)

pTX	Primary tumor cannot be assessed
pT0	No evidence of primary tumor
pTis	Melanoma in situ
pT1	Tumor 1.0 mm or less in thickness, a: without ulceration and level II/III; b: with ulceration or level III/IV
pT2	Tumor more than 1.01 mm but less than 2.0 mm in thickness, a: without ulceration; b: with ulceration
pT3	Tumor more than 2.01 mm but not more than 4.0 mm in thickness, a: without ulceration; b: with ulceration
pT4	Tumor more than 4.01 mm in thickness, a: without ulceration; b: with ulceration

Lymph node (N)

NX	Regional lymph nodes cannot be assessed
N0	No regional lymph node metastases
N1	1 lymph node, a: micrometastasis; b: macrometastasis
N2	2–3 lymph nodes, a: micrometastasis; b: macrometastasis; c: in-transit met(s)/satellite(s) *without* metastatic lymph nodes
N3	4 or more lymph nodes, matted lymph nodes, or combinations of in-transit met(s)/satellite(s) or ulcerated melanoma *and* metastatic lymph nodes

Distant metastases (M)

MX	Presence of distant metastases cannot be assessed
M0	No distant metastases. Normal LDH
M1a	Distant metastases to skin, subcutaneous tissue or lymph nodes. Normal LDH
M1b	Lung metastases. Normal LDH
M1c	All other visceral or other distant metastases. Elevated LDH

Note: LDH, serum lactate dehydrogenase.

(*b*) Stage grouping

	Clinical staging				Pathological staging		
Stage	T	N	M	Stage	T	N	M
0	Tis	N0	M0	0	Tis	N0	M0
IA	T1a	N0	M0	IA	T1a	N0	M0
IB	T1b	N0	M0	IB	T1b	N0	M0
	T2a	N0	M0		T2a	N0	M0
IIA	T2b	N0	M0	IIA	T2b	N0	M0
	T3a	N0	M0		T3a	N0	M0
IIB	T3b	N0	M0	IIB	T3b	N0	M0
	T4a	N0	M0		T4a	N0	M0
IIC	T4b	N0	M0	IIC	T4b	N0	M0
IIIA	Any T	N1b	M0	IIIA	T1-4a	N1a	M0
IIIB	Any T	N2b	M0	IIIB	T1-4a	N1b	M0
					T1-4a	N2a	M0
IIIC	Any T	N2c	M0	IIIC	Any T	N2b-c	M0
	Any T	N3	M0		Any T	N3	M0
IV	Any T	Any N	M1-3	IV	Any T	Any N	M1-3

addition, the central nervous system and spine are not infrequently affected, often with devastating neurological consequences. Although the risk of relapse decreases over time, late relapses are not uncommon.

Staging investigations for patients with advanced disease

This pattern of spread largely dictates the staging investigations that are required for patients with advanced melanoma. For patients with thick (more than 1.0 mm) primary tumors or local recurrence our standard investigations include complete blood count (CBC), serum LDH, chest x-ray and an ultrasound of the abdomen (some centers will prefer a computed tomography (CT) scan of the thorax and abdomen). For patients with nodal disease our standard investigations include CBC, LDH and a CT scan of the thorax and abdomen. In addition, for patients in whom the inguinal nodes are involved the CT scan should include the pelvis. For patients with involved cervical nodes a magnetic resonance imaging (MRI) scan of the head and neck should also be performed.

For patients with evidence of metastatic disease, staging should include CBC, differential, liver function tests, LDH, creatinine, CT scan of thorax and abdomen (+/− pelvis) and an MRI of the brain (as this is more sensitive than a CT scan). The role of positron emission tomography (PET) scanning for metastatic melanoma remains unclear and is not currently recommended outside of a clinical trial. If symptoms dictate, then a bone scan and MRI scan of the whole spine should also be arranged. In this case it is important to image the whole spine as patients may have disease at multiple levels. In certain circumstances, for example when looking for extrahepatic duct dilatation, an ultrasound scan of liver may be preferred to a CT scan.

Therapeutic approaches for advanced disease

The management of a patient with advanced melanoma depends very much on the clinical situation, especially the condition of the patient and the site and volume of the disease. Different modalities of treatment all have important roles to play. Each will be discussed separately with indications, practical details, and the possible advantages and disadvantages of each approach.

Surgery

Surgery has an extremely important role in the management of locally advanced disease, loco-regional recurrence and metastatic disease. Indeed, surgery is the treatment modality of choice wherever possible.

Loco-regional disease

For a patient with clinically obvious nodal disease the primary management is adequate surgery of the primary site and lymph node dissection. It is important when undertaking surgery in a patient with stage III disease that the whole draining basin/s are dissected wherever possible.

Local recurrence

For the patient with locally recurrent disease, surgery is also extremely important. In this situation timely surgery offers the opportunity of achieving local control and occasional long-term remission.

Palliation and prevention of ulceration

Surgery can offer useful palliation for symptomatic disease almost wherever the site. For skin and subcutaneous deposits it should preferably be performed at an early stage to prevent the ulceration that is such a difficult feature of this disease to manage.

Metastatic disease

More aggressive surgery for metastatic disease is of particular benefit in those patients with long disease-free intervals (greater than 12 months) and who have one or two metastases only. Before embarking on metastectomy for asymptomatic disease it may be worth offering a "trial of time" with imaging being repeated after an interval of 6–12 weeks to ascertain that the disease is not moving into a rapidly progressive phase for which surgery would not confer any benefit.

Neurological disease

Surgery should also be considered for resectable brain metastases and metastatic disease causing cord or corda-equina compression.

Disadvantages of surgery

Melanoma can be a particularly vascular tumor and hemorrhage, poor wound healing, and infection can complicate surgery. Radical nodal dissections can be complicated by lymphedema in up to 10% of patients. Wherever possible, melanoma surgery should be carried out by a specialist surgical oncologist with the support of a plastic surgeon as appropriate.

Radiotherapy
Indications

Radiation therapy has a limited but important role in the palliative treatment of metastatic melanoma, particularly in the management of cerebral and vertebral metastases. In one retrospective study, patients with symptomatic and radiographic evidence of bone metastases showed a palliative response rate of 85%. For patients with symptomatic cord compression the overall palliation response rate for neurological symptoms was 71%. Melanoma is relatively radio-insensitive and therefore high-dose-per-fraction (often greater than or equal to 400 cGy) schedules are often employed. In addition, for some patients with mucosal disease for whom surgery is not feasible, radiotherapy may offer local control.

Disadvantages of radiotherapy

As well as the problem of lack of response, radiation causes toxicities including skin reactions, fatigue, and nausea and vomiting. In addition, the responses to radiotherapy are often short-lived.

Chemotherapy

Indications

For the patient with symptomatic, or soon to be symptomatic, unresectable disease at multiple sites, chemotherapy should be considered. Importantly however, chemotherapy should be reserved for patients with good performance status.

Choice of agent and schedule

Although many cytotoxic agents have been shown to have activity against metastatic melanoma, no single agent has been found to have a response rate of greater than 25%. Dacarbazine (DTIC) is probably the most active agent. There is a long list of other drugs with reported activity against melanoma including methotrexate, the platinums cisplatin and carboplatin, ifosfamide and other alkalating agents, the vinca alkaloids, the taxanes, the DTIC analog temozolamide, as well as carmustine (BCNU), fotomustine, and the other nitrosoureas. None of these has been shown to be more effective than DTIC. For patients with CNS disease, both temozolamide and fotomustine can cross the blood–brain barrier and can offer palliative benefit in a minority of patients.

DTIC is generally well tolerated but causes the side effects of nausea, vomiting (largely prevented when given with selective 5-HT$_3$ antagonists and dexamethasone) and myelosuppression. The usual dose is 800 mg/m^2 delivered every 21 days. Patients should be given two cycles of treatment before evaluation of the objective and symptomatic response. For responding patients, up to six cycles of DTIC are commonly given.

Even combinations of the most active drugs, with or without biological agents, have generally been disappointing; with durable 5-year responses being seen in only 1–2% of patients. However, such aggressive regimens should be considered for younger fitter patients in the context of clinical trials. Randomized trials have shown that there is no additional benefit of adding anti-estrogens such as tamoxifen to standard chemotherapy regimens.

Disadvantages of chemotherapy

As indicated above, the major disadvantages of chemotherapy are the poor response rates and the toxicities associated with treatment.

Immunotherapy

For a number of reasons much of the work in the field of tumor immunology and immunotherapy has focused on melanoma. It has long been recognized that melanoma has a particular propensity to induce an immune response. There have been many case reports of spontaneous tumor regressions occurring in patients with melanoma and when such regressing tumors have been biopsied marked lymphocytic infiltrates have been found. This has led to the suggestion that the lymphocytes were mediating tumour regression. Tumor regression has also been observed in a proportion of patients receiving immunotherapy. More recently, a number of the antigens expressed on melanoma cells and recognized by lymphocytes have been identified.

For many years the nonspecific stimulation of the immune system with microbial products such as bacille Calmette–Guérin (BCG) or *Corynebacterium parvum* has been tried in melanoma and although anecdotal responses have been reported no overall benefit has been seen in controlled trials. However, the identification and cloning of several cytokines was shortly followed by their trial in a number of cancers including melanoma. Of these cytokines, interleukin-2 (IL-2) and interferon-alpha (IFN-α) have been shown to have consistent antimelanoma activity and can now be included amongst the orthodox therapies for this disease.

Indications

Like chemotherapy, immunotherapy should again be reserved for fit patients with good performance status. Patients should have no evidence of CNS disease, as tumor responses to immunotherapy can be associated with edema. In addition, patients should have low tumor burdens and a low LDH as these are good indicators of the overall immunocompetence.

Systemic cytokines

IFN-α

The average response rate for IFN-α as a single agent against metastatic melanoma is 16%. In a meta-analysis examining data from 1164 patients treated with biochemotherapy, regimens containing IFN-α were found to have a higher response rate than those without (24% versus 17%). The observation was made in the original studies that some of these responses were durable in contrast to the short-lived responses seen with chemotherapy. The median duration of response, however, is still only approximately 4 months. Side effects include fever, myalgia, fatigue, and flu-like symptoms with up to 30% of patients being unable to tolerate treatment.

IL-2

Like the type I interferons, IL-2 has effects on a number of cells in the immune system and has been shown to have powerful antitumor effects in animal models. IL-2 has been investigated in human trials in a number of different cancers. In metastatic melanoma high dose IL-2 alone or in combination with tumor-infiltrating lymphocyte cells has a response rate of 15–20%. A number of the responses have been durable. When given systemically IL-2 can cause a number of severe side effects including hypotension, pulmonary edema, and renal failure.

Other cytokines and biochemotherapy

Tumor necrosis factor (TNF), IFN-γ, IL-4, IL-6, and IL-12 have all been shown to be disappointing as systemic agents in metastatic melanoma. There has been a lot of interest in combinations of cytotoxic drugs with biological agents. The cytokines most widely studied in this setting are IL-2 and IFN-α. It appears from published trials that the addition of interferon to chemotherapy confers little if any benefit. A large number of patients have been treated with IL-2 in combination with chemotherapy. Although the regimens have significant toxicities and require prolonged inpatient stay a recent report suggests the overall response rate from pooled trials is of the order of 50% with 10–20% complete responses, some of which have been durable. Therefore, for the fit patient the use of biochemotherapy regimens in the context of a clinical trial would seem a reasonable approach.

Vaccines

Vaccines for melanoma can be broadly divided into cellular and acellular approaches. In the latter category, the vaccination of patients with ganglioside analogs leading to the development of antiganglioside antibodies has been reported. In addition monoclonal antibodies specific for melanoma have also been tested. The peptides identified as melanoma-associated T-cell epitopes have been used, either alone or in combination with adjuvants, for the vaccination of patients with metastatic melanoma. In patients immunized with a single peptide, tumor regression followed by progression with a tumor that has lost the presenting HLA allele has been seen. Therefore investigators are looking at vaccination with combinations of peptides tailored to the haplotype of the patient.

A number of studies have examined the use of cellular vaccines for melanoma. These can broadly be divided into the adoptive transfer of cells of the immune system or the use of tumor-cell vaccines. Rosenberg's group has pioneered adoptive therapy for melanoma with tumor-infiltrating lymphocytes combined with IL-2.

Significant response rates, above those seen with IL-2 alone, have been reported (Rosenberg et al. 1994). It is now possible to isolate and expand peptide-specific high-avidity CTL clones but again panels of CTL clones, tailored to the individual patient, may be needed.

Unmodified allogeneic tumor, often in conjunction with an immunological adjuvant, has also been investigated as a vaccine for patients with melanoma. Morton and colleagues have vaccinated large numbers of patients with a mixture of allogeneic melanoma cell lines. They have reported increased survival and immune responses in some patients although no randomized trial of this vaccine has as yet been performed. Newer cellular vaccines include dendritic cells, dendritic cell-tumor cell fusions and modified tumor-cell vaccines. All these strategies remain very much in the experimental setting, but fit and willing patients should be considered for such studies.

Isolated limb perfusion

For patients with multiple sites of disease confined to an extremity regional hyperthermic perfusion with melphalan $+/-$ TNF-α can be considered. This treatment has been shown to offer palliative but not survival benefit in randomized studies and can be repeated.

Laser therapy and other local treatments

For the palliation of symptomatic melanoma deposits laser therapy can be considered, although this remains an experimental tool. For patients with large liver metastases local treatment with radiofrequency ablation or focused ultrasound can be considered.

Palliative care and symptom control

Good palliative and symptom control is vital to the management of the patient with advanced melanoma. Melanoma poses specific problems for palliative care. The CNS metastases of melanoma can typically be very vascular and bleed, often with devastating consequences. If not controlled at an early stage skin metastases can fungate and ulcerate, becoming unsightly, painful, and smelly. In this regard, the advice of a specialist wound-care nurse, appropriate topical antibiotics and dressings are important. There may be sufficient melanin production by the tumor to produce global discoloration of the skin known as melanosis. Although melanosis is asymptomatic it may be distressing for the patient and their relatives. Abdominal disease may cause ascites requiring drainage. Multiple metastases to the gastrointestinal tract and bronchial tree may also hemorrhage and may require endoscopic palliation or sclerosis.

Table 34.2. Management of specific problems in the patient with advanced melanoma

Problem	Management
Stage III disease	Surgery to primary tumor and resection of lymph node basin. Consider entry into a clinical trial for adjuvant therapy
Local regional recurrence	Surgery for local control
Skin and subcutaneous metastases	Consider early surgery before ulceration develops. Laser can be considered for small multiple metastases
Multiple symptomatic recurrence in an extremity	Consider isolated limb perfusion
Stage IV disease with one or two slow growing metastases	Consider metastectomy
Stage IV disease with multiple symptomatic or soon-to-be symptomatic metastases in a good performance status patient. No CNS disease	Consider chemotherapy with single agent DTIC or biochemotherapy preferably in the context of a clinical trial
Stage IV disease with multiple symptomatic or soon-to-be symptomatic metastases in a good performance status patient who fails to respond to conventional chemotherapy or biochemotherapy. No CNS disease, low tumor burden and LDH.	Consider entry into a vaccine trial or phase 1 study of new drugs
Vertebral metastases with cord or corda-equina compression	Consider urgent neurosurgery and/or radiotherapy
Symptomatic bony metastases	Consider palliative radiotherapy
CNS metastases	Consider resection and/or radiotherapy. Temozolemide and fotomustine are drugs that can cross the blood–brain barrier
Tumor ulceration and fungation	Topical antibiotics, dressings and specialist wound care advice

Note: CNS, central nervous system; LDH, serum lactate dehydrogenase; DTIC, dacarbazine

Table 34.2 is a summary of some specific problems encountered and their management.

Conclusion

Advanced melanoma requires the judicious use of many modalities of treatment and the involvement of many professionals. This chapter outlines how the prevention of problems before they arise and the palliation of symptoms can be achieved in a majority of patients and that long-term remission can be achieved in a minority.

REFERENCES

Sentinel articles

Balch CM, Buzaid AC, Atkins MB et al. A new American Joint Committee on Cancer staging system for cutaneous melanoma. *Cancer* 2000;88:1484–91.

Balch CM, Soong SJ, Gershenwald JE et al. Prognostic factors analysis of 17,600 melanoma patients: validation of the American Joint Committee on Cancer Melanoma Staging System. *J Clin Oncol* 2001;19:3622–34.

Ellerhorst J, Strom E, Nardone E, McCutcheon I. Whole brain irradiation for patients with metastatic melanoma: a review of 87 cases. *Int J Radiat Oncol Biol Phys* 2001;49:93–7.

Hernberg M, Pyrhonen S, Muhonen T. Regimens with or without interferon-alpha as treatment for metastatic melanoma and renal cell carcinoma: an overview of randomized trials. *J Immunother* 1999;22:145–54.

Hsueh EC, Gupta RK, Qi K, Morton DL. Correlation of specific immune responses with survival in melanoma patients with distant metastases receiving polyvalent melanoma cell vaccine. *J Clin Oncol* 1998;16:2913–20.

Kirkwood JM, Strawderman MH, Ernstoff MS, Smith TJ, Borden EC, Blum RH. Interferon alfa-2b adjuvant therapy of high-risk resected cutaneous melanoma: the Eastern Cooperative Oncology Group Trial EST 1684. *J Clin Oncol* 1996;14:7–17.

Livingston PO, Wong GYC, Adluri S et al. Improved survival in AJCC stage III melanoma patients with GM2 antibodies: a randomised trial of adjuvant vaccination with GM2 antibodies. *J Clin Oncol* 1994;12:1036–44.

Minasian LM, Yao TJ, Steffens TA et al. A phase I study of anti-GD3 ganglioside monoclonal antibody R24 and recombinant human macrophage-colony stimulating factor in patients with metastatic melanoma. *Cancer* 1995;75:2251–7.

Riker A, Cormier J, Panelli M et al. Immune selection after antigen-specific immunotherapy of melanoma. *Surgery* 1999;126:112–20.

Rosenberg SA, Yannelli JR, Yang JC et al. Treatment of patients with metastatic melanoma with autologous tumor-infiltrating lymphocytes and interleukin 2. *J Natl Cancer Inst* 1994; 86:1159–66.

Review articles

Agarwala SS, Kirkwood JM. Adjuvant therapy of melanoma. *Semin Surg Oncol* 1998;14:302–10.

Atkins MB. Immunotherapy and experimental approaches for metastatic melanoma. *Hematol Oncol Clin N Am* 1998;12:877–902.

Boon T, Coulie PG, Van den Eynde B. Tumor antigens recognized by T cells. *Immunol Today* 1997;18:267–8.

Byers HR, Bhawan J. Pathologic parameters in the diagnosis and prognosis of primary cutaneous melanoma. *Hematol Oncol Clin N Am* 1998;12:717–35.

Cooper JS. The evolution of the role of radiation therapy in the management of mucocutaneous malignant melanoma. *Hematol Oncol Clin N Am* 1998;12:849–62.

Landis SH, Murray T, Bolden S, Wingo PA. Cancer statistics, 1998. *CA Cancer J Clin* 1998;48: 6–29.

Legha SS. Durable complete responses in metastatic melanoma treated with interleukin-2 in combination with inteferon alpha and chemotherapy. *Semin Oncol* 1997;24:S39–43.

MacKie RM. Incidence, risk factors and prevention of melanoma. *Eur J Cancer* 1998;34:S3–6.

McCarthy WH, Shaw HM. The surgical treatment of primary melanoma. *Hematol Oncol Clin N Am* 1998;12:797–806.

McClay EF, McClay M. Systemic chemotherapy for the treatment of metastatic melanoma. *Semin Oncol* 1996;23:744–53.

Internet sites

http://cancer.gov/cancer_information/cancer_type/melanoma

A very good site from the National Cancer Institute with relevant information on the treatment of all stages of melanoma.

http://hiru.mcmaster.ca/ccopgi/guidelines/mel/cpg8_1f.html

The question of adjuvant therapy for melanoma is examined in depth with guidelines from a large Canadian oncology group.

http://www.mpip.org/

The melanoma patients' information page. An informative site for both patients and researchers.

35

Primary brain tumors

Paul M. DesRosiers and Robert D. Timmerman

Indiana University School of Medicine, Indianapolis

Introduction

The presentation and management of primary brain tumors has been one of the more frustrating experiences in oncology. While good outcomes are certainly possible, the intricacy of the affected organ and the poor tolerance of therapy often spell significant debilitation for patients, dramatically affecting quality of life. Unlike most cancers in the body where metastatic disease most frequently leads to patient death, primary brain tumors rarely metastasize. Still, malignant brain tumors are rarely cured due to limitations of effectiveness and tolerance of local therapies. Even benign tumors in the brain constitute a profound threat to both a patient's quality of life and survival. As such, management strategies for primary brain tumors must be equally sensitive to quality of life issues as survival since the therapy ultimately will often fail the patient for controlling the tumor.

Natural history

There are four types of glial cells that give rise to a variety of brain tumors: astrocytes, oligodendrocytes, ependyma, and microglia. Tumors arising from astrocytes are called *astrocytomas* including pilocytic astrocytoma (grade I), fibrillary astrocytoma (grade II), anaplastic astrocytoma (grade III) and glioblastoma multiforme (GBM, grade IV). Oligodendrocytes give rise to oligodendrogliomas, which are usually low grade but can be anaplastic. Ependymomas occur in and around the ventricles, commonly in the fourth ventricle of the posterior fossa. Although ependymomas are only occasionally malignant, they are often infiltrative at the primary site and may disseminate through the cerebrospinal fluid (CSF). Microglia are phagocytic cells responsible for some aspects of immune modulation in the CNS. These cells may give rise to gliosarcomas, which are usually aggressive high-grade tumors.

Primary CNS lymphoma may occur anywhere within the brain and can masquerade as infection, glioblastoma, or metastatic tumor. Primary germ cell tumors of the brain are always midline, typically occurring above the sella or in the pineal region. Primitive neuroectodermal tumors (PNET) are malignant small round cell tumors of childhood that occur anywhere within the brain. When they occur in the posterior fossa, they are often called medulloblastoma.

Meningiomas arise from the tough fibrous coating that surrounds the brain called the dura. Tumors that arise from the myelin or insulation around the nerves are called schwannomas or neuromas. Tumors arising in the pituitary gland, pituitary adenomas, cause displacement of normal brain structures including the optic nerves, resulting in partial blindness. A significant fraction of these tumors will secrete excessive levels of a particular hormone resulting in potentially life-threatening endocrine dysfunction. All of these tumors are typically benign, but have malignant variants.

Patterns of spread and recurrence

Meningiomas, schwannomas, pituitary tumors, and pilocytic gliomas advance from their site of origin along an advancing or "pushing" border. This results in a pressure effect on adjacent normal structures causing direct injury or loss of blood supply. Grade II or greater gliomas and other malignant primary brain tumors may advance in this "pushing" fashion but more commonly by infiltration (e.g., "tentacles"). Finally, cells from the tumors such as medulloblastoma, ependymoma, and germ cell tumors may be shed into the spinal fluid and circulate within and around the brain and spinal cord. These cells may be implanted far away from the primary site. Distant spread of brain tumors through blood vessels to other organs in the body is possible but rare.

Benign tumors, such as meningiomas and pilocytic astrocytomas are not expected to recur if completely resected. Subtotal resection is associated ultimately with high rates of recurrence. It is well known that grade II gliomas may transform to higher grade tumors over time. Recurrence after radiotherapy and surgery most often occurs within close proximity to the site of the original tumor.

Prognosis

Important prognostic factors for low-grade glioma include performance status, tumor grade, patient age at diagnosis, seizure, and in some instances, extent of tumor resection. Median survival figures for groups of patients with low-grade glioma range from 1–10 years, averaging around 7 years. Similar analysis of data from patients with high-grade gliomas indicates performance status to be the most important factor followed by grade, age, and mental status. Median survival for grade III and IV astrocytomas is around 3 years and 1 year respectively.

While localized lymphomas arising outside the CNS are highly curable, CNS lymphomas are rarely cured despite aggressive chemotherapy and radiotherapy with median survival typically around 12–18 months. Primary CNS germ cell tumors are more curable malignancies using chemotherapy and radiotherapy combinations. Despite the propensity to disseminate within the CSF, the cure rate for PNETs using surgery, radiation therapy, and chemotherapy is currently 60–85% and continues to improve over the past several decades. Ependymoma recur at the primary site, warranting as complete a resection as possible and adjuvant radiation.

Therapeutic approaches

Corticosteroids are the first-line therapy for tumor-induced inflammatory effects in normal brain tissue, often providing relief of the symptoms of headache, nausea, emesis, and focal deficits. Relief is typically immediate, in the range of hours to days. If no improvements with adequate doses of steroids are noted in this period, strong consideration should be made to discontinuing the steroids to avoid the many drug-related side effects. Tapering and weaning of the steroids should proceed as symptoms permit. About one in ten brain-tumor patients on steroids experience hyperglycemia often requiring "sliding scale" insulin dosing in order to continue with necessary steroid therapy. Chronic steroid therapy suppresses adrenal function, and abrupt discontinuation may result in an addisonian crisis. Normal immune response to infection is also suppressed, and opportunistic infections (e.g., oral thrush, urinary tract infections, etc.) occur frequently. While mild personality changes are common, occasionally patients suffer from steroid psychosis with suicidal ideation. Steroid myopathy presents as bilateral proximal extremity weakness. Discontinuation of steroids will allow most of the side effects to slowly resolve, usually over a 2–3-month period.

Craniotomy is the standard neurosurgical approach to the brain, allowing tissue biopsy and resection of tumor. The goal of craniotomy with resection is to remove as much tumor-bearing tissue as possible without exposing the patient to excessive risk of further neurological debilitation. *Fractionated radiation* usually involves a series of daily radiation treatments directed either at the tumor, postoperative tumor cavity, or tissues at risk of infiltration. This therapy has the advantage of being able to treat areas of tumor infiltration prophylactically. *Stereotactic radiosurgery* delivers a single fraction of high-dose radiation to an intracranial target defined by a three-dimensional coordinate system. Radiosurgery is useful for ablative therapy of either benign or malignant lesions and is typically an outpatient procedure. Limitations of radiosurgery techniques include a relative inability to treat large lesions or those in close proximity to dense optic pathways. *Chemotherapy* may be indicated for certain malignant primary brain tumors. Agents that cross into the brain tissue include the nitrosoureas (BCNU and CCNU), the vinca alkaloids, procarbazine, and temozolomide.

Rehabilitation issues

Both inpatient and outpatient rehabilitation programs are appropriate for brain tumor patients, especially during the recovery period after surgery. Ongoing physical therapy should be directed at reversing or adapting to neurological deficits. Occupational therapy should concentrate on regaining ability for self-care. It has been shown that brain-tumor patients are at particularly high risk for deep venous thrombosis and its complications. Lack of ambulating and long car rides to and from medical appointments cause extremity blood pooling leading to clots. Seizures should be particularly avoided since they often result in long-term setbacks. However, long-term use of anti-epileptics is not necessarily required in patients with no history of seizures. Hearing and vision loss have the potential to be corrected if recognized and screening exams should be routinely performed.

Emphasis on strengthening immune function and vigor should be championed in the brain-tumor patient's rehabilitation. A balanced diet provides the best source of nutrition necessary for healing damaged tissue, obviating any need for expensive dietary supplements. Patients should avoid dehydration, preferably by drinking pure water over juices and caffeinated products. A proper balance of rest and exercise should be encouraged. Emphasis on self-care and maintaining personal decision making allows patients to retain self-esteem. Finally, depression should be treated aggressively since it dramatically interferes with all rehabilitation efforts.

Palliative care issues

Focal motor deficits such as hemiparesis, foot drop, and facial palsy would benefit from both ongoing physical therapy and adaptive measures. Measures should be taken to avoid injury from falls. Sensory deficits, particularly of the distal extremities, put patients at risk for burns and other injury. Patients with speech motor deficits and expressive aphasia should have access to speech pathology professionals experienced with these problems. As tumors progress, the neurological abnormalities become more global or not attributable to a specific region in the brain. Lack of ambulating may result in pulmonary atelectasis and infection, blood clots, constipation, muscle atrophy, and bedsores.

Death from CNS disease varies in its progression depending on the part of the brain predominantly affected. As a tumor grows and exerts mass effect on normal brain, patients typically experience headache with nausea and vomiting. Corticosteroids are the most likely beneficial therapy. Narcotic pain medicines and anti-emetics are indicated for pain and nausea not controlled by steroids. Routine blood sugar checks are reasonable, even in the hospice patient, since steroid-induced hyperglycemia can make patients feel extremely uncomfortable. Appropriate measures to avoid seizure activity include using anti-epileptics and monitoring their blood levels. In the end stages of a neurological death, patients often become obtunded with shallow irregular breathing. Alternative routes of pain and other medicine administration should be considered (such as transdermal patches) since intake by mouth could lead to aspiration.

Conclusions

Primary brain tumors are a heterogeneous group of benign and malignant neoplasms that affect a wide variety of age groups. The distinction between benign and malignant, which is so critical in the majority of tumors in the body, is blurry for primary brain tumors. Treatments are effective for certain types of tumors, but fail to ultimately control the tumor in the majority. Supportive care aimed at improving quality of life in this difficult-to-manage population is paramount.

BIBLIOGRAPHY

Sentinel articles

Bauman G, Lote K, Larson D et al. Pretreatment factors predict overall survival for patients with low-grade gliomas: recursive partitioning analysis. *Int J Radiat Oncol Biol Phys* 1999;45:923–9.

Curran WJ, Scott CB, Horton J et al. Recursive partitioning analysis of prognostic factors in three Radiation Therapy Oncology Group malignant glioma trials. *J Natl Cancer Inst* 1993;85:704–10.

Review articles

Nieder C, Nestle U. A review of current and future treatment strategies for malignant astrocytomas in adults. *Strahlenther Onkol* 2000;10176:251–8.

Prados MD, Levin V. Biology and treatment of malignant glioma. *Semin Oncol* 2000;27(Suppl. 6): 1–10.

Schmandt SM, Packer RJ. Treatment of low-grade pediatric gliomas. *Curr Opin Oncol* 2000;12: 194–8.

Internet sites

Maxine Dunitz Neurosurgical Institute
    http://www.cedars-sinai.edu/mdnsi/

National Cancer Institute
    http://www.cancer.gov/cancer_information/cancer_type/brain_tumor

36

Thyroid and adrenal cancer

Rae Zyn H. Brana and Douglas B. Evans

U.T. M.D. Anderson Cancer Center, Houston

Thyroid cancer

Thyroid cancer is a heterogenous group of diseases that accounts for most of endocrine cancer-related deaths. It is the most common endocrine malignancy; however its relative incidence and death rate compared with other cancers is low, representing only 1% of all cancers and only 0.05% of all cancer-related deaths. The American Cancer Society estimates that 18 400 new cases of thyroid cancer will occur in the United States in 2000; 13 700 in women and 4700 in men. An estimated 1200 deaths related to thyroid cancer occurred in 2000; 700 in women and 500 in men. The median age at diagnosis is 45 to 50 years but it does occur in the very young as well as in the elderly. The cause of thyroid cancer is not known but childhood exposure to radiation and iodine deficiency have been identified as risk factors.

The various types of thyroid cancers have different pathologic features, disease courses, and patterns of recurrence. Thyroid cancers are commonly categorized as well-differentiated thyroid cancer (papillary and follicular), medullary thyroid cancer, and anaplastic thyroid cancer. Less common are thyroid lymphoma and metastatic disease to the thyroid.

Well-differentiated thyroid cancers

Papillary and follicular thyroid cancers are well-differentiated malignant neoplasms that arise from follicular cells. In general, they are considered indolent malignancies with favorable long-term survival rates; however, certain patient subsets such as elderly patients with advanced disease may experience rapid tumor progression. Hurthle cell carcinomas are variants of follicular thyroid cancers, but are now considered a separate entity because they exhibit biologic behavior distinct from that of papillary and follicular cancers.

Papillary thyroid cancer is the most common among the well-differentiated types comprising approximately 75–80% of all thyroid cancers. It is usually an encapsulated tumor that spreads to the lymphatics within the thyroid and to the regional lymph nodes. It could present as an asymptomatic thyroid nodule or as an enlarged neck lymph node in the absence of a palpable thyroid nodule. There is high incidence of multifocality within the gland and while regional lymph node involvement is common, distant metastasis is infrequent at initial presentation. Regional lymph node metastasis is not strongly correlated with overall survival but does predict an increased risk for local recurrence. Patients with distant metastasis have a 50–90% rate of disease-specific death while patients with locally recurrent disease have long-term survival rates of 70–90%. The most common metastatic site is the lung.

Follicular thyroid cancer comprises approximately 10% of all thyroid cancers. It is less likely than papillary thyroid cancer to occur as a consequence of prior radiation exposure to the head or neck. It is usually unifocal and encapsulated. Invasion of the thyroid capsule increases the risk for distant metastasis, which occurs via hematogenous spread. If invasion of the tumor capsule is present without vascular invasion, prognosis is good with 85–100% of patients surviving at least 10 years. Prognosis is worse for men over the age of 50. Metastatic potential is generally a function of primary tumor size so distant metastasis with occult disease is rare. The common metastatic sites are the lungs and bones.

Hurthle cell thyroid carcinoma is considered to be more aggressive than follicular thyroid cancer, with a higher incidence of intraglandular and lymph node spread. Its inability to sufficiently concentrate radioiodine also makes diagnostic imaging and treatment more challenging. Hurthle cell carcinomas can recur in the cervical lymph nodes but in general, loco-regional recurrence is uncommon for well-differentiated thyroid cancers.

Initial treatment for well-differentiated thyroid cancer is surgery, with the extent of operation dependent on prognostic factors and stage of disease. Adjuvant radio-iodine ablation often follows surgery with the objective of ablating residual thyroid tissue and microscopic residual carcinoma. Local recurrence is treated with surgery, which is also used with palliative intent to treat metastatic disease such as osseous metastasis where there is high risk for orthopedic or neurologic complications. Lung metastases are often multiple and diffuse and surgery is therefore inappropriate. Radioiodine is also used for distant metastasis and can be effective with small volume disease. External beam radiation therapy is used for bone metastasis that is not amenable to surgery especially in sites where a pathologic fracture would cause serious disability. If there is radioiodine uptake by the tumor, iodine can be given first followed by external beam irradiation. Chemotherapy with single agent doxorubicin has shown response rates of 0–33% with all responses being partial. Bleomycin, cisplatin, mitoxantrone, and etoposide have also been studied but because advanced well-differentiated thyroid cancer is uncommon, there are few meaningful trials reported that compare single-agent versus multiple-agent regimens to treat this disease.

Treatment options for metastatic Hurthle cell carcinoma are limited. Surgical resection and external beam radiation can be used for bone metastasis but radioiodine ablation and chemotherapy for metastatic Hurthle cell carcinoma have generally been ineffective.

Medullary thyroid cancer

Medullary thyroid cancer (MTC) arises from the calcitonin-producing thyroid parafollicular C cells. It is uncommon and is unique among the various types of thyroid cancers in its strong association with familial syndromes. MTC is classified as either sporadic or familial with sporadic being more common (75% of cases). Familial MTC can occur as part of multiple endocrine neoplasia 2 (MEN2) or as a non-MEN2 familial process. Sporadic MTC is unifocal without suggestion of C cell hyperplasia in the rest of the gland. Distant metastasis from MTC usually involves the mediastinal lymph nodes, lungs, liver, and bones. Combined survival rates for both types are 80–90% for 5 years and 70–80% for 10 years.

Initial treatment for MTC is total thyroidectomy accompanied by lymph node dissection because of the high incidence of regional nodal involvement associated with this disease. Surgery is also used for local and regional recurrence. External beam irradiation is used with patients who have locally progressive disease and is a consideration with patients who have elevated postoperative calcitonin levels.

Management of advanced metastatic disease is symptomatic; patients with diarrhea, flushing, and pain are treated medically. Surgery is used in rare cases when there is a single lesion in the bone, lungs, or liver. External beam irradiation is used with painful bone involvement, and chemotherapy with single-agent doxorubicin or with 5-FU/dacarbazine or 5-FU/streptozocin is used for refractory disease.

Anaplastic thyroid cancer

Anaplastic thyroid cancer (ATC) is one of the most aggressive cancers and could present as the final stage in the dedifferentiation of follicular or papillary disease or of a long-standing thyroid tumor. The mean age at diagnosis is reported to range from 57 to 67 years. It commonly presents as a rapidly enlarging neck mass with compressive symptoms of the trachea or esophagus such as hoarseness, dyspnea, cough, dysphagia, and cervical pain. Nearly 80% of patients will have tumors greater than 5 cm in diameter at presentation and at least 50% will have distant metastasis most often to the lungs (80%), bone (15%), and brain (13%). Most patients will die from complications of aggressive local tumor invasion. Survival after diagnosis is very poor with mean survival times ranging from 2.5 to 7.4 months and median survival reported as 4–12 months.

Survival is not affected by a single treatment modality be it surgery, radiotherapy, or chemotherapy alone. Radical surgery has not been shown to be more effective than a less radical approach, and radiotherapy has failed to induce regression. Airway management however is critical; all patients require careful assessment of the adequacy of their airway and tracheostomy is performed in many patients. The most effective treatment for ATC is combination doxorubicin and radiation to the neck and upper mediastinum to help avoid significant respiratory distress or death by suffocation from tumor invasion. Occasional patients who respond to chemoradiation become candidates for surgery. Chemotherapy using paclitaxel has recently been studied for ATC and has shown a notable response rate of 64%. Supportive care for symptoms caused by tumor invasion is paramount in the care of patients with this lethal disease.

Adrenal cancer

Cancers arising from the adrenal gland are uncommon and this section will focus on adrenal cortical carcinoma (ACC). ACC is a rare malignancy with a worldwide incidence of approximately 2 million. It comprises 0.05–0.2% of all cancers. Tumors may be nonfunctional or functional; producing cortisol, aldosterone, androgens, or estrogens. Nonfunctional tumors are more common in men and functional tumors are more common in women. The etiology is unknown but studies of chromosomal alterations and growth factor production have recently been done to investigate possible causes.

The presenting symptoms are usually associated with excess hormone production in functional tumors along with abdominal pain or pressure in nonfunctional tumors. Functional adrenal cancers usually produce cortisol; clinical manifestations of which are apparent in about 30% of patients. A mixed pattern of multiple hormone overproduction is noted in 35% of patients. The rapid onset of hirsutism and virilization is characteristic of cortisol excess produced by ACC.

Diagnosis is often delayed especially in nonfunctional tumors. On diagnostic imaging studies, the size of the mass can be best evaluated with computed tomography or magnetic resonance imaging. Mass size is the best single indicator for malignancy with a size greater than 5 cm usually indicative of an invasive ACC.

Surgical resection is the primary and only curative treatment for ACC. The strongest predictor of outcome is surgical resectability of the primary tumor. Five-year actuarial survival rates range from 32–48% in patients who undergo complete resection.

Recurrent and metastatic disease is treated with surgery when complete resection of isolated metastasis is possible. Radiation therapy has not shown effectiveness in ACC and is generally not recommended except in palliating painful osseous metastasis. Most studies of treatment for recurrent or metastatic ACC involve mitotane (o,p'DDD), a minor component of a commercial insecticide with adrenolytic activity. Reports regarding the efficacy of mitotane for treatment of locally unresectable or metastatic disease have been inconsistent, with some showing benefit at high serum levels and some showing no effect on survival. Systemic chemotherapy for disease that is refractory to mitotane may be given using etoposide, cisplatin, and doxorubicin (EDP).

Care of patients with advanced ACC involves management of the adverse neurologic, endocrine, and gastrointestinal effects of mitotane as well as toxicities of other chemotherapeutic agents. The most common metastatic sites for ACC are retroperitoneal lymph nodes (68%), lung (71%), liver (42%), and bone (26%), and supportive care is geared towards control of symptoms arising from the specific metastatic site that is involved.

BIBLIOGRAPHY

Ain KB. Anaplastic thyroid carcinoma: behavior, biology, and therapeutic approaches. *Thyroid* 1998;8:715–26.

Bi J, Lu B. Advances in the diagnosis and treatment of thyroid neoplasms. *Curr Opin Oncol* 2000;12:54–9.

Cady B, Rolla, AR. Neoplasms of the thyroid. In *Cancer Medicine*, ed. JF Holland, E Frei, RC Bast, DL Morton, DW Kufe, RR Weichselbaum.

Didoklar MS, Bescher A, Elias EG, Moore RH. Natural history of adrenal cortical carcinoma: a clinicopathologic study of 42 patients. *Cancer* 1981;47:2153–61.

Evans DB. The surgical treatment of sporadic medullary thyroid carcinoma. *Ann Surg Oncol* 2000;7:393–8.

Fleming JB, Lee JB, Bouvet M et al. Operative strategy for the treatment of medullary thyroid carcinoma. *Ann Surg* 1999;230:697–707.

Fraker DL, Skarulis M, Livolsi V. Thyroid tumors. In *Cancer: Principles and Practice of Oncology*, 6th edn, ed. VT Devita, S Hellman, SA Rosenberg, pp. 1740–63. Philadelphia: Lippincott-Raven, 2001.

Haak HR, Hermans J, van de Velde CJH et al. Optimal treatment of adrenocortical carcinoma with mitotane: results in a consecutive series of 96 patients. *Br J Cancer* 1994;69:947–51.

Lubitz, JA, Freeman, L, Okun, R. Mitotane use in inoperable adrenal cortical carcinoma. *J Am Med Assoc* 1993;223:1109.

Norton JA, Le HN. Adrenal tumors. In *Cancer: Principles and Practice of Oncology*, 6th edn, ed. VT Devita, S Hellman, SA Rosenberg, pp. 1770–88. Philadelphia: Lippincott-Raven, 2001.

Osamah A, Orlo CH. Familial thyroid cancer. *Curr Opin Oncol* 2001;13:44–51.

Schlumberger MJ. (1998). Medical progress: papillary and follicular thyroid carcinoma. *N Engl J Med* 1998;388:297–306.

Stanford PA, Evans DB. Endocrine cancer: the thyroid, parathyroid, adrenal glands and pancreas. In *Primary Care Oncology*, ed. KL Boyer, MBF Ford, AF Judkins, D Levin, pp. 98–110. Philadelphia: Saunders, 1999.

Thompson NW. Hurthle cell neoplasms. *Ann Surg Oncol* 2000;7:388–90.

Vassilopoulou-Sellin R, Guinee VF, Klein MJ et al. Impact of adjuvant mitotane on the clinical course of patient with adrenocortical cancer. *Cancer* 1993;71:3119.

Venkatesh S, Hickey RC, Sellin RV, Fernandez JF, Samaan NA. Adrenal cortical carcinoma. *Cancer* 1989;64:765–9.

Wooten MD, King DK. Adrenal cortical carcinoma. Epidemiology and treatment with mitotane and review of literature. *Cancer* 1993;72:3145.

Zidan J, Shpendler M, Robinson E. Treatment of metastatic adrenal cortical carcinoma with etoposide (VP-16) and cisplatin after failure with o,p'DDD: Clinical case reports. *Am J Clin Oncol* 1996;19:229–31.

37

HIV-related cancer

Julia Ladd Smith

University of Rochester School of Medicine and Dentistry, Rochester

There were estimated to be 422 000 persons with HIV/AIDS in the US in the year 2000. Over the past 20 years, acquired immunodeficiency syndrome (AIDS) has changed from a rapidly fatal disease to a controllable, chronic disease. Among people with HIV-positive status, the presence of CD4 T-cell counts ≤ 400 and the co-diagnosis of any one of three cancers upgrade the diagnosis to AIDS. These cancers are Kaposi's sarcoma, non-Hodgkin's lymphoma, and invasive cancer of the uterine cervix. This chapter will address information on these cancers as they relate to AIDS patients including the complexities of managing two coexisting serious diseases. There are issues related to the need for numerous anti-AIDS drugs as well as prophylactic antibiotics and potential drug–drug interactions when adding chemotherapy or radiation therapy. AIDS patients are at risk for opportunistic infections and chemotherapy drugs also increase the risk of infection, both by lowering the white cell count and sometimes by direct suppression of the immune system.

In the early 1980s, medical researchers described a new syndrome associated with opportunistic infections, lymphadenopathy, primary brain lymphoma, and Kaposi's sarcoma. The infections include oral esophageal and pulmonary candidiasis, pneumocystis carinii, extrapulmonary cryptococcosis, cryptosporidiosis-induced diarrhea, cytomegalovirus of nonreticuloendothelial organs, prolonged herpes simplex infections of the mouth, esophagus or bronchi, or multiple bacterial infections during a 1-year period. The human immunodeficiency virus (HIV) was isolated in 1983 and is known to infect T lymphocytes called helper cells. Initially homosexual men predominated the affected population. Currently intravenous drug abuse and heterosexual transmission cause infection in both developed and developing countries. Thus both heterosexual men and women are increasingly contracting the virus.

Direct anti-HIV treatment has evolved over the years since AIDS was first described. Multiple antiviral drugs have been developed. Currently, HIV-positive people are treated with combinations of agents with different mechanisms of action.

Table 37.1. Complications of HIV/AIDS

Opportunistic infections	*Systemic*
Candidiasis	Cachexia
Coccidiomycosis	Delirium
Cryptococcosis	Dementia
Cytomegalovirus	Diarrhea
Herpes simplex	Dyspnea
Molluscum contagiosum	Fatigue
Mycobacterium avium intracellurae	Mucositis
Pneumocystis carinii	Nausea and vomiting
	Neuropathic pain
Hematologic complications	Weight loss
Anemia	
Thrombocytopenia-ITP or decreased production	
Leukopenia	

These combinations are collectively known as highly active antiretroviral therapy (HAART). HAART has maintained CD4 counts and reduced the rate of progression from viral positive to full-blown AIDS status. In effect it has made HIV a chronic disease. This change is likely to affect the incidence and prevalence of cancers among the HIV-positive population. Multiple conditions associated with HIV/AIDS increase the risks of treating malignancies in these patients. Untreated, HIV infection leads to severe compromise of the immune system and development of otherwise unusual infections involving so-called opportunistic infections (Table 37.1). Even if infection is not already present, chemotherapy and radiation therapy increase the risk of infection. Marrow suppression by the HIV itself or related to antiviral therapy may reduce blood counts, making further myelosuppression by anti-neoplastic treatment riskier. AIDS-associated physical compromise of performance status makes chemotherapy- and radiation therapy-associated nausea, vomiting, fatigue, mucositis, or diarrhea less tolerable. In all, the HIV/AIDS patient with cancer may have less ability to tolerate standard treatments for cancer. For these reasons, close monitoring of the patient by experienced oncologic and infectious disease professionals is mandatory.

Specific cancers associated with HIV/AIDS

Kaposi's sarcoma

In the past, Kaposi's sarcoma (KS) was known to occur primarily as an indolent disease in older men of Jewish or Italian descent and as an endemic disease in parts of Africa. More recently it developed in immunosuppressed renal transplant patients. With the onset of the AIDS epidemic, KS rates increased, especially among HIV-infected homosexual men. KS is an AIDS-defining illness when associated with HIV infection. AIDS-associated KS is a more rapidly progressive disease than the classic or endemic forms. Among HIV-positive individuals, KS is 73 000 times more likely than among HIV-negative individuals. Epidemiologic trends reveal that HIV-related KS is declining in incidence. This may be a combination of the benefits of HAART, education among the ultrahigh-risk homosexual population or other factors.

KS most commonly involves the skin. Lesions may be macular or papular and are usually reddish or violacious in color. In contrast to the classic KS seen in elderly men, HIV/AIDS-associated KS is more likely to be multifocal at diagnosis and is more likely to occur on the face and upper body. Lesions may also occur in the mouth, intestine, lung, lymph nodes, and more rarely the liver and spleen. The skin lesions may be subtle and asymptomatic or disfiguring by their presence on exposed skin and can also cause edema. Histologic analysis reveals that KS is due to proliferation of endothelial spindle cells. An interaction between human immunodeficiency virus-derived proteins and human herpes virus type 8 (HHV-8) is believed to be the cause of HIV/AIDS-associated KS. HHV-8 is also found in classic and endemic KS lesions.

Treatment for KS can include topical or intralesional therapy, systemic therapy, and localized radiation therapy. Intralesional treatments include locally injected vinblastine and interferon-alpha. Alitretinoin gel (9-*cis*-retinioic acid) was recently approved for topical treatment. It can be applied by the patient and is useful for skin lesions as they first appear or those remaining after other treatments have been used. Radiation therapy palliates locally disfiguring lesions or ones that are causing edema to the face, extremities or genitals.

Systemic therapy has evolved over the two decades of HIV/AIDS-associated KS. Initially, single-agent chemotherapy prevailed and response rates were low and of short duration. Antineoplastic agents used include etoposide (Vepesid), vinblastine or vincristine. Doxorubicin (adriamycin) and bleomycin were also used. Typical chemotherapy-related alopecia, gastrointestinal side effects, myelosuppression, and potential for neuropathies from the vinca alkaloids made these options primarily for patients with good performance status and thus early in the AIDS trajectory. Recent availability of liposomal doxorubicin (Doxil) and daunorubicin (daunoXome) provides high response rates with much lower toxicity. These agents cause much less alopecia, nausea and vomiting, and myelosuppression at doses required. This makes liposomal doxorubicin the current first-line systemic treatment. Liposomal doxorubicin is associated with risk for hand–foot syndrome, painful redness, and skin sloughing of the palms of the hands and soles of the feet. Paclitaxel (Taxol) has also been approved for use in HIV/AIDS-associated KS. A current trial is comparing liposomal doxorubicin with paclitaxel.

Systemic use of interferon-alpha gives high response rates but at the expense of treatment-related malaise, fatigue, weight loss, and risk of neutropenia and liver toxicity. The response rate is also slower. These factors make interferon likely to be of benefit to patients with lesions not requiring rapid response and in patients with few HIV-related symptoms. Typical survival rates of KS in HIV/AIDS patients are less than 2 years. No currently available treatment is associated with definite life prolongation. Death is likely to be due to pulmonary involvement or to infection.

Non-Hodgkin's lymphoma

Like KS, non-Hodgkin's lymphoma (NHL) is an AIDS-defining illness. NHL in HIV-infected patients occurs about 15 years earlier than the typical non-HIV-associated lymphomas where the median age is 55–60 years. Evidence suggests that the incidence of NHL in HIV-infected individuals is rising despite successful delay of full-blown AIDS through use of HAART. The overall incidence of NHL in the HIV-positive population is 113 times the incidence in non-HIV-infected populations. Primary central nervous system (CNS) lymphomas account for roughly 20% of AIDS-related NHL. Yet primary CNS lymphoma is otherwise rare. Systemic lymphomas and so-called "body cavity-based" lymphomas are the other common types. The latter present as effusions in chest, pericardial sac and/or abdomen and, like KS, are associated with co-infection of HHV-8. Unlike KS, the mode of HIV infection does not correlate to the risk of NHL. In other words, these lymphomas occur in heterosexual as well as homosexual HIV-infected individuals. CNS lymphomas in AIDS patients are uniformly associated with Epstein–Barr virus (EBV).

Lymphomas have a wide variety of histologic types and clinical behavior in non-HIV-infected individuals (see Chapter 38). Typically, HIV/AIDS-associated NHL are intermediate or high-grade B-cell types. Burkitt's or Burkitt's-like lymphoma with diffuse, small noncleaved cells, diffuse large cell type and diffuse large cell immunoblastic type account for most of the cases in roughly equal proportions.

Systemic chemotherapy is the treatment of choice for systemic NHL in people with AIDS. Since chemotherapy lowers blood counts, causes gastrointestinal symptoms, and is itself immunosuppressive, the risks of infection and lower tolerance of chemotherapy doses are significant in HIV-infected individuals. Prophylaxis for infection should be continued when indicated. When possible antiretroviral therapy should be maintained although some regimens halt HAART temporarily to improve patient tolerance of the chemotherapy. It is imperative to maintain a high index of suspicion for atypical infections, as listed in Table 37.1.

Chemotherapy regimens for AIDS-related NHL generally contain lower doses of standard medications. Thus half-dose CHOP (cyclophosphamide, hydroxydauno-rubicin (doxorubicin), Oncovin (vincristine) and prednisone) or reduced doses of methotrexate, bleomycin, doxorubicin, cyclophosphamide, vincristine, and dexamethasone (m-BACOD) are given. Patients with higher CD4 counts, absence of AIDS-related infection and good performance status may tolerate full doses of these regimens. Patients with bone marrow involvement may require CNS prophylaxis. Growth factors (GCSF and GMCSF) may minimize need for dose reductions or delays. Complete remissions occur but half relapse and die of lymphoma or infection. Recently, a continuous infusion regimen of cyclophosphamide, doxorubicin and etoposide along with the antiviral didanisine and intrathecal cytosine arabinoside has had a high response rate in a small group of patients. Ongoing trials will evaluate the ability to continue HAART during chemotherapy.

As with non-AIDS associated NHL, prognosis is influenced by stage of disease, extranodal involvement, especially CNS and marrow involvement, and performance status. Higher stage of disease and elevated LDH are poor prognostic markers. In people with AIDS, CD4 counts < 100 and previous opportunistic infection, history of intravenous drug abuse, and age > 35 adversely affect outcome. B symptoms, fever, and weight loss may be difficult to separate for AIDS infection-related symptoms. Overall survival for AIDS-related NHL is short, approximately 6 months.

Primary CNS lymphoma is extremely rare in the population without HIV-infection. The risk is over 1000 times greater in HIV infection. Initial diagnosis using CT or MR imaging should be confirmed by biopsy. Where available, PET scanning may be specific enough to avoid the need for biopsy. The symptoms of CNS lymphoma may mimic CNS toxoplasmosis or progressive multifocal leuko-encephalopathy. Patients with CNS lymphoma require whole brain radiation therapy. Due to low survival rates with radiation alone, patients with good performance status should be considered for combined modality therapy to include chemotherapy that crosses the blood–brain barrier.

Cancer of the uterine cervix

Cervical cancer is considered an AIDS-defining diagnosis in an HIV-infected patient. The relative risk is not nearly so great as for KS and NHL comparing HIV-infected with uninfected populations of women. Cervical cancer is about three times more common in HIV-infected women. The association is largely due to both HIV and cervical cancer being sexually transmitted. Cervical cancer is associated with human papilloma virus. Preinvasive cervical neoplasia (cervical intra-epithelial neoplasia or CIN) is largely a curable disease with local treatment. Its detection should prompt HIV screening and screening with Pap smears is mandatory among women with known HIV infection.

In HIV-positive women, those with lowered CD4 counts have a higher relapse rate of CIN. Surgery is curative in early stage invasive cervical cancer. Radiation therapy with sensitizing chemotherapy is used for more advanced stage II and III lesions. Palliative treatment for advanced stage IV disease can reduce symptoms of pelvic tumor and slightly prolong survival. Healthier women with HIV-positive status should be offered the same aggressive options as uninfected women. Among AIDS patients with low CD4 counts, presence of opportunistic infection and low performance status, response to treatment and survival of cervical cancer is reduced. Treatment decisions should be individualized.

Other cancers

Other cancers have an increased incidence in the HIV-positive population but are not considered AIDS defining. Among them are Hodgkin's disease, which is 7.5 times more likely than in the non-HIV population. There is controversy about the association of Hodgkin's disease and HIV infection. Epidemiologic series suggest an increased incidence in intravenous drug users with HIV infection. HIV-infected patients with Hodgkin's disease are more likely to have bone marrow involvement and have a poorer prognosis than non-HIV-infected patients.

Anal and conjunctival squamous cell cancers are greatly increased. Multiple myeloma is somewhat increased. Most other cancers are not increased with HIV infection. As antiviral treatments continue to prolong the lives of HIV-infected individuals, cancer rates will increase with age as they do in the general population. The status of the patient's HIV infection should influence the treatment approach when a codiagnosis of cancer occurs. Treatment should be planned according to the patient's stamina and goals of care. As a general rule, in a fit patient, with high CD4 counts, good nutrition and performance status, standard treatment protocols can be used. A person with full-blown AIDS is less likely to tolerate standard doses of chemotherapy. Gastrointestinal and neurological side effects of antineoplastic therapy may be less well tolerated in already ill AIDS patients. Early use of growth factors to support white cell counts may be considered. Treatment-induced myelosuppression increases the risk of infection. When fever or other signs of infection occur, evaluate for both routine and unusual bacterial and viral agents.

Supportive therapy

A discussion of symptom management is beyond this chapter. It is important to point out that many symptoms of cancer and cancer therapy overlap with symptoms of HIV/AIDS. Gastrointestinal symptoms of diarrhea may be due to opportunistic infection, neuropathic enteritis, chemotherapy, or abdominal radiation. Anorexia, cachexia, and fatigue are all associated with AIDS, cancer, and cancer treatments. Mucositis from herpes or chemotherapy compromises nutrition as well as comfort. Neuropathic pain syndromes are common among AIDS patients. All symptoms require evaluation and palliative measures. When specific therapy is available, such as antivirals for herpetic mucositis, that should be offered. When specific therapies are not available or not effective, symptom control with general measures must be administered to comfort.

AIDS and cancer both are potentially fatal illnesses. Sensitive planning for end-of-life care must be based on the goals and values of the patient. The emotional needs of both the patients and their social networks need to be addressed. Often, AIDS patients have the additional burden of poor social networks due to lifestyle habits or due to the still prevalent stigma and fear associated with the HIV virus. Health professionals must be able to access help from social service agencies and faith groups to address the needs of patients with cancer and AIDS.

Conclusion

The AIDS epidemic has challenged the medical community to manage complex medical illness in novel ways. The disease often leads to codiagnoses of infection and cancer. Treatment of the cancer increases the probability of infections. As the use of HAART improves life expectancy for HIV-infected individuals there is likely to continue to be a shift in the epidemiology of related cancers. KS may continue to decline. NHL may decline or, as the affected population ages, may rise as it does in the uninfected population. Cervical cancer is not as strongly increased as the other two indicator cancers. Surveillance strategies and aggressive treatments will be necessary for cervical cancer as it is detectable in pre-invasive phases. The general incidence of all cancers among HIV-positive populations is likely to increase as the affected population survives longer due to HAART. Few cancer treatment centers will see sufficient numbers of AIDS-related cancer patients to independently, prospectively assess alternative treatment strategies. For that reason, collaboration among cooperative oncology treatment groups such as the AIDS Clinical Trials Group (ACTG) remain important to evaluate new treatments in this highly complex patient population. Optimal treatments must always include attention to symptom management and the psychosocial and spiritual needs of the affected individuals and their families.

BIBLIOGRAPHY

Centers for Disease Control and Prevention. *AIDS Surveillance in the Americas.* Washington, DC: CDC, 2000.

Dezube BJ. Acquired immunodeficiency syndrome-related Kaposi's sarcoma: clinical features, staging, and treatment. *Semin Oncol* 2000;27:424–30.

Goedert JJ. The epidemiology of acquired immunodeficiency syndrome malignancies. *Semin Oncol* 2000;27:390–401.

Levine AM. Acquired immunodeficiency syndrome-related lymphoma: clinical aspects. *Semin Oncol* 2000;27:442–53.

Robinson W. Invasive and preinvasive cervical neoplasia in human immunodeficiency virus-infected women. *Semin Oncol* 2000;27:463–70.

Von Gunten CF, Von Roenn JH. Supportive care of patients with AIDS. In *Principles and Practice of Supportive Oncology*, ed. AM Berger, RK Portenoy, DE Weisman, pp. 861–72. Philadelphia: Lippincott-Raven, 1997.

Welsby PD, Richardson A, Brettle RP. AIDS: aspects in adults. In *Oxford Textbook of Palliative Medicine*, ed. D Doyle, GWC Hanks, N MacDonald, pp. 1121–48. New York: Oxford University Press, 1998.

38

Hodgkin's and non-Hodgkin's lymphoma

Craig R. Nichols

Oregon Health & Science University, Portland

Introduction

The lymphomas are historically divided into non-Hodgkin's lymphoma and Hodgkin's disease. In 1998, there were approximately 57 000 cases of non-Hodgkin's lymphoma in the US, with about 7500 cases of Hodgkin's disease. The incidence of non-Hodgkin's lymphoma appears to be rising steadily at approximately 1% per year whereas the incidence of Hodgkin's disease appears to be stable or declining slightly.

The incidence of lymphoma does not seem to vary widely over racial subsets and geographic boundaries. There is growing evidence of association of the development of non-Hodgkin's lymphoma with organopesticides. Non-Hodgkin's lymphoma and to a lesser extent Hodgkin's disease does appear to be associated with some viral infections including human immunodeficiency virus (HIV), hepatitis B, and Epstein–Barr virus. As well, non-Hodgkin's lymphoma is associated strongly with intense immunosuppression usually given for solid organ transplantation. Such patients have a 10–1000-fold increase to incidence of lymphoma depending on the type and intensity of immunosuppression.

Anatomy and histology

Non-Hodgkin's lymphoma is usually a disease that involves lymph node tissues, spleen and, in later stages, bone marrow. Extranodal sites are also seen in non-Hodgkin's lymphoma. The most common extranodal sites are stomach, testis, CNS, and bone. The non-Hodgkin's lymphoma represents a spectrum of subtypes ranging from extraordinarily indolent diseases to some of the most explosive virulent malignancies known.

Hodgkin's disease is almost always a disease of nodal origin. Over 90% of the time the patients present with disease above the diaphragm, particularly cervical lymphadenopathy and mediastinal involvement. The disease seems to have an orderly pattern of spread in most patients, spreading from one lymph node-bearing area to the next in a relatively indolent fashion. It is this predictable pattern of behavior that has allowed radiation therapy to be the mainstay of treatment for Hodgkin's disease for many years. Extranodal involvement in Hodgkin's disease is extremely uncommon.

Non-Hodgkin's lymphomas primarily are of B cell variation. About 90% of patients with non-Hodgkin's lymphoma are B cell in origin. For practical purposes, non-Hodgkin's lymphoma is divided into low-grade (indolent) lymphoma, intermediate-grade lymphoma, and high-grade lymphoma. The low-grade lymphomas are primarily the follicular histology lymphomas and these patients, while not felt to be curable, with conventional therapy, have a very indolent natural history and live oftentimes a decade or longer with simple intermittent management. The intermediate- and high-grade lymphomas are more explosive in onset and pace. All of these patients require immediate treatment with a goal of cure. It is the intermediate- and high-grade lymphomas that tend to involve extranodal sites and be associated with HIV infections. Virtually all of these patients require immediate initiation of aggressive combination chemotherapy.

Hodgkin's disease is a disease primarily of younger patients. The most common histologic subtype, nodular sclerosing variant, has a peak incidence in the third decade of life. Hodgkin's disease is now felt to be of B-cell origin. The pathognomic histologic finding is the presence of the Reed–Sternberg cell. Immunohistochemistry and microdissection have identified these cells as B cells.

Symptoms

Hodgkin's disease

The vast majority of Hodgkin's disease patients present with painless adenopathy usually with cervical adenopathy. Occasionally, patients present with symptoms related with anterior mediastinal lymphadenopathy with chest pressure, cough, and shortness of breath and superior vena cava syndrome. There are three classic "B" symptoms associated with Hodgkin's disease – fever, weight loss, and night sweats. The designation of fever is an unexplained fever greater than 101 °F for a period of 2–3 weeks without other explanation. This fever can be quite chaotic and have waxing and waning periods. This episodic fever is eponymously dubbed as Pell–Epstein fever. Weight loss is gauged as a significant "B" symptom if greater than 10% of body weight is lost. Night sweats require drenching night sweats on a regular basis. Night sweats probably represent occult breaking of fevers.

Secondary symptoms of Hodgkin's disease that do not qualify as classic "B" symptoms are itching and alcohol intolerance. The pruritus is often intense and generalized. Very occasionally this is the presenting symptom of Hodgkin's disease.

Alcohol intolerance is usually manifest with pain in the area of involvement with Hodgkin's disease after imbibing. It occurs less than 5% of the time. With the successful treatment of Hodgkin's disease, all "B" symptoms as well as pruritus and alcohol intolerance disappear.

There are symptoms of specific organ involvement as described above. Superior vena cava syndrome is the most common consequence of nodal growth. Less common is back pain from retroperitoneal involvement. Splenomegaly can lead to early satiety and left upper quadrant fullness and pain.

Non-Hodgkin's lymphoma

The presenting symptoms of non-Hodgkin's lymphoma depend largely on the histologic subtype. The low-grade (indolent) lymphomas tend to present with painless diffuse adenopathy without "B" symptoms. The intermediate- and high-grade lymphomas are much more commonly associated with fevers, night sweats, and weight loss as well as symptoms of rapid nodal expansion. Superior vena cava syndrome, retroperitoneal pain, symptoms of splenomegaly and other manifestations of bulky nodes are much more common in intermediate- and high-grade lymphoma. As well, patients with intermediate- and high-grade lymphoma occasionally present with impressive systemic illness. These patients are manifestly unwell with profound asthenia, cachexia, and hypermetabolic symptoms.

Hematologic and bone marrow manifestations are much more common in non-Hodgkin's lymphoma. Two categories of hematologic abnormalities are usually encountered. Immunologic destruction of either red cells or platelets are relatively common with low-grade lymphomas and such patients manifest symptoms much as patients with immune thrombocytopenia or autoimmune hematolytic anemia would manifest. These such patients usually have a solitary cell lineage affected, with relatively normal other lineages. Occasionally these patients do present with high numbers of circulating lymphoma cells. Rarely do they cause leukostasis.

Bone marrow failure from marrow infiltration is more commonly seen with intermediate- and high-grade lymphomas. Such patients can present with pancytopenia and associated manifestations of bleeding, infections, and symptoms of anemia.

Treatment of lymphoma

Hodgkin's disease

For many years the paradigm of treatment of Hodgkin's disease was dependent on precise anatomic staging, frequent utilization of exploratory laparotomy, and extensive radiation therapy. In part, this approach was developed because of lack of effective systemic therapy and the morbidity of chemotherapy treatments. While advances in radiation therapy in precise mapping of disease presentations resulted in disease control in a larger number of patients, extensive radiation therapy, exploratory laparotomy and older style chemotherapy have resulted in significant long-term morbidity and mortality for cured Hodgkin's disease patients. The primary consequences of extensive radiation therapy such as cardiac disease, second malignancies, hyperthyroidism, and pulmonary toxicity will be discussed separately.

The recognition of an increased incidence of late toxicities has resulted in a marked paradigm shift in management of patients with early- and late-stage Hodgkin's disease. For patients with localized supradiaphragmatic disease, the US standard is brief chemotherapy with three to four cycles of ABVD (adriamycin, bleomycin, vinblastine, DTIC). Such therapy is followed by involved field radiation therapy at restricted doses. Early estimates suggest that this results in disease control in over 90% of patients. Ten-year follow-ups also suggest that there appears to be a lesser incidence of secondary side effects; particularly secondary malignancies, cardiac disease, and gonadal functional impairment. Long-term follow-up is awaited but it is anticipated that such therapeutic advances would not be associated with a high incidence of secondary complications. It is also noteworthy that the above results are obtained without the necessity of exploratory laparotomy and its attendant morbidity and occasional mortality. Patients are treated promptly, effectively and cured reliably with a single brief intervention.

Advanced-stage Hodgkin's disease is primarily managed with systemic chemotherapy alone. The worldwide standard is six to eight cycles of ABVD. There is insufficient evidence to recommend the addition of radiation therapy, in advanced nonlocalized disease. Overall, approximately 65–70% of such patients are cured with extended systemic chemotherapy.

For those patients recurring after primary treatment, there are successful salvage treatments. Approximately 50% of patients relapsing after primary treatment of Hodgkin's disease will be successfully salvaged with high-dose chemotherapy and stem cell transplantation.

Those patients who have recurrent disease after high-dose chemotherapy still have significant opportunities for palliation. Judicious use of radiation therapy, single-agent chemotherapy with new agents such as Navelbine, gemcitabine, and taxane can offer significant palliation for long periods of time.

Non-Hodgkin's lymphoma

Low-grade non-Hodgkin's lymphoma

Most patients with low-grade non-Hodgkin's lymphoma are elderly and present with advanced albeit asymptomatic disease. There is scant evidence that early initiation of treatment results in better palliation, survival, or improvement in clinical symptomatology. Thus, many patients are suitable for watch and wait strategies and reservation of chemotherapy or radiation therapy for such time as the patient develops symptomatic or rapidly progressive disease. When the patient has either symptomatic or cosmetically unacceptable disease, usual management is initiation of therapy with either single-agent alkylating treatment or simple intravenous combinations with regimens with CVP (cyclophosphamide, vincristine, and prednisone). Alternatives include fludarabine or the use of the monoclonal antibody rituximab. There is no high-grade evidence suggesting superiority of newer treatments over standard treatment. Ongoing trials are poised to answer these questions. In general, patients are treated with chemotherapy until symptom control is established and lymphadenopathy is minimal. Thereafter periods of observation ensue that may extend for years. If and when the patient relapses, subsequent therapies can offer significant palliation including fludarabine, Rituximab, repeat alkylating agent-based therapies or other simple chemotherapeutic combinations. There are newer monoclonal antibodies, both naked and radiolabeled, that have shown significant activity in early investigational trials.

Intermediate-grade lymphoma

Approximately one-third of patients with intermediate-grade lymphoma present with localized disease. Such patients enjoy a high cure rate with combined modality therapy. Standard management includes three to four cycles of CHOP chemotherapy (cyclophosphamide, doxorubicin, vincristine, and prednisone), followed by involved field radiation therapy. With such treatment for clinical stage I and II disease, the expectation is that in excess of 80% of patients will be cured with brief combined-modality therapy.

For the two-thirds of patients with advanced disease, the prognosis is significantly less optimistic. However, fully 40% of patients with advanced staging of intermediate-grade lymphoma, can be expected to be cured. Standard management includes six to eight cycles of CHOP. Investigations of newer combinations of therapy have failed to demonstrate a superior combination to CHOP. Likewise, the early incorporation of high-dose chemotherapy has not uniformly demonstrated benefit in this group of patients with advanced intermediate-grade non-Hodgkin's lymphoma.

For those patients failing primary treatment, there again is a significant chance of long-term disease control and cure with high-dose chemotherapy and bone marrow transplantation. Depending on the timing of relapse and degree of chemotherapy refractiveness somewhere between 20–40% of patients will be cured with high-dose chemotherapy and autologous stem cell support.

For those patients who are either too old or too frail to be considered for high-dose chemotherapy and stem cell rescue, there are a number of alternative salvage therapies that provide significant palliation with acceptable side-effect profiles. "Kinder and gentler" regimens such as CEPP (cyclophosphamide, etoposide, prednisone, and procarbazine), single-agent chemotherapy with new active agents such as gemcitabine and vinorelbine and combinations of judicious use of radiation therapy can provide significant palliations or a surprising amount of time. When considering salvage therapy, one must consider the consequences of treatment measured against the alleviation of symptoms and improved survival. All of these regimens are associated with significant potential for myelosuppression, nausea and vomiting, and a decline of performance status. As with all palliative treatments, one must constantly reassess to gauge the quality of symptom relief versus therapeutic side effects.

Most recently, investigators have begun to add monoclonal antibodies targeted at B-cell antigens as therapy in intermediate- and high-grade lymphomas. A very promising report from the French Lymphoma Study Group demonstrated superiority of CHOP plus Rituximab versus CHOP alone in elderly patients with intermediate- and high-grade lymphoma. This is a particularly difficult group to provide effective treatment for, as they are frequently frail. The addition of Rituximab in preliminary analysis improved response rate and overall survival at 1 year. Longer follow-up on this trial and results of a confirmatory Eastern Cooperative Oncology Group are eagerly awaited. It is of note that the addition of monoclonal antibody Rituximab did not significantly add to the toxicity of the chemotherapy regimen. Additional iterations of this approach are being investigated using radiolabeled monoclonal anti-CD20 antibodies (Ibritumomab tiuxetan).

Symptom management and long-term follow-up

Fever

Fever is an extremely common symptom in patients with Hodgkin's and non-Hodgkin's lymphoma. The differential diagnosis in this group of patients is long and may be related to cryptic infections related to underlying immunosuppression, infections related to chemotherapy-induced neutropenia, or a paraneoplastic phenomenon related to the lymphoma itself. One must be vigilant in analyzing fever in these patients and rule out causes treatable by antimicrobial interventions. If infectious causes have been ruled out, the most effective management of lymphoma-associated fever is effective management of the underlying disease. As addressed in the therapeutic section, such patients should receive standard management, and it is often the case that the fevers disappear promptly with effective treatment of the underlying disease. In the setting where effective therapeutic options have been exhausted, one must consider palliation of fevers as an important goal.

Antipyretics, nonsteroidal anti-inflammatories, and judicious use of corticosteroids frequently provide significant comfort for such patients. Night sweats are usually an occult manifestation of breaking fever and can be managed similarly with evening antipyretic programs. The availability of well-tolerated long-acting nonsteroidal anti-inflammatories, such as celecoxib and rocicoxib, may provide significant relief for such patients.

Weight loss

Weight loss is again a very frustrating symptom for patients and physicians. One must again be diligent about assessing less obvious causes of weight loss such as bacterial overgrowth syndromes, radiation enteritis, mucositis, ill-fitting dentures, and other subtle causes of weight loss. One particular caveat is that many patients with Hodgkin's disease have received radiation therapy to the thyroid. Frequently, thyroid abnormalities manifest with weight loss and lethargy and in all such patients, evaluation of the thyroid is appropriate. For those patients who are felt to have weight loss as a consequence of progressive lymphoma, and for whom there are no significant therapeutic options, again, corticosteroids, megestrol acetate, and cannabinoids are useful in a small subset of patients (see chapter 45).

Itching

Itching related to lymphoma is an extremely unpleasant symptom. Itching is particularly prevalent after hot showers and temperature changes. Patients should be cautioned regarding this. Standard antipruritics, again including corticosteroids, diphenhydramine, and hydroxyzine are useful adjuncts in many patients.

Late complications

As the relative effectiveness of chemotherapy and radiation therapy has improved the cure rate for patients with Hodgkin's and non-Hodgkin's lymphoma, a number of long-term complications of treatment have become apparent in follow-up. Physicians seeing such patients in family practice and internal medicine practices should be aware of such late consequences, as effective preventive and early diagnostic interventions can be most fruitful.

Listed below are the primary consequences of radiation therapy as given frequently for Hodgkin's disease and mediastinal and non-Hodgkin's lymphoma. Such patients frequently experience dental caries, hypothyroidism, thyroid cancer, pulmonary fibrosis related to radiation therapy, accelerated atherosclerosis related to cardiac radiation therapy, pericardial disease, esophageal dysfunction and strictures (rarely), and increased related peptic ulcer disease. Accordingly, such patients should in follow-up have intense dental hygiene, yearly thyroid assessment, monitoring and interventions for cardiac disease including smoking cessation, aggressive management of cholesterol and triglycerides, and weight management.

Second malignancies

The incidence of second malignancies related to chemotherapy include early onset of acute leukemias and secondary non-Hodgkin's lymphomas. Patients should have monitoring of their blood counts and assessment of nodal stations on physical exam on a regular basis in follow-up. Second malignancies related to radiation therapy characteristically are late findings. There is a significantly increased incidence of second solid tumors in the irradiated portals. Primary-care physicians following such patients should be cognizant of such possibilities and vigorously investigate symptoms in these areas early on. Again, smoking prevention and smoking cessation is critical in management of such patients.

Conclusions

The management of Hodgkin's disease, and to a lesser extent non-Hodgkin's lymphoma, has been an important validation of the concept of chemotherapy-curable malignancies. In Hodgkin's disease, the vast majority of patients are cured with brief combined modality inventions. In non-Hodgkin's lymphoma, successful management occurs in a significant portion of patients and control of disease in patients with low-grade non-Hodgkin's lymphoma can extend for decades. New immunologic and molecular oncologic research is in the process of yielding significantly improved targeted therapies that will likely result in even more favorable outcomes for such patients and therapies associated with fewer side effects. We are on the cusp of significant immunologic understanding that likely will yield effective vaccine treatments for patients with non-Hodgkin's lymphoma, and it is anticipated that over the next decade major new therapeutic approaches will become available. Nonetheless, our current therapy is largely effective, well tolerated and curative in a surprisingly high number of patients. Significant palliation can be achieved in most of the remaining patients. Treating and following physicians must be aware of the short- and long-term consequences of treatment and aggressively managed symptoms.

BIBLIOGRAPHY

Bonnadonna G, Zucali R, Monfardini S et al. Combination chemotherapy of Hodgkin's disease with adriamycin, bleomycin, vinblastine and imidazole carboxamide versus MOPP. *Cancer* 1975;36:252–9.

DeVita V, Serpick A, Carbone P. Combination chemotherapy in the treatment of advanced Hodgkin's disease. *Ann Intern Med* 1970;73:881–95.

Fisher R, Gaynor E, Dahlberg S et al. Comparison of a standard regimen (CHOP) with three intensive chemotherapy regimens for advanced non Hodgkin's lymphoma. *N Engl J Med* 1993;328:1002.

Hauke RJ, Armitage JO. Treatment of non-Hodgkin lymphoma. *Curr Opin Oncol* 2000;12:412–18.

Hoppe RT. Hodgkin's disease: complications of therapy and excess mortality. *Ann Oncol* 1997;8(Suppl. 1):S115–18.

Kaplan HS. Role of intensive radiotherapy in the management of Hodgkin's disease. *Cancer* 1966;19:356.

39

Leukemia, myelodysplastic syndrome and myeloproliferative disorder

Larry D. Cripe and Cheryl Rutledge

Indiana University Medical Center, Indianapolis

Overview

Leukemia and myelodysplastic syndromes (MDS) are malignant disorders of normal hematopoiesis. The complications of leukemia or MDS are due to either the excess accumulation of morphologically immature cells (blasts) or the reduced or absent production of leukocytes, red blood cells, or platelets, i.e., pancytopenia. Myeloproliferative disorders (MPD) are distinct disorders of hematopoiesis that initially involve excess production of mature blood cells. Table 39.1 summarizes the estimated incidence, median survival, and likelihood of cure with contemporary treatment. Untreated leukemia is uniformly and rapidly fatal due to the infectious or hemorrhagic complications of the pancytopenia. Treatment produces a relatively modest prolongation of life for the majority of patients with leukemia. The prolonged median survival of certain subtypes of MDS and MPD is due to their relatively benign behaviors. However, except for the uncommon individual cured of the disease or who dies of unrelated causes, patients with leukemia, MDS, or MPD will succumb to complications of progressive pancytopenia either due to leukemia refractory to chemotherapy or marrow fibrosis. The complications are enumerated in the section entitled "Caring for the individual with advanced leukemia."

We define the term, advanced leukemia, as the phase of the disease when the likelihood of benefit from conventional therapy does not justify the potential toxicity of therapy. The likelihood of benefit is influenced by factors such as age, overall health, characteristics of the disease, and whether the disease is newly diagnosed or recurrent. The goal is to eradicate or suppress the malignant hematopoiesis sufficiently to allow partial or complete restoration of normal hematopoiesis. In general, this is possible in leukemia but not in advanced MDS or MPD. However, the potential toxicity of chemotherapy for leukemia is considerable. Thus, the timely recognition

Table 39.1. Incidence and overall survival (OS) of leukemia and related disorders. The figures are illustrative of the relative incidence as the epidemiology of uncommon disorders may be inaccurate

Disease	Incidence	Median OS	Cure?
AML/ALL (including RAEB-t and poor-risk RAEB)	3 per 100 000. Increases to 12/100 000 in patients > 65 years	8–12 months	≤ 25% of patients ≤ 60 years of age; < 5–10% in patients >60 years of age
MDS RA/RARS	1–2 per 100 000	4–7 years	No for vast majority. Possible in rare patients eligible for allo-BMT
MPD CML, chronic phase	1.5 per 100 000	4–5 years	Allo-BMT may produce benefit in 60–75% of eligible patients
MPD PRV, ET, AMM	0.5–1 per 100 000	7–10 years	No

Note: AML, acute myeloid leukemia; ALL, acute lymphoblastic leukemia; MDS, myelodysplastic syndromes; MPD, myeloproliferative disorders; RAEB-t, refractory anemia with excess blasts in transformation; RAEB, refractory anemia with excess blasts; CML, chronic myeloid leukemia; PRV, polycythemia rubra vera; ET, essential thrombocythemia; AMM, agnogenic myeloid metaplasia; RA, refractory anemia; RARS, refractory anemia with ringed sideroblasts; BMT, bone marrow transplant.

of advanced leukemia may prevent burdensome side effects of chemotherapy, radiation, or surgery when such therapy is likely futile. We may then provide affected individuals a greater opportunity for comfort and dignity as life ends.

The timely recognition of advanced leukemia may be accomplished by repeatedly posing two fundamental questions. First, what are the available options for treatment? Second, what are the goals of treatment and how likely is the desired outcome? Table 39.2 provides an overview of the treatment options and goals for newly diagnosed disease and features of advanced disease. In general, the treatment of advanced disease emphasizes supportive care such as transfusions and avoids intensive chemotherapy.

Presentation and patterns of progression

The most common presentation of leukemia and the related disorders is the discovery of some combination of anemia or erythrocytosis, leukopenia or leukocytosis and thrombocytosis or thrombocytopenia on a complete blood count performed during routine healthcare. The more common symptoms include bruising, fatigue, fever, weight loss, dyspnea, or early satiety due to splenomegaly. Uncommon but noteworthy presentations include signs of vascular insufficiency due to

Table 39.2. Overview of natural history of leukemia and related disorders (for definitions of diseases see Table 39.1)

Disease	At time of initial diagnosis		Recognition of advanced disease
	Goals of care	Options	
AML/ALL (including RAEB-t and poor-risk RAEB)	Remission Cure in younger patients with low-risk features Palliation in older adults with poor health or poor-risk features End-of-life care	Intensive myelosuppressive therapy (induction and consolidation) Minimally myelosuppressive therapy (low-dose, palliative) Transfusions of blood products Antibiotics Hematopoietic CSFs Therapeutic cytapharesis Comfort measures	Concurrent health problems reduce likelihood of surviving rigors of therapy Failure to achieve remission after two or more treatments Relapse in less than 6 months Multiply relapsed disease Relapse after BMT
MDS RA/RARS	Amelioration of complications of cytopenia or need for transfusions	Transfusions of blood products Hematopoietic CSFs Investigational therapy	Development of AML Progressive decline in performance status Increasingly frequent transfusions
MPD CML, chronic phase	Maintain in chronic phase Cure (if allogeneic BMT possible)	Hydroxyurea Interferon Allogeneic BMT Imatinib mesylate	Blast crisis or accelerated phase CML Relapse after BMT
MPD PRV, ET, AMM	Reduction in erythrocytosis or thrombocytosis Reduce risk of thrombosis Reduce degree of splenomegaly	Therapeutic cytapharesis Minimally myelosuppressive therapy Antiplatelet agents Radioactive phosphorus Splenectomy	Development of AML (rare) Development of transfusion requirement Progressive decline in performance status

Note: CSF, colony-stimulating factor; BMT, bone marrow transplant.

hyperleukocytosis, a variety of skin rashes due to leukemic infiltration of the skin, and neurologic syndromes such as radiculopathy or spinal cord compression due to leukemic infiltration of the meninges, or mass lesions.

The diagnosis of leukemia, MDS, or MPD requires, in the vast majority of cases, the morphologic and cytogenetic analysis of a sample of bone marrow. Rarely an individual will present with a localized mass of leukemia cells (granulocytic sarcoma) and the diagnosis is made on biopsy of the mass. The traditional morphologic examination of bone marrow is supplemented by analysis of cellular antigen expression with immunologic techniques. Leukemia may be broadly subdivided based upon the anticipated course of the disease if untreated (i.e., acute or chronic) and whether the cells are of myeloid or lymphoid origin. The term acute implies that survival beyond three months is extremely unusual without treatment or a response to treatment. Death most frequently results from hemorrhage or infection. The term chronic implies that prolonged survival (greater than 12 months) is frequently observed. Initially the symptoms and complications relate to the excess production of leukocytes.

The development of advanced phase disease implies the progressive accumulation of blasts in the marrow or occasionally other tissues and/or worsening anemia, leukopenia, and thrombocytopenia. The consequences include a steady decline in overall health without specific complications or increasingly severe and frequent infections, episodes of hemorrhage, or cardiopulmonary insufficiency due to the reduced delivery of oxygen to the tissues. The benefit of transfusions and antibiotics decreases over time for identified reasons, such as alloimmunization or emergence of resistant bacteria, and for poorly understood reasons.

Treatment options

Except for the unusual situation of radiation for leukemic meningitis, the treatment of leukemia requires chemotherapy. The dose and schedule of chemotherapy may be broadly defined as conventional or myeloablative. Myeloablative therapy indicates that a supplemental source of marrow is required to assure recovery of peripheral blood counts after the period of myelosuppression, i.e., bone marrow transplantation (BMT). If the marrow is from a donor the process is labeled an allogeneic bone marrow transplant (allo-BMT). Autologous BMT (auto-BMT) indicates that the marrow is from the individual with the disease. Table 39.3 is a summary of the treatment options with an overview of the clinical situations for which each option is most appropriate.

There are several options for the treatment of the individual with acute myeloid leukemia (AML)/acute lymphoblastic leukemia (ALL) or the RAEB/RAEB-t subtype of MDS: intensive induction chemotherapy with the intent of achieving

Table 39.3. Treatment options for the individual with leukemia and related disorders (for definitions of diseases see Table 39.1). The progression to advanced leukemia implies that the more aggressive or intensive therapies are probably not appropriate

Treatment	Action	Appropriate usage/comments
Conventional dose chemotherapy	Intensively myelosuppressive	Used in treatment of AML, ALL, blast crisis of CML. Goal is remission
	Moderately myelosuppressive	Used in control of myeloproliferative disorders. Remission is not achieved. Hydroxyurea is classic example
	Low-dose (palliative)	May slow rate of progression of AML or provide temporary reduction in symptoms or frequency of transfusions
	Molecularly targeted	Examples include all trans-retinoic acid (ATRA) and Imatinib mesylate
Myeloablative-dose chemotherapy	*Followed by infusion of:* Allogeneic HLA-matched sibling stem cells	Used in first or second or greater remission of AML. Rarely used in treatment of MPD or MDS
	Allogeneic HLA-matched nonsibling stem cells	Used in first or second or greater remission of AML. Rarely used in treatment of MPD or MDS
	Cryopreserved autologous stem cells	Used in first or second or greater remission of AML
Biologic agents	Hematopoietic colony-stimulating factors	Used to reduce complications of chemotherapy and occasionally to ameliorate cytopenias
	Interferon	Used in chronic phase CML and other MPDs
Antibody-based therapies	Anti-CD33	Possibility of outpatient salvage therapy in relapsed AML
Surgery	Splenectomy	May palliate symptoms of splenomegaly
Therapeutic cytapharesis	Physical removal of excess blood elements	Reasonable strategy in PRV and useful emergently in ET or hyperleukocytosis of AML
Radiation	Craniospinal electron beam	Leukemic meningitis
Investigational approaches	Variety of options	Eligibility is restricted. Overall PS must be fairly good
Best supportive care	Red cell or platelet transfusions and oral antibiotics	Goal is to prolong life by compensating for lack of marrow function
Hospice		

a complete remission; palliative-intent chemotherapy with the goal of reducing symptoms, transfusion requirements or rate of disease progression; best supportive care with the intent of providing transfusions or hematopoietic colony stimulating factors to reduce symptoms; or hospice care. Typically, a prolonged hospitalization (4–6 weeks) is necessary to safely administer treatment and support the individual during the period of profound myelosuppression that occurs with intensive induction therapy. The concept of palliative intent chemotherapy is discussed further in the section on AML and ALL.

The treatment options for the RA/RARS subtypes of MDS or the advanced form of ET, AMM, or PRV that occurs because of fibrosis are essentially best supportive care, investigational trials, or, for the rare younger individual with an allogeneic donor, an allo-BMT.

Prognostic factors: Predicting progression and likelihood of benefit to treatment

Individuals with leukemia or the related disorders deserve the opportunity to experience the improvement in quality of life or life expectancy possible with antineoplastic therapy. However, if such therapy is unlikely to produce benefit then they are equally deserving of receiving expert palliative care. The counseling of patients with advanced leukemia, MDS, or MPD involves communicating the low likelihood of benefit from therapy. Consideration of the following prognostic factors may assist the clinician in estimating the likelihood of benefit (Table 39.4).

Age

Retrospective studies of results of treatment and prevalence of other poor-risk characteristics suggest that 60 years of age serves as a reasonable dividing point between likely to benefit and unlikely to benefit from chemotherapy. The explanations for the poor outcome include the different biology of the disease and poor tolerance to the complications of cytopenias or to therapy. Epidemiologic studies suggest approximately half the older patients diagnosed with AML/ALL, CML, or advanced stage MDS or MPD are not treated with chemotherapy.

Performance status

In the era of sophisticated laboratory analysis, the predictive value of performance status should not be overlooked. Unless the decline in performance status is directly attributed to the disease, it in general predicts for a poor outcome.

Antecedent hematologic disorders

People with AML/ALL who have received prior chemotherapy or radiation for an unrelated malignancy or who have had a prior MDS or MPD fare extremely poorly

Table 39.4. Prognostic factors in leukemia and related disorders (definitions as in Table 39.1)

General features	Comments
Age	Older patients less tolerant of intensive therapy
	Disease tends to be more resistant to therapy
Performance status	Reasonable marker of likelihood of tolerating therapy
Antecedent hematologic disorders	Predicts for chemotherapy resistance: low likelihood of CR and short remission duration
Relapsed or refractory disease	Predicts for chemotherapy resistance: low likelihood of CR and short remission duration
	Each time likelihood of CR less than prior therapy
	CR duration less than preceding CR
Karyotype	Predictive of outcome in AML/MDS
	Favorable: inv 16, t8;21, t15;17
	Intermediate: normal and others
	Unfavorable: 5/del(5q), -7/del(7q), abn of 11q,
	Acquisition of other abnormal chromosomes is unfavorable
Immunophenotype	Certain patterns poor outcome, e.g., CD34 expression
Basophilia	Poor outcome in CML
Degree of splenomegaly	Poor outcome in CML

with conventional chemotherapy. The older individual may wisely choose to forgo the rigors of induction chemotherapy. Younger individuals may receive allo-BMT once in remission or rarely as primary therapy.

Relapsed or refractory disease

The failure to respond to chemotherapy is a very grave prognostic feature (see discussion under AML). Typically, patients with MPD will initially experience control with moderately myelosuppressive chemotherapy. The development of pancytopenia or difficult to control erythrocytosis or thrombocytosis may indicate the diagnosis of advanced disease.

Karyotype

Numerical or structural abnormalities of chromosomes can be identified by the examination of metaphase preparations of dividing cells in marrow aspirates. It has been well established that the karyotype at the time of diagnosis may be predictive of outcome. Three subgroups have been routinely discussed in acute leukemia: favorable, intermediate, and poor risk. Similar findings are also applicable to MDS.

The MPD, CML, has a hallmark translocation between chromosome 9 and 22. The acquisition of further chromosomal abnormalities in CML is a predictive factor for progression to the accelerated phase or blast crisis.

Discussion of specific disorders

Acute leukemia

The diagnosis of acute leukemia requires the demonstration of more than 20% blasts (WHO criteria) on a marrow specimen that is typically hypercellular. The distinction between AML and ALL depends on cytochemical reactions (AML is myeloperoxidase or esterase positive) and the demonstration of lymphoid antigens. The treatment options include conventional induction chemotherapy, palliative chemotherapy, supportive care with transfusions and antibiotics, or strictly palliative end-of-life care during which time supportive care is progressively withdrawn.

Acute myeloid leukemia (including poor-risk RAEB and RAEB-t)

The median age at the time of diagnosis of AML is 65–70 years of age, so concurrent health problems frequently limit treatment options. Conventional induction chemotherapy for AML utilizes one or more courses of cytarabine and an anthracycline or an anthracycline derivative. The dose of cytarabine is 100 or 200 mg/m^2 as a continuous intravenous infusion over 24 hours × 7 days. The traditional anthracycline is daunorubicin administered at a dose of 30–60 mg/m^2 as a brief intravenous infusion daily on the first 3 days. The goal of the intensive treatment of acute leukemia is to produce a remission defined as normal peripheral blood counts and less than 5% blasts in the marrow. Palliative chemotherapy is reduced-dose chemotherapy. The intent is to reduce the leukocytosis and suppress leukemic hematopoiesis to allow some normal hematopoiesis. In general, remissions are not achieved with palliative dose chemotherapy. In our opinion, the complications and inconvenience of the low-dose palliative chemotherapy do not justify the meager results. We encourage affected individuals to decide between full-dose induction chemotherapy or palliative supportive care.

The major adverse prognostic factors are older age, the presence of certain chromosomal abnormalities, a high leukocyte count, and a history of a pre-existing hematologic abnormality or prior chemotherapy. Table 39.5 lists the likelihood of achieving a remission for adults with AML. It is apparent that the likelihood of a remission varies between less than 25% (older adult with poor-risk cytogenetics) to greater than 80% (younger than age 40 with good risk cytogenetics). Death during induction therapy and refractory AML are the reasons for failure to achieve a remission. The second phase of treatment is postremission therapy. In general, there

Table 39.5. Representative outcomes to the treatment of acute myeloid leukemia (AML) based upon time of treatment

AML	Possible outcome (%)		
	Remission	Death	Overall survival
Newly-diagnosed			
<60 years of age	70	<5	25
≥60 years of age	50	20	<10
Relapsed			
CR >12 months	60	20	20
CR 6–12 months	50	20	15
CR <6 months	<25	25	<5

Note: CR, complete response.

is no difference in overall survival whether the person receives further conventional therapy, or an autologous or allogeneic BMT.

The majority of patients in remission will relapse; the median survival is 8–14 months. However, approximately 25% of younger individuals may experience cure. It is uncommon to see an older individual survive longer than 2 years and most relapse within 10–12 months. The prognosis at the time of relapse is strongly influenced by the length of the preceding remissions and whether it is the first or subsequent relapse. People with a remission less than six months are very unlikely to experience another remission of significant duration. If the remission was greater than 18–24 months, then treatment is likely to be successful. Conventional salvage chemotherapy typically includes the administration of higher doses of cytarabine (1000–3000 mg/m^2 once or twice daily for 6–12 doses) with or without other chemotherapy agents. If a second or subsequent remission is achieved an allo-BMT or auto-BMT is the preferred postremission therapy. Otherwise prolonged survival is unlikely. Palliative care or investigational trials may be more appropriate options for people with remissions less than 6–12 months.

What are reasonable times to advise the individual of the advanced nature of the disease, and that therefore strong consideration of a more palliative approach is warranted? Patients who fail to achieve a remission after two induction attempts have an extremely poor prognosis. Many older adults at the time of diagnosis may be considered to have advanced phase disease due to the presence of multiple adverse prognostic factors and poor-risk health conditions. Older adults who relapse within 6 months and younger adults with multiply-relapsed disease have a similar dismal outcome. The greatest challenge is to counsel the younger individual with an allogeneic donor about the risks and small but definite benefit to proceeding to an allo-BMT.

Acute lymphoblastic leukemia (ALL)

ALL is much less common than AML. The prognosis in older adults is extremely poor. ALL may respond temporarily to prednisone and vincristine which may be administered as an outpatient. The adverse prognostic features and course of ALL are similar to AML.

Myelodsyplastic syndromes

The myelodysplastic syndromes are characterized by the inadequate production of blood cells. The classification is based upon the presence of morphologic evidence of abnormal blood cell production (dysplasia) and the percentage of marrow blasts. The details of the subtypes are beyond the scope of this chapter. The natural history of the disorder is characterized by progressive pancytopenia and a risk of transformation to AML. The subtypes of MDS with the greater likelihood of transformation are refractory anemia with excess blasts (RAEB) and refractory anemia with excess blasts in transformation (RAEB-t). The clinical course of RAEB and RAEB-t is similar to AML. The other subtypes, refractory anemia (RA) and refractory anemia with ringed sideroblasts (RARS), typically are not rapidly fatal diseases. The management is usually restricted to the use of hematopoietic colony-stimulating factors and transfusions. There is no curative therapy for the vast majority of patients.

Myeloproliferative disorders

The myeloproliferative disorders are characterized by the excess production of blood cells and are subdivided based upon the predominant overproduced cell type. Chronic myeloid leukemia (CML) is the excess production of mature appearing white blood cells; it has a unique and more predictable natural history and is discussed in more detail below. Polycythemia rubra vera (PRV) is the excess production of red blood cells; essential thrombocythemia (ET) is the excess production of platelets; and agnogenic myeloid metaplasia (AMM) is the excess production of abnormal megakaryocytes that leads to progressive marrow fibrosis. Many individuals will experience no major complications and succumb to other illnesses typical of an older population. The goals of treatment initially are to reduce the complications of the excess production by phleobotomy or chemotherapy such as hydroxyurea or anegrelide. There is no evidence that the induction chemotherapy similar to that described for AML is of value. A rare individual may benefit from allo-BMT. Relatively few individuals with PRV will develop AML. Treatment, however, of secondary AML is quite difficult and most patients should be enrolled into hospice care at that point. The other common cause of advanced MPD is progressive marrow fibrosis and loss of normal blood cell production. Transfusions and splenectomy represent the limited treatment options.

Chronic myeloid leukemia (CML)

The natural history of CML may change dramatically with the recent introduction of an oral medication (STI-571, marketed as Gleevec) that specifically inhibits the pathogenic molecular defect of CML, the bcr-abl tyrosine kinase. The only known curative option for CML is allo-BMT. Individuals without a donor or who are too old to receive an allo-BMT are treated with interferon, hydroxyurea or Imatinib mesylate. The goal of treatment is to control symptoms of leukocytosis and spleno-megaly and to maintain the disease in the chronic phase. However, uniformly the disease progresses to the blast crisis. The blast crisis is essentially uniformly fatal within several months. Individuals in the blast crisis may be offered conven-tional induction chemotherapy similar to AML or ALL, investigational chemo-therapy, allo-BMT, or palliative care. The vast majority are better served with pal-liative care or investigational chemotherapy. The median survival of individuals with CML is 4.5 years. Relevant prognostic factors include the relative numbers of blasts, promyelocytes, and basophils; the degree of splenomegaly; the presence of additional cytogenetic abnormalities; and the absolute platelet count.

The care of the individual with advanced leukemia

The judicious use of transfusions and oral antibiotics to reduce the complications of the anemia, thrombocytopenia, and neutropenia is of value early on in the care of advanced leukemia. However, inexorably people will decline. The goal is to discuss the gradual discontinuation of supportive measures to allow life to end with as much comfort as possible. The following discussion enumerates common problems of advanced leukemia and provides guidance into the management.

Decline in performance status

The decline in performance status most people with advanced leukemia experience is multifactorial. Therefore, a formal review of systems may be helpful in determin-ing if an underlying cause can be determined and ameliorated. It is also important to pay close attention to the individual's assessment of daily life. There are decisions involved in the care of people with advanced cancer such as when to forgo transfu-sions. If quality of life has declined to an unacceptable level, then there may be little rationale for transfusions. Thus, we pose two questions. First, overall, is the indi-vidual doing activities that are of value to him or her? We identify specific activities that he or she cannot perform. Second, has the current care improved the likelihood of the individual doing what he or she wants? Is the care too burdensome relative to the benefit? It is important to not increase the rate of decline by the toxicity associated with therapy. We also use the decline in performance status to guide decisions such as discontinuing transfusion support or not administering antibiotics. For example, transfusions may not improve the symptoms sufficiently to warrant continuation. Or we may deliberately choose to not treat an infection or fever if overall the performance status implies an unacceptable quality of life.

Anemia

The cause of anemia in advanced leukemia is most commonly impaired red cell production. The patient should be evaluated for immune-mediated destruction by red cell serologic assays or blood loss. The mainstay of treatment is transfusion of packed red blood cells. A trial of erythropoietin may be reasonable in selected cases. However, the utility of erythropoietin is limited because of a low response rate. On occasion, significant splenomegaly will worsen the degree of anemia or reduce the benefit to transfusions. In those cases splenectomy may be warranted. The physician should anticipate a time when the symptomatic improvement associated with transfusion is minimal and/or the burden of transfusion therapy is great. Counseling patients to forgo red cell transfusions is appropriate at that time. The dyspnea of progressive anemia is responsive to narcotic analgesics.

Neutropenia

The major risk of neutropenia is infection. Prophylactic antibiotics are of little value and may produce diarrhea or colitis. The use of the myelopoietic colony-stimulating factors (G-CSF or GM-CSF) may produce a beneficial rise in the absolute neutrophil count (ANC). Typically, we will try daily injections for 1 or 2 weeks. We monitor blood counts to avoid an increase in the leukemic cells and to see if any improvement in the ANC occurs. The ANC may only modestly increase (300–400 per microliter) but that may be of clinical benefit. We try to administer injections at a reduced frequency and observe if the response is maintained. The most problematic infection from a symptom standpoint is breakdown of the oral mucosal membranes with chronic ulcers. In that case we use a short course of G- or GM-CSF to attempt to improve the neutrophil count. It is important to discuss the strategy in the event of a high fever with systemic symptoms. In the setting of advanced leukemia the administration of empiric broad-spectrum intravenous antibiotics is probably not warranted; especially if the decline in performance status has been substantial.

Thrombocytopenia

Transfusions of platelets are the mainstay of therapy. The practical limitations of platelet transfusions are the relatively brief increase in platelet counts (usually 3–7 days) and the likelihood of a progressive decline in the posttransfusion increase in platelet count in the multiply transfused subject. The latter limitation is termed platelet refractoriness. Transfusions are administered to prevent or treat bleeding episodes. We tend to transfuse if the platelet count falls below 5000 per microliter. However, the overall clinical condition is considered. It is important to monitor coagulation parameters periodically to avoid vitamin K deficiency due to poor nutrition or use of antibiotics. Hemorrhage that persists despite platelet transfusions may respond to the use of the antifibrinolytic agent, aminocaproic acid. In the event of hemorrhage as a terminal event, sedation is most humane.

Splenomegaly

The causes of splenomegaly include extramedullary hematopoiesis, infiltration by the leukemic process, or portal vein thrombosis. Splenomegaly may produce pain and early satiety; it may exacerbate the pancytopenia or impair the response to transfusions; and it may represent the major site of disease. The treatment options include chemotherapy such as hydroxyurea, splenic irradiation, or splenectomy. Splenic irradiation controls the splenomegaly for at most several months typically. The concern with surgical splenectomy besides the operative risk is whether the spleen is a site of significant blood cell production. This is especially relevant in the MPD. In general, we favor splenectomy. If an individual is too moribund to undergo splenectomy then perhaps the disease process is more advanced than appreciated.

Leukemic meningitis

The syndrome of most clinical concern is the development of meningeal leukemia. In general, we treat with intrathecal chemotherapy and craniospinal irradiation depending on the extent of disease. It is unlikely that overall survival is affected. However, the preservation of nerve function appears to significantly improve the quality of life and lessens the distress of individual and family during the end of life.

Bone pain

Pain is an uncommon problem in individuals with advanced leukemia. Perhaps the most common syndrome is diffuse bone pain due to expansion of the marrow space and bone destruction. Corticosteroids, narcotic analgesics, radiation, and chemotherapy may improve the pain. We have observed responses to the infusion of pamidronate. The administration of hydroxyurea or radioactive phosphorus may also be of value. The latter options will almost certainly exacerbate the pancytopenia.

Hyperleukocytosis

On occasion the peripheral leukocyte count may be sufficiently high to impair the flow in the microcirculation. The symptoms typically reflect the vascular congestion.

Especially problematic are ischemic neurologic events, symptoms of dyspnea due to pulmonary vascular congestion, and priapism. If the disease has been refractory to chemotherapy, then a strictly palliative approach is more appropriate. A transient reduction in the circulating leukocyte count may be achieved by leukapheresis.

Hypermetabolism

Some individuals with MPDs will experience complications related to the tremendous proliferation of blood cells. This may manifest as weight loss sometimes despite a good appetite, fatigue, fevers or night sweats, or metabolic complications such as gout from hyperuricemia.

Pruritus

MPD's may be complicated by itching especially after hot showers. Typically the use of antihistamines will control the pruritus.

BIBLIOGRAPHY

Sentinel articles

Cassileth P, Harrington D, Appelbaum FR et al. Chemotherapy compared with autologous or allogeneic bone marrow transplantation in the management of acute myeloid leukemia in first remission. *N Engl J Med* 1998;339:1649–56.

Greenberg P, Cox C, LeBeau MM et al. International scoring system for evaluating prognosis in myelodysplastic syndromes. *Blood* 1997;89:2079–88.

Grimwade D, Walker H, Oliver F et al. The importance of diagnostic cytogenetics on outcome in AML: Analysis of 1,612 patients entered into the MRC AML 10 trial. *Blood* 1998;92:2322–33.

Gruppo Italiano Studio Policitemia. Polycythemia vera: the natural history of 1213 patients followed for 20 years. *Ann Intern Med* 1995;123:656–64.

Löwenberg B, Suciu S, Archimbaud E et al. Mitoxantrone versus daunorubicin in induction-consolidation chemotherapy – the value of low-dose cytarabine for maintenance of remission, and an assessment of prognostic factors in acute myeloid leukemia in the elderly: final report. European Organization for the Research and Treatment of Cancer and the Dutch-Belgian Hemato-Oncology Cooperative HOVON Group. *J Clin Oncol* 1998;16:872–81.

Mayer RJ, Davis RB, Schiffer CA et al. For the Cancer and Leukemia Group B: Intensive post-remission chemotherapy in adults with acute myeloid leukemia. *N Engl J Med* 1994;331:896–903.

Reviews

Heaney ML, Golde DW. Myelodysplasia. *N Engl J Med* 1999;340:1649–60.

Messinezy M, Pearson TC. Polycythaemia, primary (essential) thrombocythaemia and myelo-fibrosis. *Br Med J* 1997;314:587–90.

Tefferei A. Myelofibrosis with myeloid metaplasia. *N Engl J Med* 2000;342:1255–65.

Internet site

National Cancer Institute
http://www.cancer.gov/cancer_information/cancer_type/

40

Multiple myeloma

Letha E. Mills

Southwestern Vermont Cancer Center, Bennington

Multiple myeloma is a malignant proliferation of plasma cells that is not curable with standard therapy. The disease can cause significant disability and tends to occur in older individuals, so the care must be comprehensive with palliation of symptoms a major goal. This chapter will review the supportive care recommended for patients with myeloma, after providing basic information regarding the biology and available standard chemotherapy.

Biology/natural history

Plasma cells differentiate from B lymphocytes and normally function to produce antibodies. Antibodies are plasma proteins produced to help the cellular immune system fight foreign matter such as bacteria. Antibodies are found in the gamma globulin fraction on serum protein electrophoresis (SPEP). One clone of plasma cells produces one specific antibody (idiotype) so that when one plasma cell becomes malignant the clone of abnormal cells all produce the same idiotypic protein. As these cells proliferate, more antibody is produced and this leads to a monoclonal ("M") spike on the SPEP. Plasma cells normally comprise less than 5% of bone marrow cells.

A number of staging systems have been developed for myeloma. Criteria to make a diagnosis of multiple myeloma include marrow plasmacytosis of greater than 10%, presence of an M-protein (for IgG usually greater than 3 g/dl) in the serum on SPEP, and at least one of the following: (1) anemia; (2) M-protein (or light chains only greater than 1.0 g/24 hour) in the urine (usually measured by a 24-hour urine collection); (3) lytic bone lesions demonstrated on a skeletal survey, or osteoporosis only but with greater than 30% plasma cells in the bone marrow; (4) renal insufficiency; or (5) hypercalcemia. It is important to distinguish myeloma requiring treatment from smoldering myeloma, where more than 10% plasma cells are present in the bone marrow and the M spike may be greater than 3 g/dl, but there is no other disease requiring therapy. Monoclonal gammopathy of undetermined significance (MGUS) patients have an M protein usually less than 3 g/dl, less than 10% plasma cells and no other criteria for myeloma. These patients do not require therapy and may never progress to overt myeloma.

Current therapy

Treatment of myeloma is determined by the age of the patient, the extent of disease and the presence and extent of comorbid disease. However, patients under the age of 70 without significant comorbid disease should be considered as potential candidates for a clinical trial employing peripheral blood stem cell transplantation (PBSCT). Patients in otherwise good health have been successfully treated with high-dose chemotherapy and PBSCT. Single-center data have reported up to 50% complete remissions with some sustained responses for as long as 10 years. This does not appear to be curative therapy and the morbidity of the treatment is much higher than with standard-dose chemotherapy.

Patients requiring treatment who are not candidates for clinical trials will receive either oral therapy with melphalan and prednisone or combination chemotherapy with multiple alkylators. Combination therapy yields higher response rates but has no significant survival advantage and is therefore often reserved for patients considered to have "high risk" disease. Patients who relapse may be treated with second-line chemotherapy or with more novel therapies such as thalidomide.

Supportive therapies

Anemia

Anemia is often the presenting sign of multiple myeloma. As many as 80% of patients may have anemia at diagnosis. Fatigue is a common symptom and in part may be due to the anemia. When the hematocrit is less than 30%, patients may be treated with recombinant erythropoietin. This can be administered subcutaneously once per week. It has been shown to improve quality of life and a sense of well-being for patients.

Skeletal fractures

Patients with multiple myeloma are at high risk for fractures due to bone loss. Lytic lesions most often occur in the axial skeleton and proximal long bones where bone marrow production occurs in the adult. Lytic lesions at sites important for weight-bearing can lead to fractures causing significant pain and disability. To maintain functional mobility it may be necessary to intervene surgically with intramedullary rod placement for stabilization and prevention of pathologic fractures. Lesions in the femur involving more than 50% of the cortex have a 50% or higher risk of fracture. Post-operative therapy with radiation is usually indicated with the aim to eliminate the myeloma cells and allow healing. Radiation therapy should always be considered for pain relief for any painful site of disease.

Spinal cord compression

This is a complication that should be prevented if at all possible by early evaluation and treatment. The possibility of cord compression should be entertained in any patient with myeloma complaining of significant back pain. The patient should be asked about any weakness, paresthesias, or bowel or bladder dysfunction. A magnetic resonance imaging (MRI) or computed tomography (CT) scan should be immediately obtained when suspicion is high. Treatment with steroids followed by radiation therapy to the involved site should be instituted rapidly. A comprehensive plan for effective pain management must also be put in place.

Bone pain

Bone pain is another common presenting symptom of myeloma, occurring in 80% of patients at diagnosis. Bone pain may be caused by bone loss leading to pathologic fractures or due to bone infiltration with malignant plasma cells. The bone loss is caused by stimulation of the bone-resorbing osteoclasts and cannot be reversed easily with chemotherapy or radiation aimed at eradicating myeloma cells. However, bony infiltration with plasma cells can have an associated soft tissue mass leading to nerve or spinal cord impingement and can be more effectively treated with radiation and or chemotherapy. Corticosteroid therapy in this situation may be used both as a means to decrease local soft tissue swelling as well as an agent capable of killing myeloma cells. It is important to determine the etiology of the bone pain so that appropriate therapy can be implemented.

Bisphosphonates are potent inhibitors of bone resorption. Their use in the treatment of multiple myeloma has become important as adjunctive therapy both for bone pain and for bone healing. Orally administered agents are not absorbed well and therefore have not been demonstrated to be clinically useful in myeloma patients. Intravenous pamidronate 90 mg given over at least 2 hours and administered monthly has been shown to decrease skeletal complications. Administration in less than 2 hours may contribute to nephrotoxicity. There is no effect on bone marrow function and so can be given in conjunction with chemotherapy. Recent studies in the laboratory suggest bisphosphonates may also have direct antimyeloma effects and clinical data are beginning to emerge suggesting there may be survival benefit. A more potent bisphosphonate, zoledronic acid, has shown superiority in treating tumor-induced hypercalcemia and is undergoing study for use adjunctively. Its advantage for the patient is not only the higher potency but administration takes only

5–15 minutes, greatly reducing the time the patient will have to spend in the clinic each month.

Hypercalcemia

High serum calcium levels are a common complication associated with myeloma. Thirty percent of patients with myeloma present with hypercalcemia as the initial manifestation of their disease. Bone resorption causes increased calcium in the extracellular fluid. Patients with decreased renal function will be more susceptible to hypercalcemia. Obligate fluid loss with the high calcium causes further problems, as dehydration will develop.

Treatment begins with normal saline hydration of three liters or more per day depending on the cardiac status of the patient. Diuresis with furosemide may be used to enhance calcium excretion and to prevent fluid overload in the elderly or in those with compromised cardiac function. The mainstay of therapy has become the prompt administration of an intravenous bisphosphonate such as pamidronate or zoledronic acid. Outpatient treatment instituted quickly may avoid hospitalization. More resistant hypercalcemia may be treated with calcitonin. This agent is effective but patients rapidly develop tachyphylaxis and it is therefore of limited usefulness.

Renal failure

Approximately one-fifth of patients with myeloma have a creatinine of at least 2.0 mg/dl at diagnosis. A number of factors may contribute to this: hypercalcemia, dehydration, hyperuricemia, use of nonsteroidal anti-inflammatory agents (NSAIDs) or roentgenographic contrast material, as well as infiltration of the kidney with plasma cells ("myeloma kidney"), tubular damage due to light chain precipitation, or deposition of amyloid within the kidney. Deposition of amyloid is associated with nephrotic syndrome.

General treatment of renal insufficiency involves fluid and electrolyte replacement, maintenance of high urine output, prompt recognition and correction of high serum calcium or uric acid levels. Avoidance of dehydration, use of contrast agents during evaluation, and limiting exposure to NSAIDs if the creatinine is elevated are important for prevention.

If renal failure is determined likely to be due to plasma cell infiltration, treatment with more aggressive chemotherapy may be warranted after alkalinization of the urine and administration of allopurinol to prevent uric acid precipitation. For treatment of acute renal failure a trial of plasmapheresis may be considered, especially if gamma globulin levels are high. Hemodialysis or peritoneal dialysis may be necessary if renal insufficiency is severe.

Hyperviscosity

Symptoms of hyperviscosity include headache, blurred vision, epistaxis and other spontaneous bleeding. It is often caused by elevated gamma globulin, more often occurring with an IgA monoclonal protein than IgG. Measurement of serum viscosity is of limited usefulness, as symptoms do not correlate well with the measured values. Symptoms will respond temporarily to decreasing the immunoglobulin level through plasmapheresis. Treatment with effective therapy aimed at decreasing the production of the protein must be done at the same time. Repeated plasmapheresis is to be avoided given the time involved, the potential for side affects associated with the procedure, the risk of infection with the venous access lines required, the cost, and the temporary nature of the response.

Bone marrow abnormalities

About 60% of patients present with leukopenia at the time of diagnosis and one-quarter to one-third will have thrombocytopenia. Some patients appear particularly liable to persistent problems with bone marrow dysfunction leading to delays in therapy. The use of cytokines such as erythropoietin for anemia and colony-stimulating factors such as granulocyte colony-stimulating factor (G-CSF) for neutropenia may permit more aggressive chemotherapy. Despite this treatment, a subset of patients with myeloma progress to bone marrow failure. This may be due to progressive infiltration with plasma cells, the development of a myelo-dysplastic syndrome or myelofibrosis. Rarely, acute leukemia can occur. A bone marrow aspirate and biopsy may be necessary for accurate diagnosis. The time from bone marrow failure to death is often short, usually occurring in the range of 1–9 months.

Infection

Infection in patients with myeloma are a major cause of morbidity and mortality; 20–50% of patients die due to infection. Patients may present with leukopenia or develop it over time, either due to progressive bone marrow failure or secondary to myelosuppressive therapy. Patients also have decreased levels of normal immunoglobulins and a poor to no primary antibody response to immunizations. Patients given pneumococcal vaccination have been shown to respond with increased antibody titers, but the end result was suboptimal due to very low pre-immunization titers. It is recommended that vaccinations be done early after diagnosis.

Abnormalities in cellular immunity, complement function and granulocyte function have all been reported and also contribute to the increased risk of both the development of infection and the difficulty in the resolution of infection even in the absence of leukopenia. Prompt treatment of infection with appropriate antibacterial or antifungal therapy is essential. Patients with recurrent defined infection may benefit from prophylactic antibiotics, but in general this therapy has not been shown to benefit.

Psychosocial support

It is important to recognize that psychosocial support for patients as well as family members is an essential element of supportive care. Patients may live for years with myeloma and can suffer considerable disability with bone fractures and the consequences of therapy. Learning to live with pain or the fear of recurrent pain may lead to clinical depression, and having a high index of suspicion is important to allow for early evaluation and intervention. Repeated infections may lead to multiple hospitalizations. Patients tend to be elderly, making the likelihood of comorbid disabling disease high.

Conclusions

Patients with multiple myeloma can develop debilitating complications while surviving months to years with their disabilities. Prompt identification of the etiology of problems, and early intervention are important for optimizing the quality of life. Clinical trials aimed at improving our therapy for this disease are important, not only with the aim to cure but also to enhance the supportive care we give to these patients.

BIBLIOGRAPHY

Sentinel articles

Berenson JR, Lichtenstein A, Porter L et al. Long-term pamidronate treatment of advanced multiple myeloma patients reduces skeletal events. *J Clin Oncol* 1998;16:593–602.

Desikan R, Barlogie B, Sawyer J et al. Results of high dose therapy for 1000 patients with multiple myeloma: durable complete remissions and superior survival in the absence of chromosome 13 abnormalities. *Blood* 2000;95:4008–10.

Durie BGM, Salmon SE. A clinical staging system for multiple myeloma. *Cancer* 1975;36:382–91.

Garton JP, Gertz MA, Witzig TE et al. Epoetin alpha for the treatment of anemia of multiple myeloma. *Arch Intern Med* 1995;155:2069–74.

Johnson WJ, Kyle RA, Pineda AA et al. Treatment of renal failure associated with multiple myeloma. Plasmapheresis, hemodialysis and chemotherapy. *Arch Intern Med* 1990;150:863–9.

Singhal S, Mehta J, Desikan R et al. Antitumor activity of thalidomide in refractory multiple myeloma. *N Engl J Med* 1999;341:1565–71.

Review articles

Alexanian R, Barlogie B, Dixon D. Renal failure in multiple myeloma. Pathogenesis and prognostic implications. *Arch Intern Med* 1990;150:1693–5.

Bataille R, Harousseau JL. Multiple myeloma. *N Engl J Med* 1997;336:1657–64.

Hallek M, Bergsagel PL, Anderson KC. Multiple myeloma: increasing evidence for a multistep transformation process. *Blood* 1998;91:3–21.

Myeloma Trialists' Collaborative Group. Combination chemotherapy versus melphalan plus prednisone as treatment for multiple myeloma: an overview of 6633 patients from 27 randomized trials. *J Clin Oncol* 1998;16:3832–42.

Internet sites

http://myeloma.org
http://www.multiplemyeloma.org
http://myeloma.med.cornell.edu

Part III

Management of specific symptoms and syndromes

41

Assessment of pain

Larry Driver

U.T. M.D. Anderson Cancer Center, Houston

A major fear of cancer patients is the fear of uncontrolled pain. As disease progresses so does the prevalence of pain, with up to 90% of those with advanced disease suffering from severe pain, and as many as 25% of those dying with their pain unrelieved. Despite these disheartening statistics, currently available pharmacologic therapies can mitigate up to 90% of cancer pain. Why the apparent disconnect?

If the capstone goal of an effective pain management regimen is decreased pain and concomitant symptoms, and hence improved quality of life, the underlying cornerstone must be disciplined, thorough, and ongoing assessment. However, 76% of physicians admit that their own inadequate assessment is the predominant barrier to adequate cancer pain management. We must develop systematic approaches to pain assessment in the context of overall symptom burden, coupled with knowledge of common pain syndromes affecting cancer patients, expertise in the pharmacology of available opioids and adjuvants, and education and reassurance of patients and their families. We then can prescribe rational pain management plans that can enhance the quality of life for as long as there is life.

In addition to acquiring information for diagnosis and treatment, clinical assessment offers the opportunity to develop a relationship with the patient that sets the stage for improved therapeutic success. A sound initial assessment will provide the benchmark for measuring that success. Pain staging may also be prognostic for clinical course. Certainly a comprehensive history and physical examination are mandatory for the proper assessment of any patient, but our focus will be on pain and associated problems.

Cancer history

Delineating the cancer diagnosis and history are prerequisite to pain assessment. Important aspects to consider include the extent and status of disease, treatment

Table 41.1. Key questions in the assessment of pain

Where does it hurt?
How bad is it? (intensity rating scale)
What is it like? (descriptors)
Duration? Temporal variation?
What makes it better? . . . worse?
What treatments have been tried? . . . worked? . . . not worked?
Were there any side effects?
What is the impact of the pain on activity, function, mood, quality of life?
What concurrent symptoms are there?
What is the context of the pain? (interpersonal, psychosocial, spiritual aspects)

history with attention to sequelae, concurrent medical problems, and further plans and goals for treatment.

Pain history

The patient's self-report and description of pain and other symptoms is the framework upon which systematic assessment is built. This offers the clinician an opportunity to establish rapport and build a relationship with the patient, to gather information that will guide the plan of care, to establish mutual goals of care, and to foster patient satisfaction with their management. An approach analogous to the investigative reporter's "Who? – What? – When? – Where? . . . " will provide the essential information upon which to build a rational regimen, as illustrated in Table 41.1.

Where does it hurt? The anatomic site (or sites) of origin and patterns of radiation or referral offer the first clue regarding the pathophysiology of the pain. Remember that most cancer patients will have more than one site or type of pain.

How bad is it? Pain intensity rating scales reveal the perceived severity of pain (least, worst) at specific points in time (current, past 24 hours, past week), and help the patient and physician agree upon realistic goals (acceptable level of pain). The tool for reporting pain intensity should be easy to administer and easy for the patient to understand and use, and should validly measure pain severity and reveal changes in severity due to treatment or clinical situation. The tool helps translate a subjective symptom into an objective scale that can be administered repeatedly by nonphysician caregivers. Table 41.2 lists several validated and, for most purposes, interchangeable pain rating scales that fit the above criteria.

What is the pain like? How would you describe the pain? Qualitative verbal descriptors (sharp, dull, stabbing, aching, squeezing, burning, tingling, etc.) reveal

Table 41.2. Common pain intensity rating instruments

Numerical scale: 0–10
Visual analog scale (VAS): 0–100
Verbal scale: None–Mild–Moderate–Severe–Unbearable
Wong–Baker Faces scale
Color scale
Currency scale
Fruit scale

more about the pathophysiology – somatic or visceral nociceptive pain, neuropathic pain.

When did the pain start? How long have you had it? Does it change over the course of the day? These are further clues delineating the perpetration of the pain.

What makes it better? What makes it worse? What treatments have been tried and what were their effects and side effects? Aggravating and alleviating factors, and previous therapy will influence the plan of care.

What impact does the pain have? Quality of life impact may include effects on relationships, activities, cognition, mood, emotions, appetite, sleep, and overall enjoyment of life. In addition to the burden of chronic pain, the functional impairment may be of great distress for the patient.

What other symptoms accompany the pain? In the patient with advanced cancer, no symptoms exist in isolation from others. Pain is a part of a constellation of problems that burden the patient. Fatigue is a near universal problem among cancer patients. Symptoms of anxiety and depression may aggravate the impact of pain, or may be provoked by unrelieved pain. Chronic nausea may be due to advanced disease, or to pain medications. Constipation is a constant battle for the patient on opioids and other drugs. Appetite and sleep disturbances due to pain take their toll. Concurrent symptoms can be readily assessed using a numeric 0–10 scale for each problem, with outcomes of treatment strategies then followed over time.

Contextual factors include aspects of psychosocial distress and coping strategies, history of chemical abuse, family issues, spiritual suffering and existential angst – all of which may influence the plan of care and response to treatment.

Assessment tools

Various assessment tools are available. The clinician should survey, become familiar with, and choose the tools that best fit the needs of one's particular practice. Available tools include the Brief Pain Inventory (BPI), the McGill Pain Questionnaire, the Memorial Pain Assessment Card (MPAC), the Edmonton Symptom Assessment Scale (ESAS), the Edmonton Staging System for Cancer Pain, and the Memorial Symptom Assessment Scale. These validated tools assist the clinician in formulating the plan of care for pain and symptom management, and then in revising that plan as indicated by clinical response. Just as progress can be tracked by observing serial vital signs and other physical findings, so too the graphic charting and display of symptom intensity ratings reveals the degree of success of a particular treatment regimen, and guides adjustment of that regimen to enhance the response. As a visible part of the patient's chart, pain and symptom tools reinforce the importance of addressing problem areas that might otherwise be overlooked and lost in the clinical milieu, and may be helpful as quality improvement or research measures.

Physical examination

In addition to the overall examination, attention should be focused on the painful area and surrounding region, with special attention given to appropriate musculoskeletal and neurologic evaluation. This may yield important information regarding progression of disease or metastasis. Thorough examination leads to better localization of somatic pain, and definition of neurologic deficits and levels. This may be of crucial importance in those patients with spinal involvement or disease of a neural plexus.

Psychosocial evaluation

The patient's understanding of and reactions to the disease, pain, and other symptoms revolve around the meaning of the problems, the overall impact and effect on the patient, adaptive and maladaptive coping strategies, and the external support structure of family and friends. Attitudes about pain management are influenced by level of knowledge, previous experience, anecdote, expectations, and concerns about pain medication's effects and side effects. The psychosocial evaluation provides an opportunity to gather information, and also to educate the patient.

Imaging

In the patient with advanced disease, imaging studies may play a less prominent role than earlier in the course of illness. However, situations such as spinal metastasis with impending spinal cord compression that may be amenable to palliative radiation warrant evaluation.

Table 41.3. Difficult clinical situations affecting assessment

Altered sensorium, impaired cognition
Communication problems, cultural issues
Psychosocial distress (e.g., anxiety, depression)
Alcohol or other substance abuse
Opioid tolerance
Neuropathic, incidental, or excessive breakthrough pain

Initial empiric therapy

Some patients may present with severe pain that proves difficult to assess and diagnose. This should not preclude the physician from initiating an empiric pain management regimen while further assessment proceeds. Compassion and beneficence demand this. Such a treatment strategy should be based upon a working diagnosis and knowledge of prior therapies' effects and side effects.

Difficult clinical situations

Some situations and syndromes provide challenges in assessment and treatment. Impaired sensorium or cognition may hinder communication, and hence behaviors such as vocalizations, facial expressions, physical postures or movements may provide important clues about pain. Difficult-to-treat pain syndromes include some neuropathic pain states, incident or movement-related pain, underlying psychosocial distress from anxiety or depression, alcohol or other substance abuse, rapid development of opioid tolerance, rapidly progressing disease, and some ethnic and cultural issues. These difficult clinical situations in themselves portend a negative prognosis which should be factored into the assessment (see Table 41.3).

Follow-up assessment

Pain and associated symptoms are dynamic problems in the advanced cancer patient. Reassessment may be frequently necessary as the course of disease progresses. By disciplined use of assessment tools, outcomes can be measured and treatment plans adjusted to fit the clinical situation. Assessment of pain and collateral symptoms should be done at every follow-up visit, and certainly whenever the patient's condition changes. For patients who have been clinically stable on a fairly constant pain medication regimen, worsening pain heralds disease progression until proven otherwise.

A daily pain diary may help the patient put the pain in perspective, better communicate concerns about the pain and its impact, and assist the physician in refining the management regimen.

Solid foundational pain and symptom assessment should provide a framework upon which to build a rational plan of care with effective improvement in symptom relief and quality of life. Proactive assessment helps build the relationship between patient and clinician, works toward maximizing control of burdensome symptoms with improvement in function, and seeks to optimize the patient's quality of life. We hope that this brief overview will prompt the reader to develop a clinical approach of disciplined initial and ongoing assessment that will serve as that framework.

BIBLIOGRAPHY

Abrahm JL. Assessing the patient in pain. In *A Physician's Guide to Pain and Symptom Management in Cancer Patients*, ed. JL Abraham, pp. 79–121. Baltimore: Johns Hopkins University Press, 2000.

Caraceni A, Portenoy RK. An international survey of cancer pain characteristics and syndromes. IASP Task Force on Cancer Pain. *Pain* 1999;82:263–74.

Foley KM. Pain assessment and cancer pain syndromes. In *Oxford Textbook of Palliative Medicine*, 2nd edn, ed. D Doyle, GWC Hanks, N MacDonald, pp. 310–31. Oxford: Oxford University Press, 1998.

Gonzales GR, Elliot KJ, Portenoy RK et al. The impact of a comprehensive evaluation in the management of cancer pain. *Pain* 1991;47:141–4.

Nekolaichuk CL, Maguire TO, Suarez-Almazor M, Rogers WT, Bruera E. Assessing the reliability of patient, nurse, and family caregiver symptom ratings in hospitalized advanced cancer patients. *J Clin Oncol* 1999;17:3621–30.

Shannon MM, Ryan MA, D'Agostino N, Brescia FJ. Assessment of pain in advanced cancer patients. *J Pain Symptom Manage* 1995;10:274–8.

Internet sites

The following Internet sites contain virtual libraries, CME activities, links to other sites, and other features pertinent to pain medicine and palliative care.

American Pain Society
    www.ampainsoc.org
Department of Pain Medicine and Palliative Care at Beth Israel Medical Center
    www.StopPain.org
Department of Palliative Care and Rehabilitation Medicine at University of Texas M. D. Anderson Cancer Center
    www.palliative.mdanderson.org

42

Drugs for managing cancer pain

Barry A. Eagel

Beth Israel Medical Center, New York

Assessment of the severity and causes of pain dictate the type of drugs used for treatment. The choice of drugs and route of administration is dependent on

1. The severity of the pain.
2. The frequency and duration of the pain.
3. The source or cause of the pain.

Drugs used to treat pain can be broadly divided into analgesics and adjuvant drugs. Adjuvant drugs are not considered analgesics per se, however, they can augment the analgesic properties of analgesics for specific pain syndromes, for instance corticosteroids for spinal cord compression or antidepressants for neuropathic pain. In addition, adjuvant drugs include those which can be used to manage undesirable but expected adverse effects of analgesics.

The goal of pain management is to achieve the best possible pain relief with the least side effects. Choices of drugs, doses, and routes should be tailored to meet these goals for the individual patient.

The WHO three-step ladder is useful for establishing the class of drug to start with depending on the severity of the pain at initial assessment, or if there is a failure to achieve adequate pain control with less potent drugs.

Step 1. Analgesics for mild pain include aspirin, acetaminophen and NSAIDs. These drugs have a ceiling effect (beyond a certain dose range, increasing the dose does not provide for greater analgesic effect), and have specific organ toxicities at high doses. Acetaminophen is the only drug in this group which has no antiplatelet activity, which may be important postsurgery and in patients with thrombocytopenia or thrombopathy. Hepatotoxicity occurs when the daily dose of acetaminophen exceeds 4 grams per day in patients with normal liver function. The maximum dose that can be used is diminished in patients with impaired liver function. Nonsteroidal anti-inflammatory drugs are useful for managing pain associated with bone metastases. The newer COX-2 selective inhibitors, celecoxib and rofecoxib have a lower incidence of gastrointestinal side effects compared with older, nonselective NSAIDs. However, they also have a ceiling effect and have similar effects on platelet and renal function.

Step 2. Analgesics for moderate pain. Drugs in this class include opioids such as codeine, dihydrocodeine, hydrocodone, propoxyphene and tramadol, as well as combinations of these opioids with acetaminophen, aspirin, or NSAIDs. Although there is no ceiling effect for the opioids in this group, when combined with acetaminophen or aspirin combination the daily maximum dose is limited by the aspirin or acetaminophen content of the combination drug. All dosed drugs in this group are generally given every 4–6 hours.

Step 3. Drugs used to manage moderate to severe pain include the pure agonist opioids. These drugs include morphine, oxycodone, fentanyl, hydromorphone, methadone, levorphanol, and meperidine. Pure opioid agonists do not have a ceiling effect, and with the exception of meperidine, there is no "maximum" dose that can be given in order to achieve adequate analgesia.

Opioid drugs used for cancer pain management

Tramadol inhibits serotonin reuptake and its primary metabolite binds to the mu-opioid receptor. Tramadol 50 mg is approximately equivalent to 60 mg of codeine. Tramadol has recently become available in combination with acetaminophen (tramadol 37.5 mg/ ACAP 500 mg). Seizures have been reported when the dose of tramadol is rapidly escalated, so it must be gradually titrated, and may be relatively contraindicated in patients taking medications which may lower the seizure threshold or who may be prone to seizures due to intracranial malignancy or metabolic derangement.

Several step-2 agents deserve special mention because of some of their adverse effects. Codeine is associated with a higher incidence of nausea and constipation compared with other weak opioids. Propoxyphene has no greater analgesic potency than aspirin, but it has a neurotoxic metabolite norpropoxyphene which can accumulate in patients with renal impairment. It is not recommended for repeated dosing for chronic pain. Mixed agonist-antagonists and partial agonists should not be used for repeated dosing in patients with chronic pain. These drugs may cause a withdrawal syndrome when repeat doses are given.

Meperdine is not recommended for managing chronic pain, since a neuro-excitatory toxic metabolite, normeperidine can bioaccumulate with repeated dosing.

Methadone is a useful strong opioid for management of chronic cancer pain. However, the dosing of methadone must be carefully titrated to the individual patient. When used for analgesia (as opposed to for management of substance abuse), the dosing frequency ranges from 4–24 hours (usually 6–8 hours) and must be tailored to the individual patient. One effective approach is to use prn dosing for several days in order to determine the correct dosing interval for an individual patient. Equianalgesic ratios between methadone and other opioids do not appear to be linear as is the case with other opioid conversion ratios. This may be due to the binding of the L-isomer of methadone to the mu-opioid receptor while the D-isomer binds to the NMDA receptor. Thus, when converting from another opioid to methadone, the calculated equianalgesic dose of methadone should be decreased by 75–90% (i.e., use 10–25% of the calculated oral morphine equivalent daily dose). For example, a patient who has been using sustained release morphine at 100 mg every 8 hours (300 mg/day) would be appropriately switched to methadone at a dose of 10 mg every 8 hours (30 mg/day). After the initial switch, close follow-up is needed to titrate the dose (usually upwards) to obtain the best results.

Initial dosing, dose titration, and dose conversion

For patients who have not been receiving opioids, the recommended starting doses of drugs for pain relief can be found in the literature (e.g., Portenoy and Frager 1999). For patients that are being converted from one opioid to another drug or route, equianalgesic dosing charts are useful for approximating the correct dose when converting from one opioid drug or route to another (see Table 42.1). Incomplete cross-tolerance refers to differential binding affinities to mu-receptor subtypes. Because of incomplete cross-tolerance, rotating (switching) to another opioid can alleviate some of the adverse effects while retaining effective analgesia. When converting from one opioid drug to another, the calculated dose is decreased by 50% in patients who have effective analgesia, or by 25% in patients who are still experiencing moderate to severe pain (> 4–6 out of 10). This rule does not apply to transdermal fentanyl, which was developed with dose recommendations that already incorporated this safety factor. In general, dosages should be titrated by determining the effectiveness of pain relief achieved after plasma steady state is achieved (generally after three half-lives of the drug). The rule of thumb in opioid dosing is: "The dose that is needed by the patient is the dose the patient needs." There is no ceiling effect for opioids, and the dosing titration proceeds based on the balance between efficacy and side effects as described in Table 42.2.

Opioid rotation

Pure agonist opioid analgesics should be increased in dose until adequate analgesia is achieved without excessive side effects. If side effects occur with good analgesia, the side effect should be managed. However, if a patient has poor pain relief with the concomitant occurrence of unmanageable side effects, the drug should be changed. Because of incomplete cross-tolerance, a lower dose of another opioid may afford better analgesic relief with lower incidence of side effects.

Table 42.1. Equianalgesic doses for opioids

Drug	Intramuscular	Oral[a]	Half-life (hours)	Duration of action oral route (hours)
	Route			
Buprenorphine	0.4		30–40	6–8
Butorphanol	2		2.5–3.5	
Codeine	120	200	2–3	2–4
Dihydrocodeine[b]		200	2–3	2–4
Fentanyl	0.1		4–8	1–3
Transdermal fentanyl[c]	(0.25)		14.7–19.3	48–72
Transmucosal fentanyl[d]	0.8		1.7–12.9	5–60
Heroin	5	30		
Hydrocodone[e]		200		2–4
Hydromorphone	1.5	7.5	2–3	2–4
Levorphanol	2	4	12–16	4–8
Meperidine	75	300	3–4	2–4
(Normeperidine)			12–14	
Methadone[g]	10	20	13–50	4–8
Morphine	10	30	3–4	
Controlled-release morphine		30		8–24
Nalbuphine	10		5	
Oxycodone[e]	15	30	2–3	2–4
Controlled-release oxycodone		30		
Oxymorphone	1	10 (p.r.)	2–3	3–4
Pentazocine	60	180	2–3	
Propoxyphene[e]	50	100	2–3	2–4
(Norpropoxyphene)			30–40	
Tramadol[f]		~ 167	5.1	1–3
(M1 metabolite)			9	

Source: Eagel BA, Foley KM. Opioid analgesics. Chapter 8. In *Current Neurological Drugs*, ed. L Rowland, et al. Philadelphia: Current Medicine, 2000. Adapted from Foley KM. The treatment of cancer pain. *N Engl J Med* 1985; 313:84–95.

[a] Oral (p.o.) dose equivalency is for repeated dosing schedules.

[b] Dihydrocodeine is available in combination with caffeine and acetaminophen or aspirin.

[c] Transdermal fentanyl is available in 25, 50, 75 and 100 μg/hour patches. Fentanyl 100 μg/hour ~4 mg/hour morphine sulfate IV.

[d] Transmucosal fentanyl is available in dosage formulations, ranging from 200–1600 μg (Actiq). Dose and titration must be individualized to the patient since dose conversion from other opioid or other formulation fentanyl may not correlate linearly (Streisand JB, Varvel JR, Stanski D et al. Absorption and bioavailability of oral transmucosal fentanyl citrate. *Anesthesiology* 1991;75:223–9. Sevarino FB, Ginsberg B, Lichtor JL, et al. Oral transmucosal fentanyl citrate compared with IV morphine for acute pain in patients following abdominal surgery. *Anesth Analg* 1997;84:S330).

[e] These drugs are available in combination with acetaminophen and/or aspirin. When converting to or from these preparations, it is important to account for the analgesic effect of the nonopioid component.

[f] Tramadol 50 mg p.o. is equivalent to codeine 60 mg p.o. (Sunshine A. New clinical experience with tramadol. *Drugs* 1994; 47:(Suppl. 1):8–18.)

[g] This equianalgesic ratio for methadone applies only to opioid-naïve patients. When converting from another opioid to methadone, the calculated equianalgesic dose should be decreased by 75–90% to account for incomplete cross-tolerance.

Table 42.2. Balancing opioid side effects and efficacy

	No side effects	Side effects
Good pain control	Ideal	Treat side effects
Poor pain control	Increase opioid dose	Switch to another opioid or route

Routes of administration

The oral, transdermal, and transmucosal routes are the easiest and least invasive routes of administration of opioids. Intramuscular injections should be avoided for repeated dosing due to pain associated with this route as well as the increased risk of bleeding in patients who may be predisposed to hemorrhagic diatheses due to their underlying malignancy or treatment effects. Rectal administration should be avoided in patients at risk for neutropenia, although it may be useful in certain settings where the oral and parenteral routes cannot be used. Although the bioavailability of rectally administered opioids approximates oral administration, it may be more highly variable due to hydration status and bowel function. Subcutaneous injection can be used for repeated dosing where rapid onset is desired without the need for intravenous access. The subcutaneous route can also be used for continuous infusion as long as the infusion rate does not exceed 2 cc/hour. Intravenous analgesia is the preferred route for rapid relief of pain. Permanent intravenous access may be used for prolonged dosing, either via a peripheral (PICC-line) or central venous catheter. The intrathecal and epidural routes have the advantage of lower systemic dosage (~10% of the IV dose) and concomitantly fewer systemic side effects such as nausea, constipation and altered sensorium. Combinations of opioids with anesthetic agents can be employed via this route. However, they should be used by clinicians trained in the placement and maintenance of epidural or intrathecal placed catheters. Patient-controlled analgesia can be used for patients receiving opioids via intravenous, subcutaneous or epidural routes using a mechanical device which allows for programming of the basal and rescue doses and the interval between rescue doses.

Adjuvant drugs for pain relief

Adjuvant drugs are medications that augment either the analgesic efficacy via a mechanism distinct from interruption of normal pain signal transmission, or are drugs which can be used to manage side effects associated with analgesic drugs. Adjuvant drugs are particularly useful in managing neuropathic pain, pain due to

Table 42.3. Adjuvant drugs for pain relief

Antidepressants		Burning dysethetic pain
Tricyclic antidepressants	Amitriptyline	
	Desipramine	
"Newer" antidepressants	Trazodone	
	Maprotiline	
	Fluoxetine	
	Paroxetine	
Anticonvulsants	Carbamazepine	Lancinating paroxysmal pain
	Phenytoin	
	Valproate	
	Clonazepam	
	Felbamate	
Oral local anesthetics	Mexiletine	
	Tocainide	
Neuroleptics	Pimozide	
	Methtrimeprazine	
Corticosteroids	Dexamethasone	Nerve compression pain, inflammatory pain
	Prednisone	
	Methylprednisolone	
Sympatholytic drugs	Prazosin	
	Phenoxybenzamine	
Topical agents	Capsaicin	
	Local anesthetics	
Miscellaneous drugs for neuropathic pain	Baclofen	
	Clonidine	
	Calcitonin	
	Ketamine	
	Dextromethorphan	
Drugs for bone pain	Bisphosphonates	
	Calcitonin	
	Gallium nitrate	
	Strontium-89	
Drugs for bowel obstruction	Scopolamine	
	Octreotide	

Source: Adapted from Portenoy R, Frager G. Pain management: Pharmacological approaches. In *Palliative Care and Rehabilitation of Cancer Patients*, ed. CF Gunten. Boston: Kluwer Academic Publishers 1999; and from DeConno F, Caraceni A. *Manual of Cancer Pain.* Boston: Kluwer Academic Publishers, 1996. Used with permission.

bone metastases or visceral pain such as due to bowel dysfunction. Neuropathic pain describes a process of abnormal pain transmission due to injury to the nerve. Neuropathic pain is commonly due to tumor infiltration, tumor compression of a nerve, root or at the level of the spinal cord or direct damage to a nerve due to surgical trauma, transection or hypoxia. The most common symptoms are described as either burning, tingling sensations, with abnormal reaction to light touch (dyesthesia) or sharp, shooting (lancinating) paroxysms of pain. Table 42.3 describes some of the commonly used adjuvant drugs used for managing cancer pain. Overall, with careful pain assessments and skillful use of opioid and nonopioid analgesics plus adjuvants, the overwhelming majority of patients with cancer pain can feel better and live better.

BIBLIOGRAPHY

Sentinel articles

Bruera E, Pereira J, Watanabe S, Belzile M, Kuehn N, Hanson J. Opioid rotation in patients with cancer pain. A retrospective comparison of dose ratios between methadone, hydromorphone, and morphine. *Cancer* 1996;78:852–7.

Bruera E, Belzile M, Pituskin E et al. Randomized, double-blind, cross-over trial comparing the safety and efficacy of oral controlled-release oxycodone with controlled-release morphine in patients with cancer pain. *J Clin Oncol* 1998;16:3222–9.

Cleeland CS, Gonin R, Hatfield AK et al. Pain and its treatment in outpatients with metastatic cancer. *N Engl J Med* 1994;330:592–6.

Mercadante S, Casuccio A, Agnello A, Serretta R, Calderone L, Barresi L. Morphine versus methadone in the pain treatment of advanced cancer patients followed up at home. *J Clin Oncol.* 1998;16:3656–61.

Ripamonti C, Groff L, Brunelli C, Polastri D, Stavrakis A, De Conno F. Switching from morphine to oral methadone in treating cancer pain: what is the equianalgesic dose ratio? *J Clin Oncol* 1998;16:3216–21.

Review articles

Cherney NI, Arbit E, Jain S. Invasive techniques in the management of cancer pain. *Hematol Oncol Clin N Am* 1996;10:121–37.

Cherney N, Ripamonti C, Pereira J, Davis C, Fallon M, McQuay H. Strategies to manage the adverse effects of oral morphine: an evidence-based report. *J Clin Oncol* 2001;19:2542–54.

Indelicato RA, Portenoy RK. Opioid rotation in the management of refractory cancer pain. *J Clin Oncol* 2002;20:348–52.

Pereira J, Lawlor P, Vigano A, Dorgan M, Bruera E. Equianalgesic dose ratios for opioids: a critical review and proposals for long-term dosing. *J Pain Symptom Manage* 2001;22:672–7.

Portenoy RK. Issues in the economic analysis of therapies for cancer pain. *Oncology* 1995; 9(Suppl.):71–8.

Portenoy R, Frager G. Pain management: pharmacological approaches. In *Palliative Case and Rehabilitation of Cancer Patients*, ed. CF Gunter. Boston: Kluwer Academic, 1999.

Portenoy RK, Hagen NA. Breakthrough pain: definition and management. *Oncology* 1989; 3 (Suppl.):25–9.

Rowlingson JC. Interventional cancer pain management. *Anesthes Analges* 1998;Suppl.:106–13.

Internet sites

CancerNet – NCI Cancer Supportive Care guidelines
www.cancer.gov/cancerinfo/pdg/supportivecare

Agency for Healthcare Research and Quality (AHRQ) Management of Cancer Pain. Evidence Report/Technology Assessment
http://www.ahrq.gov/clinic/canpainsum.htm

Edmonton Palliative Care Program
http://www.palliative.org/pc_home.html

M.D.Anderson Cancer Center Pain Management
http://www.mdanderson.org/topics/paincontrol/

Beth Israel Medical Center, Dept of Pain Medicine and Palliative Care
http://www.stoppain.org/

American Pain Society
http://www.ampainsoc.org/

International Association for the Study of Pain
http://www.iasp-pain.org

University of Wisconsin Pain and Policy Studies Group
http://www.medsch.wisc.edu/painpolicy/

American Academy of Pain Medicine
http://www.painmed.org/

American Pain Foundation
http://www.painfoundation.org/

University of Washington Hypermedia Assistant for Cancer Pain Management Website (including AHCPR Cancer Pain Guidelines)
http://www.talaria.org/

NIH State-of-the-Science Statement on Cancer Pain, Depression, Fatigue
http://www.consensus.nih.gov/ta/022/022_statement.htm

43

Difficult pain management problems

Robin L. Fainsinger

University of Alberta, Edmonton

Introduction

In the international effort to provide better pain management around the world, it has been repeated in lectures and standard texts, that better pharmacological management and increased use of opioids in particular will go a long way to solving this problem. The "three-step analgesic ladder" has been promoted by the World Health Organization in its guidelines *Cancer Pain Relief* to enable healthcare providers to offer effective management. Reviews have often stated that this can be expected to provide effective analgesia in 70–95% of patients. Although this approach is not above criticism, lack of knowledge and restriction of opioid availability has continued to present barriers to effective pain management. Nevertheless knowledge of a basic approach to pharmacological management and access to opioids, still leaves a significant number of patients with difficult pain management problems. This is well illustrated by evidence that even though global consumption of opioids has increased dramatically, particularly in North America and Western European countries, this has not provided a complete solution. Over the last decade there have been numerous reports of toxicity associated with high opioid doses producing a constellation of problems including myoclonus, hallucinations, agitated delirium and seizures. These difficult pain management problems have resulted in a somewhat controversial discussion on the topic of neuropsychiatric toxicity and opioid rotation or sequential opioid trials.

The complexity of the human experience that may result in the failure of pharmacological management alone is recognized by both classic literature and more recent commentators: "It was true, as the doctor said that Ivan Ilych's physical sufferings were terrible, but worse than the physical sufferings were his mental sufferings, which were his chief torture." *The Death of Ivan Ilych*, by Tolstoy.

Clinicians are often under pressure to increase the number and strength of pharmacological options to achieve pain control. However, it needs to be recognized that due to the complexity of underlying issues, this will not always bring success in some patients. We live in an era where patients and families often read in the media that adequate pharmacological management should provide relief. In dealing with difficult pain problems it is essential to be aware of the poor prognostic factors that may help to lower expectations of success from pharmacological management alone, and suggest alternative approaches.

Difficult pain management issues

Consider the following alternative scenarios.

A 60-year-old female with breast cancer and bone metastases presents with pain localized to the left arm and lower back. She is able to move comfortably, and is oriented and alert. She takes 30 mg codeine approximately 3–4 times a day and feels she is very comfortable. She has a stable marriage and home life, with no psychiatric history or history of addictive behavior.

Or

A 60-year-old female with breast cancer and bone metastases presents with burning, stabbing pain down the left leg with marked tenderness to any touch in this area. She is reasonably comfortable at rest, but is unable to move without excruciating pain to the point that movement is severely limited. There is some evidence of confusion. Her morphine dose has increased from 10 mg every 4 hours to 150 mg every 4 hours over 10 days. She is also on ibuprofen, gabapentin, fluoxetine, and lorazepam. She has been divorced twice, lives on her own, and has a history of depression and suicide attempts. There is also a long history of ongoing alcohol and benzodiazepine abuse.

In the initial scenario the patient apparently has a nociceptive pain syndrome well controlled on low analgesic doses. There is also a history suggesting that the patient has probably coped well with the stress of life and work to this point. However, in the second situation the patient has a problematic neuropathic pain syndrome, a severe incidental component, difficulty in providing an accurate pain history due to some cognitive impairment, rapidly escalating opioid doses and a complicated adjuvant analgesic regime. Her history suggests that she does not cope well with stress and has very poor psychosocial support.

As we assess a patient for the multidimensional aspects of pain (Figure 43.1) it is useful to consider the following: Production, perception, and expression.

Production of pain occurs at the site of injury, and cannot be measured directly. Perception of pain occurs at the level of the central nervous system / brain, and cannot be measured in clinical settings. We use the expression of pain as the main target for assessment and planning management. Individual patients with similar

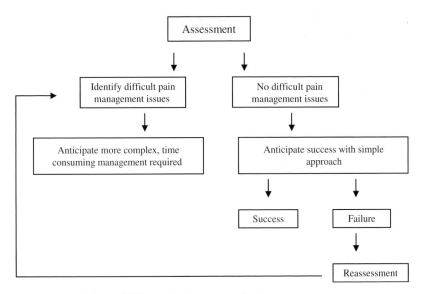

Figure 43.1 Assessment of the multidimensional aspects of pain.

injury may have similar levels of perception, but express different pain intensity levels, that require consideration of the multidimensional aspects of the individual pain experience.

Neuropathic pain

Neuropathic pain is commonly recognized as a potentially difficult syndrome. This pain arises from damage to nervous tissue that can be due to peripheral nerve injury, damage to the autonomic nervous system, the central nervous system, or a combination of these different mechanisms. It is often described as burning, stabbing, stinging, or aching and may be associated with hyperalgesia or allodynia. Although the benefit from the use of opioids in neuropathic pain syndromes has been controversial, it is now generally accepted that most neuropathic pains will be opioid responsive, but often at higher doses than typically seen for nociceptive pain syndromes. In addition to the use of sequential opioid trials including methadone for the effective management of neuropathic pain, other adjuvant analgesics suggested include corticosteroids, tricyclic antidepressants (e.g., amitriptyline), anticonvulsants (e.g., gabapentin, carbamazepine), and antiarrhythmic drugs (e.g., mexelitine).

Incidental pain

It is important to distinguish patients who have severe incidental pain with significant impairment of physical function. This is particularly relevant where the patient is comfortable at rest, and is well managed with a relatively simple pharmacological approach, which is then completely inadequate in controlling movement-related pain. The increased analgesic requirements for relatively brief movements, or sufficient to allow improved physical independence, places the patient at risk for increased side effects during the many hours of the day when they do not require this medication. Cancer-related incident pain is known to be a prevalent and heterogeneous phenomenon, that is a marker for more severe pain syndromes, and is associated with both pain-related functional impairment and psychological distress. If increasing analgesic management to control incidental pain runs the risk or causes the patient to have unacceptable side effects then alternative approaches will need to be utilized. These approaches could include limiting mobility, immobilizing limbs, radiotherapy, bisphosphonates, corticosteroids, and surgical fixation when appropriate.

Tolerance

The concern that chronic use of opioid therapy will inevitably result in dose escalation has been suggested as a barrier to early effective use of opioids. There is good evidence that opioid doses do not usually require escalation in the absence of progressive injury from the underlying cancer. However, it is accepted that there is a small subset of patients for whom true opioid analgesic tolerance results in a poor response to escalating doses and is associated with increasingly problematic side effects. The important clinical issue is whether the escalation of opioid dose, in some patients producing increasing side effects, can be avoided by changing the opioid or the route of opioid administration, using adjuvant analgesics, or blocking the tolerance mechanism.

Psychosocial distress

It is impossible to deny and dangerous to ignore the potential involvement of psychosocial distress and/or somatization that can complicate the expression of pain in cancer patients. It would be simplistic to assume that every patient asked to provide a pain score on a visual analog scale from zero to ten, is able to express their physiological pain alone. The visual analog scale is at best a unidimensional assessment, and certainly a patient expressing a large component of their psychosocial distress in this manner is at risk for being prescribed increasing opioids that will not address this component of their suffering, and certainly may provoke significant side effects. Although it is certainly wise to give patients the benefit of the doubt in prescribing adequate amounts of opioids, there are elements of the history and physical findings that may alert attending staff to unrecognized psychosocial/somatization issues. In addition to the obvious risk factors in past psychosocial history, there are some patients whose observed sound sleeping habits and good physical function may sometimes seem inappropriate in the context of rapidly escalating opioid doses.

Concern may be heightened further as the patient's physical and mental function deteriorates from apparent opioid-related side effects. Attempting to manage these problems with pharmacological means alone is doomed to failure, and requires skilled intervention from a comprehensive interdisciplinary psychosocial support team.

Alcohol/drug abuse

There is certainly ample evidence in the literature to demonstrate that patients with a past history of alcohol or other drug abuse, should still be prescribed opioids in a standard approach that will often achieve good pain management. Some pre-existing tolerance to analgesics may sometimes require that these patients are prescribed high opioid doses. Nevertheless it also needs to be recognized that an inability to cope with the stress of life prior to developing an advanced incurable illness, and heavy dependence on potentially cognitively impairing agents in order to assist coping mechanisms, may be a risk factor for some patients to replace or supplement previous addictions by the use of increasing opioid doses to achieve the same obtunding effect. It has been suggested that the use of the four CAGE questions to screen for alcohol abuse will allow not only early diagnosis, but early intervention with appropriate counseling and supportive measures that can be very effective in preventing opioid misuse in this small but problematic patient group.

Cognitive deficits

Cognitive deficits are not uncommon in advanced cancer populations for a number of reasons. Advanced cancer patients tend to be older, with the increasing prevalence of dementia widely recognized. In addition, advanced cancer patients are at risk of developing delirium from a number of potentially reversible and nonreversible causes. Patients with pre-existing dementia may go unrecognized and provide an expression of their pain that is not necessarily an accurate representation of their pain perception. In addition, pharmacological management with opioids as well as adjuvant analgesics puts these patients at increased risk for medication-induced delirium superimposed on the dementia. Patients with an element of hypoactive delirium may also go unrecognized with the same result as increasing medications allow the delirium to rapidly progress to the development of agitated symptoms. Recognition of this problem and consistent and repeated assessments of cognition are extremely useful in preventing this situation from developing, or dealing with it sooner rather than once a severe agitated delirium has developed.

Complicated analgesic regimes

A patient presenting with a history of sequential opioid trials, poorly controlled on high opioid doses with a number of other adjuvant analgesics prescribed

Table 43.1. Conditions that can cause possible pain management difficulty

Neuropathic pain
Incidental pain
Analgesic tolerance
Psychosocial distress
Alcohol/drug abuse
Cognitive problems
Complicated analgesic regimes

simultaneously, can certainly present a treatment dilemma when the pain remains poorly controlled. A careful reassessment of the clinical situation will often reveal one or more of the previously described difficult pain management issues that have gone unrecognized and resulted in an overreliance on pharmacological management. In the rare circumstances where the physiological underpinnings of the pain syndrome are truly unresponsive to routine opioid and adjuvant analgesic approaches, consideration can be given to anesthetic techniques in this minority of patients. Options would include intraspinal administration of drugs via the epidural or intrathecal space, destruction of nerve tissue by neurolytic procedures such as celiac plexus block or cordotomy, as well as a variety of other neurolytic procedures.

Conclusion

An understanding of the basic approach to pain management may bring initial success and confidence (Table 43.1). However, increasing experience will inevitably lead to failures and frustration, unless an appreciation of the possible multidimensional aspects of a patient's pain experience becomes part of routine assessment and management.

BIBLIOGRAPHY

Sentinel articles

Bruera E, Macmillan K, Hanson J, MacDonald RN. The Edmonton staging system for cancer pain: preliminary report. *Pain* 1989;37:203–9.

Bruera E, Moyano J, Seifert L, Fainsinger RL, Hanson J, Suarez-Almazor M. The frequency of alcoholism among patients with pain due to terminal cancer. *J Pain Symptom Manage* 1995;10:599–603.

Bruera E, Schoeller T, Wenk R et al. A prospective multi-center assessment of the Edmonton Staging System for cancer pain. *J Pain Symptom Manage* 1995;10:348–55.

Cohen SR, Mount BM. Pain with life-threatening illness: its perception and control are inextricably linked with quality of life. *Pain Res Manage* 2000;5:271–5.

Jadad AR, Browman GP. The WHO analgesic ladder for cancer pain management. *J Am Med Assoc* 1995;274:1870–3.

Kaplan R, Slywka J, Slagle S et al. A titrated morphine analgesic regime comparing substance users and non-users with AIDS-related pain. *J Pain Symptom Manage* 2000;19:265–73.

Lawlor P, Walker P, Bruera E et al. Severe opioid toxicity and somatization of psychosocial distress in a cancer patient with a background of chemical dependence. *J Pain Symptom Manage* 1997;13:356–61.

Lawlor PG, Fainsinger RL, Bruera ED. Delirium at the end of life. Critical issues in clinical practice and research. *J Am Med Assoc* 2000;284:2427–9.

Portenoy RK, Payne D, Jacobsen P. Breakthrough pain: characteristics and impact in patients with cancer pain. *Pain* 1999;91:129–34.

Review articles

Breura E, Pereira J. Neuro-psychiatric toxicity of opioids. In *Proceedings of the 8th World Congress on Pain, Progress in Pain Research and Management, Vol. 8.* ed. TS Jensen, JA Turner, Z Wiesenfeld-Hallen, pp. 717–38. Seattle: IASP Press, 1997.

Bruera E, Pereira J. Recent developments in palliative cancer care. *Acta Oncologica* 1998; 37:749–57.

Cherny N, Ripamonti C, Pereira J et al. Strategies to manage the adverse effects of oral morphine: an evidence-based report. *J Clin Oncol* 2001;19:2542–4.

Fainsinger RL, Tapper M, Bruera E. A perspective on the management of delirium in the terminally ill. *J Palliat Care* 1993;9(3):4–8.

Fallon M. Opioid rotation: does it have a role? *Palliat Med* 1997;11:177–8.

Foley KM. Misconceptions and controversies regarding the use of opioids in cancer pain. *Anti-cancer Drugs* 1995;6:4–13.

McQuay H. Opioids in pain management. *Lancet* 1999;353:2229–32.

Portenoy RK, Coyle N. Controversies in the long-term management of analgesic therapy in patients with advanced cancer. *J Pain Symptom Manage* 1990;5:307–19.

Sykes J, Johnson R, Hanks GW. Difficult pain problems. *Br Med J* 1997;315:867–9.

World Health Organization. *Cancer Pain Relief.* Geneva: WHO, 1986.

44

Dyspnea

Sam H. Ahmedzai and Silvia Paz

Royal Hallamshire Hospital, Sheffield

Introduction

Dyspnea or breathlessness is a normal sensation we all experience from time to time, but which becomes a serious and sinister symptom in patients with advancing malignancy. It has been described simply as "an uncomfortable awareness of breathing," but that does not convey the full impact on the patient. A more comprehensive definition is "the subjective sensation of difficulty or undue effort in breathing, which is not necessarily related to exercise, and which compels the individual to either increase ventilation or to reduce activity."

The actual words that patients use to describe the sensation may vary depending on the severity, psychological effects, and to some extent, the causes. Thus people with long-term chronic airflow limitation often speak of "tightness;" those with sudden onset of pulmonary embolism of "gasping;" a patient who has cardiac failure may feel he is "drowning." The words used, however, are not sufficiently consistent to be useful in diagnosis.

Prevalence and impact

Dyspnea is a very common symptom in patients with cancer, and in lung cancer it may be the reason for initial presentation. A recent large screening study of a mixed cancer population found the prevalence to range from 33% in sarcoma to 83% in lung cancer patients. In general, the symptom becomes more common with advancing disease – this reflects both a real increase in the pathophysiological factors which predispose to dyspnea, and also the lack of efficacy of many current treatments.

Becoming acutely short of breath is a frightening experience, and not surprisingly many patients quickly learn to restrict their activity in order to avoid provoking further episodes. This tends to lead to deconditioning of the skeletal muscles, which has been recognized as a major problem in chronic airflow limitation. The reduced activity further has the consequence of restricting the patient's social functioning, which can have a negative impact on overall quality of life. Thus, a proper assessment of the patient with dyspnea should include an inquiry of social and domestic activities, and what has been lost from the patient's daily routine. This is admittedly made rather more difficult because of the additive effects of other symptoms, such as pain and fatigue, which also tend to limit functioning.

Causes

As with many symptoms in advanced cancer, dyspnea can be the result of many discrete and interacting causes, and it is not unusual to find several factors which contribute at the same time. These causes can be divided into the following groups.

- Respiratory – e.g., bronchial obstruction leading to lobar or lung collapse; pneumonia; chronic bronchitis and asthma (often overlooked in patients with lung cancer); pleural effusion; pulmonary thromboembolism; lymphangitis carcinomatosa; diaphragmatic weakness or splinting (e.g., by ascites).
- Cardiovascular – e.g., heart failure; pericardial infiltration by tumour or effusion; superior vena caval obstruction (in this the dyspnea may be related to central vein thrombosis and pulmonary embolism).
- Anemia – e.g., resulting from chronic bleeding; secondary to bone marrow suppression by anticancer treatments; nutritional deficiency.
- Systemic causes – e.g., cachexia with weakness of chest wall muscles; steroid myopathy.

Investigations

In the advanced stages of cancer the patient has usually been already extensively investigated, and the likely causes of breathlessness may be readily apparent. If dyspnea arises anew, or if it becomes acutely worse in a previously stable patient, it may be appropriate to request limited investigations. It is important to keep these from being too invasive or requiring many hospital visits in sick patients. The tests which can give useful pointers towards the underlying cause and practical ways of helping include:

- Complete blood count.
- Chest radiograph.
- Spirometry to exclude airflow obstruction and to determine reversibility with bronchodilator.
- Chest computed tomography scan if mediastinal disease is suspected.
- Chest ultrasound if pleural effusion is suspected, and to identify the best place to insert a drain.

- Echocardiogram if pericardial effusion is suspected.
- Pulse oximetry to estimate oxygen saturation (preferable to arterial blood gases, unless carbon dioxide retention is suspected or there may be a real risk of this if sedatives are being planned.)
- Ventilation/perfusion scan if pulmonary embolism is suspected.

It must be stressed that the majority of patients with advanced cancer can be evaluated with only two or three of these tests, for rational treatments to be instituted. Several studies have also shown that the patient's complaints of breathlessness and anxiety are often not correlated with the standard pulmonary function tests such as spirometry. The maximum inspiratory pressure may be a more reliable predictor of dyspnea, because of its sensitivity to respiratory muscle weakness (Dudgeon et al. 2001*a*,*b*). However, this is not feasible to perform in routine clinical practice or with very frail patients.

Clinical assessment

It is therefore useful also to consider patient-oriented assessments of dyspnea, especially so that the effects of treatment can be monitored. Suitable instruments for this purpose include the Edmonton Symptom Assessment Scale (ESAS); the EORTC or FACT quality-of-life scales with their respective lung cancer specific questionnaires; and the recently developed Cancer Dyspnea Scale.

As stated above, the major impact of dyspnea is a reduction in activity. For patients who are ambulant, the shuttle walking test has been tested and found to be a practical, reproducible measure of exercise capability in patients with advanced cancer.

Palliative management

The best therapy in individual cases will depend partly on the cause of dyspnea, partly on the level of urgency and very much on the overall fitness of the patient. There should always be an early review of the possibility of oncological interventions, where cancer is thought to be a major factor in etiology. Usually, chemotherapy options will have been exhausted or the patient may not be fit for cytotoxics, in the advanced stage. Radiation therapy may still play a part, especially if a bronchial obstruction is accompanied by cough or hemoptysis which are readily palliated by external beam therapy. In some centers endobronchial (intraluminal) brachytherapy may be available, but patients need to be fit for bronchoscopy to consider this. Intraluminal laser or photodynamic therapy are even more restricted because of the need for specialized equipment and staff training.

Other invasive procedures which could be considered include endobronchial stenting (i.e., insertion of a tubular device to maintain the patency of the airway). Stenting can give very rapid relief of dyspnea, and the patient's airway can then be further treated by intraluminal radiation or laser.

If there is a significant pleural effusion, it is nearly always beneficial to drain this, preferably under ultrasound guidance so that the maximum amount of fluid can be removed with least risk of causing a pneumothorax. Various methods can be used to cause pleurodesis, i.e., sticking together of parietal and visceral pleura in order to prevent recurrent effusions. Pericardial effusion can cause very rapid onset of severe and potentially fatal dyspnea: This can be an indication for an emergency pericardial tap, which could be followed by the opening of a "window" into the pleural space to prevent re-accumulation.

Drug treatments form the mainstay of palliation, whether or not the invasive and anticancer measures described above may be used. The main classes of drugs that can be used are:
- Bronchodilators (and corticosteroids if there is severe airflow limitation).
- Diuretics, if there is heart failure.
- Antibiotics, if infection is thought to be contributing, and the patient is not obviously "terminally ill."
- Anticoagulants, if there is a high index of suspicion of thromboembolism and there are no contraindications.
- Sedatives.
- Opioids.

The last two classes of drugs need further description in this context. Studies in chronic lung-disease patients have shown that benzodiazepines may be useful in reducing anxiety, but they can cause unacceptable central sedation. There is a risk of respiratory depression, as with opioids discussed below, but this is not usually a problem if the doses are built up gradually and if the patient does not have a history of respiratory failure. Other sedatives such as neuroleptic agents have been studied but they are generally too toxic (sedating) for most purposes.

Opioids have been extensively researched in both chronic lung disease and cancer patients. The overall message from these is that the more potent opioids (but also dihydrocodeine) can give very useful relief of dyspnea, if titrated carefully, usually with acceptable toxicity. The oral route is preferred, but for rapid relief in a very frightened patient, e.g., with pulmonary thromboembolism or a pericardial effusion, intravenous administration may be needed. There is no reliable research evidence to point to one potent opioid being the "best," but most experience is with morphine and hydromorphone. Unlike the use of opioids in the management of pain, where regular prophylactic medication is recommended to prevent pain recurring, patients with breathlessness that is episodic or related to exertion often prefer to take these drugs on an "as needed" (prn) basis. (This also applies to benzodiazepines, e.g., lorazepam.)

If a patient is already on an opioid for pain control and then becomes breathless, it has been shown that a prn dose calculated as 25% of the normal "rescue dose" of the opioid can be helpful. As with pain control it is necessary to titrate the regime for each individual patient rather than apply a blanket policy of dosing. If opioids are used, it is essential to advise the patients about early nausea and to prescribe a prophylactic laxative.

In the final hours or days of life, some patients may experience constant and severe dyspnea. In such circumstances it may be reasonable to install a continuous subcutaneous infusion of either a benzodiazepine, preferably midazolam; or an opioid such as morphine or fentanyl; or sometimes both. The aim of this palliative sedation must always be to reduce the sensory level to the point where the patient is no longer distressed – and *not* to induce a level of unconsciousness from which it may be difficult for the patient to recover. This balance is often very difficult to implement at the bedside of a dying patient, and so it is very important for the multidisciplinary team to engage the patient – if that is still possible – and the family into discussion of the benefits and risks before embarking on palliative sedation.

Oxygen has long been thought of by patients and the public as being a "natural" and essential remedy for breathlessness. This misconception is not helped by the overuse of oxygen in sports and in oxygen bars! Some of the apparent benefit of oxygen delivered by facial masks is actually from the stimulation of nasal and cheek skin receptors to moving airflow. Even if this mechanism is not involved, it is apparent that many patients derive psychological benefit from oxygen therapy and find it hard to give up. It has been shown from research and clinical experience that cancer patients with resting hypoxia (e.g., oxygen saturation below 90%) will gain relief by oxygen administration. Usually this only needs to be given intermittently, during and after exercise, so that the mask or nasal cannulae are not constantly interfering with speech, eating and drinking, or body image.

Recently the replacement of nitrogen by helium in compressed air cylinders ("Heliox") has been shown to result in a lighter gas mixture with physical properties that can be helpful for patients with very severe airflow limitation. The place of Heliox in dyspneic cancer patients still needs to be clarified.

Psychological and behavioral methods have been shown in both cancer and chronic lung disease to be helpful for some patients. A wide range of interventions can be used, from guided relaxation to imagery. If these are combined with breathing retraining, which is usually offered by physiotherapists or trained nurses, then the combined nonpharmacological package can be effective and safe. Of the *complementary therapies*, acupuncture has been shown in one study of cancer patients to be effective in relieving dyspnea and anxiety, without affecting other aspects of objective pulmonary function.

Ideally, such a program of nonpharmacological and complementary interventions should be integrated with appropriate anticancer therapies, physical invasive procedures and pharmacological treatments. This is best done, in the care of advanced cancer patients, through a multiprofessional team that has access to relevant investigations and can offer the patient frequent monitoring and advice to the family as well as the community-based services, if the patient wishes to remain at home.

BIBLIOGRAPHY

Sentinel articles

Allard P, Lamontagne C, Bernard P, Tremblay C. How effective are supplementary doses of opioids for dyspnea in terminally ill cancer patients? A randomised continous sequential clinical trial. *J Pain Symptom Manage* 1999;17:256–65.

Booth S, Adams L. The shuttle walking test: a reproducible method for evaluating the impact of shortness of breath on functional capacity in patients with advanced cancer. *Thorax* 2001;56:146–50.

Bruera E, de Stoutz N, Velasco-Leiva A, Schoeller T, Hanson J. Effects of oxygen on dyspnea in hypoxaemic terminal cancer patients. *Lancet* 1993;342:13–14.

Bredin M, Corner J, Krishnasamy M, Plant H, Bailey C, A'Hern R. Multicentre randomised controlled trial of nursing intervention for breathlessness in patients with lung cancer. *Br Med J* 1999;318:901–4.

Dudgeon DJ, Kristjanson L, Sloan JA, Lertzman M, Clement K. Dyspnea in cancer patients: prevalence and associated factors. *J Pain Symptom Manage* 2001*a*;21:95–102.

Dudgeon DJ, Lertzman M, Askew GR. Physiological changes and clinical correlations of dyspnea in cancer outpatients. *J Pain Symptom Manage* 2001*b*;21:373–9.

Filshie J, Penn K, Ashley S, Davis CL. Acupuncture for the relief of cancer-related breathlessness. *Palliat Med* 1996;10:145–50.

Tanaka K, Akechi T, Okuyama T, Nishiwaki Y, Uchitomi Y. Development and validation of the Cancer Dyspnea Scale: a multidimensional, brief, self-rating scale. *Br J Cancer* 2000;82: 800–5.

Review articles

Ahmedzai SH. Palliation of respiratory symptoms. In *Oxford Textbook of Palliative Medicine*, ed. D Doyle, GWC Hanks, N McDonald, pp. 584–616. Oxford: Oxford University Press, 1998.

Davis CL. ABC of palliative care: breathlessness, cough and other respiratory problems. *Br Med J* 1997;315:931–4.

Internet sites

This is the internet version of the excellent resource *Palliative Care Formulary* (Twycross, Wilcock, Thorp, 1998)

http://www.palliativedrugs.net/pdi.html

This is a very useful article about endobronchial (intraluminal) palliation techniques. It needs registration with Medscape, which is free.

http://www.medscape.com/moffitt/CancerControl/ 2001/v08.n04/cc0804.04.simo/cc0804.04. simo-01.html

45

Loss of appetite and weight

Aminah Jatoi and Charles L. Loprinzi

Division of Medical Oncology, Mayo Clinic, Rochester

Introduction

Over 50% of patients with advanced cancer suffer from loss of weight and/or appetite during the course of their disease.[1] In a landmark Eastern Cooperative Oncology Group study, Dewys and colleagues found that loss of more than 5% of premorbid weight predicted a poor prognosis, independent of tumor stage, tumor histology, and patient performance status. This weight loss was also associated with a trend towards lower chemotherapy response rates.[2]

How might we explain this prognostic impact? Investigators have hypothesized that loss of lean tissue is directly tied to prognosis. Because lean tissue carries all the body's metabolic machinery, these investigators have suggested there might be a cause and effect relationship between loss of lean tissue and an early demise. In fact, an excessive loss of lean tissue is a hallmark of cancer-associated weight loss.[3] Although weight-losing cancer patients manifest loss of both fat and lean tissue, it is the loss of lean tissue that is the most dramatic and stands in stark contrast to the preferential loss of fat tissue observed in classical starvation.[4] Thus, it may be hypothesized that a reversal of loss of lean tissue might improve prognosis. To date, however, despite ongoing investigation with such agents as eicosapentaenoic acid, thalidomide, adenosine triphosphate, anticytokine therapy, and nonsteroidal anti-inflammatory agents, this hypothesis remains unproved.

Independent of lean tissue wasting, however, a strong argument can be made for diagnosing and palliating anorexia. Wolfe and others interviewed parents of deceased children who died of cancer.[5] Approximately 80% of these children had suffered from anorexia and 36% of parents identified this symptom as a cause of suffering for their child when a physician failed to identify it. These researchers concluded "greater attention to symptom control...might ease... suffering."

Treatment options

The day-to-day management of cancer-associated anorexia and weight loss should maintain "ease...[of] suffering"[5] as its primary goal.

An important first step in evaluating the cancer patient with weight loss and anorexia is deciding whether the patient is a candidate for orexigenic agents. It is important to remain cognizant of the fact that a subgroup of cancer patients may benefit from direct caloric supplementation. These patients require direct intervention with nutritional support as opposed to the more indirect use of appetite stimulants. Although controversial, studies suggest that increased caloric intake by means of nutritional support might benefit cancer patients under the following circumstances:[6-10] (1) perioperatively, (2) in the setting of stem cell or bone marrow transplantation, and (3) during treatment for head and neck cancer. Along similar lines, improvement in appetite often accompanies tumor response and under such circumstances where tumor shrinkage is anticipated with antineoplastic treatment, orexigenic agents might not be necessary. To illustrate this point, a recent study by Geels and colleagues examined 300 metastatic breast cancer patients who had received antineoplastic therapy.[11] A direct relationship was observed between tumor response and improvement in appetite: Approximately 82% of patients with a complete or partial response to cancer treatment also demonstrated an improvement in appetite. Thus, if chemotherapy is likely to yield notable tumor regression, orexigenic agents need not be prescribed.

What are the options for patients who do not fall into any of the three categories listed above and yet suffer from anorexia, advanced cancer, and a low likelihood of response to antineoplastic treatment? An important component of treating anorexia in this setting is an honest discussion with patients and family members about realistic expectations with regard to food intake. The purpose of this discussion is to assuage guilt arising from patients' failure to meet preconceived expectations. It is important to acknowledge that aggressive caloric supplementation in chemotherapy patients with advanced cancer has not improved outcome. For example, Ovesen and colleagues randomly assigned patients to receive nutritional counseling versus no nutritional counseling. Although the former group consumed significantly more calories than the latter, tumor response rates, patient survival, and quality of life did not differ between the two groups.[12] Sometimes such frank and honest discussions with patients and their family members lead exclusively to an acceptance of anorexia and a validation of realistic eating goals. At other times, they also lead to a prescription for an orexigenic agent.

Several potential orexigenic agents have been studied, most notably progesterones and corticosteroids. Megestrol acetate and medroxyprogesterone acetate are two progestational agents, which improve appetite. Mechanisms of action have not been fully elucidated. Megestrol acetate has been more extensively studied: 15 placebo-controlled trials have been published, and 13 of these demonstrate that megestrol acetate improves appetite in the cancer setting. For example, a North Central Cancer Treatment Group trial examined 133 cancer patients and found that patients who received megestrol acetate at a dose of 800 mg/day manifested both an increase in appetite as well as an increase in nonfluid weight.[13] In a follow-up study from this same group, the optimal dosing of megestrol acetate was determined at 480–800 mg/day. These doses provided better appetite stimulation than did 160 mg/day.[14] An oral suspension of megestrol acetate is associated with less cost, and improved bioavailability. A reasonable approach is to begin with 400 mg/day of oral suspension megestrol acetate and consider an escalation to 600–800 mg/day over 2–4 weeks in patients who do not receive a favorable initial response.

Megestrol acetate has few side effects. It carries a slightly increased risk of thrombophlebitis (especially with concomitant chemotherapy). In patients with a history of thrombophlebitis, we usually do not prescribe it. Suppression of the pituitary-adrenal axis has also been observed. Should a patient suffer a serious infection, trauma, or undergo surgery while on or while having recently received megestrol acetate, supplemental corticosteroids should be prescribed to prevent overt adrenal insufficiency.

Corticosteroids can also be used to palliate cancer-associated anorexia. Moertel and colleagues were the first to report that corticosteroids improve appetite in patients with advanced cancer,[15] a finding that has been confirmed by others. In a recent study, Loprinzi and colleagues found that dexamethasone at 0.75 mg qid (four times a day) and megestrol acetate 800 mg/day are relatively comparable in palliating cancer-associated anorexia. However, dexamethasone was associated with a significantly worse side-effect profile when compared with the megestrol acetate-treated arm: myopathy (18 versus 6%); cushingoid changes (6 versus 1%); and peptic ulcer disease (3 versus 0%), respectively. This toxicity profile provides guidance as to when to use which of these two agents. We generally recommend that dexamethasone be reserved for cancer patients with a poor prognosis of only a few weeks, since troublesome side effects such as myopathy are unlikely to occur over the short term. Additionally, dexamethasone is a reasonable choice in patients at higher risk for thromboembolic phenomena. Other patients might be better candidates for progestational agents should they choose to try drug therapy.

Despite relatively high rates of appetite improvement with the use of progestational agents and corticosteroids, the search for more effective orexigenic agents justifiably continues. Rates of appetite improvement have been reported to be as high as 74% with these agents among patients who continue medications for a month or more. However, such rates obscure a placebo effect, which has been as high as 40% in previous trials.[13] Promising orexigenic agents that require further testing include thalidomide, type 3 serotonergic receptor antagonists, and specific inhibitors of TNFα.

Conclusions

Loss of weight and appetite are associated with great morbidity among cancer patients. An important aspect of treating cancer-associated anorexia is embarking upon a frank discussion with the patient and family members about realistic feeding goals in the setting of advanced, refractory cancer. While several novel approaches for abrogating lean tissue wasting and improving appetite are currently being tested, progestational agents and corticosteroids, both of which primarily target appetite, have thus far provided the most palliation.

REFERENCES

Sentinel articles

1 Tchekmedyian NS. Costs and benefits of nutrition support in cancer. *Oncology* 1995; 9(Suppl. 11):79–84.

2 Dewys WD, Begg C, Lavin PT et al. Prognostic effect of weight loss prior to chemotherapy in cancer patients. Eastern Cooperative Oncology Group. *Am J Med* 1980;69:491–7.

3 Cohn SH, Gartenhaus W, Sawitsky A et al. Compartmental body composition of cancer patients by measurement of total body nitrogen, potassium, and water. *Metabolism* 1981; 30:222–9.

4 Keys A, Brozek, J, Henschel A, Michelsen O, Taylor HL. *The Biology of Human Starvation.* St. Paul: University of Minnesota Press, 1950.

5 Wolfe J, Grier HE, Klar N et al. Symptoms and suffering at the end of life in children with cancer. *N Engl J Med* 2000;342:326–33.

6 Anonymous. Perioperative total parenteral nutrition in surgical patients. *N Engl J Med* 1991;325:525–32.

7 Fan ST, Lo M, Lai ECS et al. Perioperative nutritional support in patients undergoing hepatectomy for hepatocellular carcinoma. *N Engl J Med* 1994;331:1547–52.

8 Weisdorf SA, Lysne J, Wind D et al. Positive effect of prophylactic total parenteral nutrition on long-term outcome of bone marrow transplantation. *Transplantation* 1987;43:833–8.

9 Daly JM, Hearne B, Dunaj J et al. Nutritional rehabilitation in patients with advanced head and neck cancer receiving radiation therapy. *Am J Surgery* 1984;148:514–20.

10 Nayel H, el-Ghoneimy E, el-Haddad S. Impact of nutritional supplementation on treatment delay and morbidity in patients with head and neck tumors treated with irradiation. *Nutrition* 1992;8:13–18.

11 Geels P, Eisenhauer E, Bezjak A et al. Palliative effect of chemotherapy: objective tumor response is associated with symptom improvement in patients with metastatic breast cancer. *J Clin Oncol* 2000;18:2395–405.

12 Ovesen L, Allingstrup L, Hannibal J, Mortenson EL, Hansen OP. Effect of dietary counseling on food intake, body weight, response rate, survival, and quality of life in cancer patients undergoing chemotherapy: a prospective, randomized study. *J Clin Oncol* 1993;11:2043–9.

13 Loprinzi CL, Ellison NM, Schaid DJ et al. Controlled trial of megestrol acetate for the treatment of cancer anorexia and cachexia. *J Natl Cancer Inst* 1990;82:1127–32.

14 Loprinzi CL, Bernath AM, Schaid DJ et al. Phase III evaluation of megestrol acetate as therapy for patients with cancer anorexia and/or cachexia. *Oncology* 1994;51(Suppl. 1):2–7.

15 Moertel CG, Schutt AJ, Reitemeier RJ, Hahn RG. Corticosteroid therapy of preterminal gastrointestinal cancer. *Cancer* 1974;33:1607–9.

Review articles

Baracos VE. A panoply of anabolic and catabolic mediators. *Curr Opin Clin Nutr Metab Care* 2000;3:169–70.

Gagnon B, Bruera E. A review of the drug treatment of cachexia associated with cancer. *Drugs* 1998;55:675–88.

Internet sites

http://www.cancer.org/
http://www.aicr.org

46

Fatigue

Hans Neuenschwander

Oncology Institute of Southern Switzerland

Introduction

Fatigue and asthenia are present in some extent in 70–90% of patients with advanced cancer.[1,2] Nevertheless until now this symptom has been widely neglected by clinical attention and by research, for several reasons:

- It is not reported by patients because they accept it as inevitable.
- It is therefore not identified by the physician, since it is not visible.
- Even if it is identified it is not therapeutically addressed.

Fatigue and asthenia are usually inseparably associated with the tumor by patient and caregiver. Since a well-trained palliative care team may be able to control frequent major symptoms such as pain, nausea or dyspnea, asthenia will become the most important cause of physical and psychosocial suffering.

Clinical features

The onset of fatigue may be one of the first symptoms and even precede the diagnosis of a malignancy. It may be present during the whole course of a disease and increase following anticancer treatments. However, in the palliative care setting it is usually not an issue for aggressive assessment or treatment.

Fatigue is a multidimensional symptom. It can be divided roughly into physical and mental aspects. Patients report muscle weakness and effort intolerance, in the meantime also a lack of motivation and interest, and difficulty in maintaining concentration. In a more advanced stage, patients do not start an activity since they know or fear that they will not be able to accomplish it. Other than in a physiological tiredness neither rest nor sleep may improve performance.

The affected person is often discouraged by the persistence of this highly function-impairing symptom, and also has the sensation that the physician does not pay attention to nor understand the phenomenon.

Table 46.1. Causes of asthenia in advanced cancer

Cachexia/malnutrition

Dehydration

Anemia

Infection (recurrent acute infection, chronic infection as hepatitis, tuberculosis, brucellosis, mononucleosis, herpes, etc.)

Chronic hypoxia

Neurologic disorders (autonomic dysfunction, myasthenia syndrome, parkinsonism, demyelinization)

Psychogenic causes

Metabolic and electrolyte disorders

Endocrine disorders (thyreopathy, Morbus Addison, diabetes mellitus, etc.)

Chronic insomnia

Overexertion

Pharmacologic/toxic (narcotics, sedatives, alcohol, chemotherapy, etc.)

Assessment

A number of assessment tools for asthenia have been proposed in cancer and non-cancer settings. Most of them are useful for research purposes. Irvine and colleagues have published an excellent review of these instruments and the history of the increasing awareness of the clinical importance of fatigue.[3] Recently, the Functional Assessment of Cancer Therapy (FACT-scale) and the Brief Fatigue Inventory have been recognized as useful for clinical trials.[4] In clinical practice a tool for measuring asthenia should not be energy-consuming for the patient. Since the symptom is multidimensional, for the daily work-up it seems wise to integrate a simple measurement like a VAS in a multidimensional symptom assessment tool, for example, the Edmonton Symptom Assessment System (ESAS). This allows identification of interactions and interdependence between different symptoms and their treatments.

Mechanisms

Fatigue is a typically multicausal symptom. In individual cases it is often impossible to conclude whether and in which proportion the disease itself, the therapeutic interventions, or several agents contribute to the asthenia (Table 46.1). Nevertheless, in some cases fatigue may result from one predominant etiology.

Mechanisms can be

1. Directly due to the tumor (e.g., lipolytic factors, tumor degradation products).
2. Induced by the tumor but produced by the host (tumor necrosis factors, interleukins etc.).

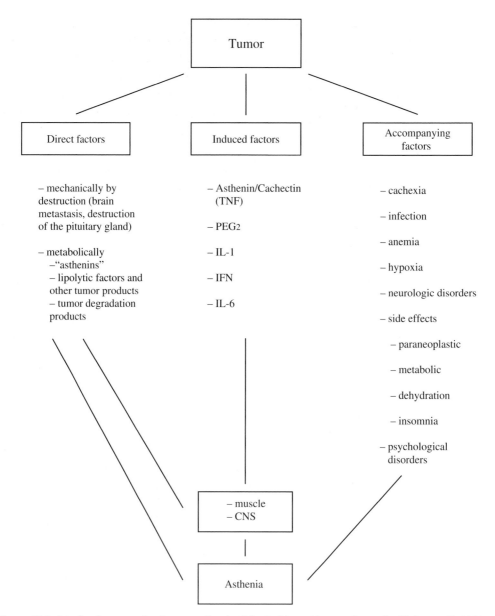

Figure 46.1 Mechanisms causing tumor asthenia. Adapted from Neuenschwander H, Bruera E, 1998.

3. They may accompany the disease.

Although quite often the therapeutic possibilities are modest, in some cases it might be worthwhile to identify the major contributing causes. The accompanying factors are briefly discussed here (Figure 46.1).

- Cachexia: Asthenia and cachexia are very often coexisting findings in advanced cancer patients. Some authors consider therefore asthenia to be just an epiphenomenon of profound cachexia. In fact, some of the mediators of the two symptoms are identical. However, we can recognize conditions where fatigue is present without cachexia. This can happen in benign conditions such as CFS or depressive disorders, and in malignancies such as early breast cancer or malignant lymphomas. Therefore it has to be assumed that asthenia may also exist independently from cachexia.
- Anemia: The role of anemia as a contributing cause to asthenia is still controversial and has been probably overvalued in the past. In fact, quite often blood supply in anemic cancer patients does not result in an improvement of asthenia. There are clinical conditions (e.g., thalassemia) where people, despite a hemoglobin value about 10 g/l, do not experience asthenia. In clinical practice it is wise to correct anemia only if the hemoglobin value is very low (beyond 8 g/l) or if it has occurred in a short time, or if in the past a patient's asthenia has improved significantly after transfusions.
- Dehydration: Dehydration is usually underestimated in the palliative situation. Patients may have a disturbed sense of thirst or their physicians may prescribe diuretic drugs in presence of hypoalbuminemic edema ("cachectic and hypoalbuminemic patients without edema are dehydrated"). In case of doubt a trial of rehydration might be worthwhile.
- Chronic oxygen hyposaturation.
- Insomnia: Lack of sleep might contribute to fatigue but less to weakness. Sleep disorders in cancer patients are however linked to a number of other factors such as pain, depression, and drugs, and may not be an independent variable.
- Neurological changes: Beside a number of functional alterations in the mid brain or other neurological syndromes associated with malignancy (e.g., Eaton–Lambert syndrome) the most important problem is probably autonomic dysfunction. This syndrome includes postural hypotension and gastrointestinal symptoms such as nausea, anorexia, and constipation. The association between autonomic failure and asthenia has not yet been adequately investigated.
- Psychological disorders: Patients presenting with an adjustment disorder or a major depression can have asthenia as one of the prevalent symptoms. The diagnosis of a major depression in the cancer patient with advanced disease is difficult because of the presentation with neurovegetative and somatic symptoms that are part of the disease itself.
- Metabolic disorders: Diabetes, electrolyte disorders such as low sodium, potassium, or magnesium and hypercalcemia should be excluded since an effective treatment is potentially available.

- Liver metastasis: Liver metastasis can contribute to the generation of asthenia even in a stage where the function of the organ is not yet clinically compromised.
- Side effects: Side effects of anticancer treatments are frequently contributors to asthenia, even though the mechanisms are not always well understood. For instance, fatigue and flu-like syndromes can be a dose-limiting side effect of some recent chemotherapeutic agents or of biological response modifiers such as interferon.[5] But even drugs prescribed exclusively for palliative purposes (opiates, benzodiazepines, etc.) may generate fatigue. Radiotherapy is also widely recognized as a potent asthenia-generator. The energy level may be impaired for months and in some cases not return to normal.

Treatment and management

Patients with far advanced malignant disease always experience a number of symptoms, which represent different levels of priority. In order to avoid side effect-bearing measures with low benefit we need to answer three questions.

1. Is asthenia a symptom of primary importance?
2. What are the major probable contributing causes?
3. Are there therapeutic interventions available with a favorable cost–benefit ratio?

Specific measures

We have learned that asthenia is almost always multicausal or in some cases only an epiphenomenon of another symptom complex (cachexia, infection, etc.)

Any measure aiming to reverse the underlying abnormality would result in an improvement of fatigue. Reversible factors, such as dehydration, metabolic disorders, and severe anemia may co-exist with nonreversible factors. The prescribed pharmacotherapy must be checked continuously in order to recognize iatrogenic fatigue (e.g., opioid accumulation in presence of renal failure). Psychological disorders can be therapeutically addressed.

We suggest making a list of the probable contributing factors. Among them we will try to identify the potentially reversible causes. Ask the patient if he feels that some of his drugs are contributing to his asthenia.

To treat a symptom successfully does not necessarily mean to eliminate it completely. A minor but significant improvement may be sufficient to shift the symptom out of the high priority range. It also can be useful to address partial factors, such as hypoxia (deliver O_2) or opioid toxicity (opioid-rotation), to make a difference.

Nonspecific measures

Nonpharmacological

First of all we will inform the patient about his situation, about the reasons for his asthenia and the therapeutic possibilities. This is crucial in order to allow the patient to develop realistic expectations and therefore avoid future conflicts and delusions.

In order to focus on the patient's own resources some suggestions can be given:

- Adapt daily activities to the residual energy (less housework, accept help of others in physical activities).
- Revise the daily time schedule. Perform important activities when feeling least fatigued.
- Increase the time dedicated to rest.
- Avoid "nonimportant" activities.
- Physical training can be helpful more in a prophylactic than in a therapeutic perspective. However, there are no clinical studies available that prove the usefulness (or the nocicivity) of physical training.

Pharmacological

Corticosteroids

A number of studies document the effect of these substances on fatigue. Unfortunately, the positive effects of steroids on asthenia vanish after a few weeks. For that reason, and because of the increasing risk of side effects (infection, steroid-induced myopathy), it is not advised that a treatment course is longer than 2–4 weeks.

Amphetamines

These drugs have shown to be useful especially in those patients in whom asthenia presented after increasing doses of opioids. Although these drugs are currently being used cautiously against asthenia it is not well established whether they have a direct effect or are just secondary to the improvement of subclinical depression. The best-documented drug is methylphenidate, which is prescribed at low doses of 5(–10) mg in the morning and an additional 5 mg at noon.

Progestagene

The prescription of progestagenes makes sense in situations where cachexia is assessed as the major contributing factor to asthenia. These drugs (e.g., medroxyprogesterone acetate) improve the appetite and also induce some weight gain. The therapeutic effect may occur only after 2–4 weeks. The use of these expensive drugs should therefore be limited to patients with a survival prognosis of at least 3 months or longer. If the prognosis is shorter, the former mentioned and rapidly effective corticosteroids should be preferred.

Conclusion

Asthenia is seen as a multidimensional syndrome. It requires a multimodal therapeutic approach including a number of drugs, exercise, and counseling for its management. However, in order to prevent excessive and unnecessary treatment, it is crucial to assimilate a decision-making framework on it as to when to initiate or renounce treatment options.

Summary

No other symptoms are so closely associated with cancer as asthenia and fatigue. Therefore they are unfortunately often accepted as unavoidable. Although they are by far the most prevalent symptoms in cancer patients, until recent years they have received only limited attention by clinicians and researchers.

New understanding of the underlying mechanisms of asthenia will hopefully change this nihilistic attitude in the near future. In the meantime, in order to engage at least the limited knowledge about effective management of asthenia, an appropriate assessment of symptom extent, the individual symptom significance and impact, and of the major contributing causes, is crucial.

BIBLIOGRAPHY

Bruera E, MacDonald RN. Asthenia in patients with advanced cancer. Issues in symptom control. Part I. *J Pain Symptom Manage* 1988;3:9–14.

Cleary JF. The reversible causes of asthenia in cancer patients. *Topics Palliat Care* 1998;2: 183–202.

Irvine DM, Vincent L, Bubela N, Thompson L, Graydon J. A critical appraisal of the research literature investigating fatigue in the individual with cancer. *Cancer Nurs* 1991; 14:188–99.

Neuenschwander H, Bruera E. Pathophysiology of cancer asthenia. *Topics Palliat Care* 1998; 2:171–81.

Portenoy RK, Thaler HT, Kornblith AB et al. Symptom prevalence, characteristic and distress in a cancer population. *Qual Life Res* 1994;3:183–9.

Yellen SB, Cella DF, Webster K, Blendowski C, Kaplan E. Measuring fatigue and other anemia-related symptoms with the Functional Assessment of Cancer Therapy (FACT) measuring system. *J Pain Symptom Manage* 1997;13:63–74.

Review articles

Neuenschwander H, Bruera E. Asthenia. In *Oxford Textbook of Palliative Medicine.* 2nd edn, ed.
Doyle, Hanks and MacDonald, pp. 573–81. Oxford: Oxford University Press, 1998.

Walker P, Schleinich MA, Bruera E. *Asthenia in Palliative Medicine*, ed. N MacDonald, pp. 29–33.
Oxford: Oxford Medical Publications, 1998.

Internet sites

NIH State-of-the-Science Statement on Cancer Pain, Depression, Fatigue
http://www.consensus.nih.gov/ta/022/022_intro.htm

47

Depression and anxiety

Michael Fisch

U.T. M.D. Anderson Cancer Center, Houston

Depression: An overview

Depression is a prevalent symptom in patients with advanced cancer. The reported rates of depression vary from less than 5% to greater than 50%, depending on how "depression" is defined and the nature of the patient population studied. The bulk of the data support an estimated prevalence in the 25–35% range. There are several inherent difficulties in diagnosing depression in this population. The most obvious problem is that sadness and grief are normal responses to the changes associated with the diagnosis of cancer and at transitional points in the disease. In addition, the physical signs of depression (such as fatigue, anorexia, sleep disturbance, etc.) may be attributable to malignancy itself. Finally, many of the medications used in advanced cancer patients may cause depression and/or physical symptoms. Due to these confounding issues, it can be difficult for cancer providers (and even behavioral health professionals) to distinguish depressed from nondepressed patients.

Distinct conceptual approaches: Symptom versus syndrome

Defining depression as a diagnostic syndrome (for example, using DSM–IV criteria) has some potential advantages and disadvantages when applied to advanced cancer patients. One of the advantages is that it enables clinicians to document the presence or absence of a depressive disorder in a reproducible fashion, and the existing data about the natural history and consequences of depression and appropriate treatment options generalize well to this population. The formal diagnosis of a depressive disorder may also be useful in order to establish appropriate reimbursement for management of this condition. The potential disadvantage of this approach is that it may deter management of depressive symptoms that do not reach the threshold for a DSM–IV diagnosis. The alternative to the syndrome-based approach is a symptom-based approach. The symptom-based approach is commonly used for phenomena such as pain and nausea. This involves ascertaining whether or not

Table 47.1. Major depressive episode findings

Depressed mood	Fatigue or loss of energy
Diminished interest or pleasure	Feelings of worthlessness or excessive guilt
Significant weight loss or gain	Diminished ability to think or concentrate
Insomnia or hypersomnia	Recurrent thoughts of death or suicide
Psychomotor agitation or retardation	

Table 47.2. Simple assessment of depressive symptoms

One-question screening:
"Are you depressed?"

Two-question screening
"Have you often been bothered by feeling down, depressed, or hopeless?"
"Have you often been bothered by having little pleasure or interest in doing things?"

Numerical rating scales

No depression ———————————————— Worst depression
          0 1 2 3 4 5 6 7 8 9 10

the symptom is present, elucidating further details about eliciting factors and the degree of suffering that is attributable to the symptom, and then taking into account other co-occurring symptoms to ultimately form a judgement about the proper management for the patient. The potential advantages of the symptom-based approach are (1) it can be applied by providers who are not behavioral health specialists, (2) it generates less stigma for patients, and (3) it can be applied in busy office settings where time and scheduling are major constraints. The disadvantage of this approach is that there are only limited data regarding its utility. One study performed by the Hoosier Oncology Group randomly assigned advanced cancer patients to an antidepressant (fluoxetine) versus placebo based on the patient's response to a two-question screening survey. In this 12-week study, patients with a minimum threshold of depressive symptoms showed improved overall quality of life and depressive symptoms with antidepressant therapy. Further research is needed to confirm these findings. Meanwhile, the preference style of the patient, the assessment and treatment "comfort zone" of the clinician, the practice setting, and availability of behavioral health resources are likely to influence the depression assessment model that is applied to any given patient.

The diagnosis of a major depressive disorder involves expression of depressed mood and/or anhedonia (diminished pleasure in doing things) for at least 2 weeks, plus the presence of at least five other depressive symptoms (Table 47.1). In contrast, symptom assessment of depression can be achieved with one or two screening questions or use of a numerical rating scale (Table 47.2). It is important to note that complicated cancer patients may present with atypical features of depression. Atypical presentations may include confusion or memory loss (pseudodementia), chronic pain unresponsive to analgesics, somatization, severe anxiety, and substance abuse. Just as depression may be obscured by other conditions, other medical problems may look like depression. For example, hypoactive delirium is frequently misdiagnosed as depression. For this reason, clinicians should pay careful attention to the timing of onset of the clinical change, and the presence or absence of features such as a fluctuating course, difficulty focusing attention, disorganized thinking, and altered level of consciousness. Appropriate reasons to refer to a behavioral health specialist include diagnostic uncertainty, significant suicidal ideations, and uncertainty about therapeutic management (particularly when patients fail initial therapy).

Depression treatment

When a patient has significant depressive symptoms and a judgement is made to initiate therapy, appropriate therapeutic options include pharmacotherapy, psychological counseling, or a combination of medication and counseling. The choice of treatment often depends as much on the patient's family and social circumstances and preferences as it does on clinical factors. For instance, individual or group counseling may require time, energy, expense, and transportation – all of which can be scarce resources for certain patients. It is important to realize that expressive-supportive counselling provided by any caring health professional can be effective at managing depression and anxiety in this population. Some providers feel inadequately trained for such counseling, but it is really the clinician's ability to allow the patient to express his/her own emotions along with the therapeutic effect of an empathetic listener that provides the value of this kind of therapy.

When an antidepressant medication is chosen, it may be chosen with the intent of providing efficacy at relieving depression with the fewest possible side effects. Alternatively, the drug may be chosen with the goal of relieving depression and/or anxiety along with some other bothersome symptom(s) by mobilizing particular side effects of the chosen drug. A list of commonly prescribed antidepressants in cancer patients is shown in Table 47.3. In general, the serotonin-selective reuptake inhibitors (particularly citalopram, paroxetine, and sertraline) are well tolerated and are often chosen due to their favorable side-effect profile. However, other medications may be chosen due to a side-effect profile that is particularly useful for a given patient. For example, a patient with a hypoactive depression may be given an antidepressant that tends to be activating. Likewise, a patient with insomnia and depression may be given a sedating antidepressant dosed at bedtime. Some

Table 47.3. Selected antidepressants

	Initial dose	Maintenance dose	Important side effects
Tricyclics			Cardiac arrhythmias; sexual dysfunction; weight gain; lower seizure threshold; caution in patients with cardiac disease, narrow-angle glaucoma, urinary retention
Amitriptyline	25–50 mg qhs	150–300 mg/day	
Nortriptyline	10–25 mg qhs	90–150 mg/day	
Serotonin selective reuptake inhibitors (SSRI)			Life-threatening reactions if SSRIs used within 2 weeks of MAO inhibitors; insomnia; sexual dysfunction
Citalopram	10 mg qAM	10–40 mg/day	Ejaculation disorder
Fluoxetine	10–20 mg qAM	20–80 mg/day	Anxiety; anorexia; weight loss; hyponatremia; photosensitivity; may alter glycemic control in diabetics; SA node slowing
Paroxetine	10–20 mg qAM	20–50 mg/day	Anxiety; anorexia; weight loss; hyponatremia; photosensitivity
Sertraline	25–50 mg qAM	50–200 mg/day	Anxiety; anorexia; weight loss; hyponatremia; photosensitivity
Combination agents (Serotonin/noradrenergic)			
Venlafaxine	37.5 mg qAM	75–225 mg/day	Somnolence; dizziness; constipation; nausea; hypertension
Mirtazapine	15 mg qhs	15–45 mg/day	Somnolence; dizziness; constipation; increased appetite; edema
Psychostimulants			
Methylphenidate	5 mg at 8 AM, 2.5 mg at noon	15–20 mg/day	Tachycardia; hypertension; nervousness; agitation; insomnia; anorexia; decreased seizure threshold; drug dependence or abuse potential

examples of side effects that may be mobilized with specific antidepressants are shown in Table 47.4.

Another important consideration when dosing antidepressants in cancer patients is the potential for drug interactions. This patient population is prone to polypharmacy, with analgesics, anticonvulsants, antibiotics, and other drugs frequently prescribed. Many antidepressants and anxiolytic agents interact with cytokine P450 enzyme system. These enzymes lie on the endoplasmic reticula in hepatocytes as

Table 47.4. Mobilizing side effects of antidepressants

Sedating agents	Activating agents	Increase appetite
Amitriptyline	Methylphenidate	Amitriptyline
Nortriptyline	Fluoxetine	Nortriptyline
Mirtazapine		Mirtazapine

well as in other sites (intestinal mucosa, brain, kidney). The interactions that may occur at the level of the enzymes are varied and complex. Some medications cause enzyme induction and a resulting decrease in the pharmacodynamic effect of other drugs. In other cases there may be inhibition of an enzyme and enhancement in the effect (or toxicity) of other drugs. Some important P450 drug interactions in the advanced cancer population are listed in Table 47.5.

Assessment and management of anxiety

Anxiety is a very common symptom in patients with advanced cancer. Like depression, anxiety occurs in 20–40% of patients and usually co-exists with depressive symptoms. Using a syndrome-based model, anxiety and depression may be characterized as the DSM–IV diagnosis "adjustment disorder with anxious mood." This refers to the development of emotional or behavioral symptoms in response to an identifiable stressor where the symptoms cause either impaired functioning and/or distress in excess of what one would expect from the stressor alone. Symptoms that are uniquely attributable to anxiety include physical symptoms such as tremor, sweating, tachycardia, hyperventilation, and restlessness. Psychological symptoms of anxiety include worry, rumination, and fear. These symptoms may cause patients to flee their environment or display avoidant behaviors.

A crucial part of the management of anxiety symptoms is to consider that the differential diagnosis of anxiety includes unrelieved physical symptoms (such as pain or dyspnea), toxic/metabolic conditions (such as hypoxia, opioid toxicity, or akathisia), agitated delirium, or an "anxious" depression. The treatment of anxiety may involve use of antidepressants, use of anxiolytics, and/or psychological counselling. Counseling is effective for treatment of anxiety and it generally involves substitution of more adaptive behaviors and problem-solving approaches for expression of anxiety (which is less adaptive). Counseling may be psychoeducational, behavioral, cognitive–behavioral, or group-oriented.

For patients with pervasive worry and autonomic hyperreactivity, pharmacotherapy may be indicated. The categories of medications used to treat anxiety are listed in Table 47.6. Benzodiazepines are the most commonly prescribed agents and

Table 47.5. Selected cytochrome P450 drug interactions

	2C9	2C19	2D6	3A4
Substrates	**Fluoxetine**	**Tricyclics**	**Tricyclics**	**Citalopram**
	Celecoxib	**Venlafaxine**	**Trazodone**	Benzodiazepines
	Warfarin	**Citalopram**	**Fluoxetine**	Theophylline
	Tamoxifen	Proton pump inhibitors	**Mirtazapine**	Methadone
	TMP-SMX	Benzodiazepines	**Paroxetine**	Rofecoxib
	Cytoxan		Haloperidol	Cyclosporine
			Phenothiazines	Donezepil
			Donezepil	Zolpidem
			Oxycodone	Tacrolimus
			Hydrocodone	Tamoxifen
			Beta blockers	Etoposide
			Ondansetron	Vinca alkaloids
				Paclitaxel
				Calcium channel blockers
				Proton pump inhibitors
Inhibitors	Amiodarone		**Fluoxetine**	**Nefazodone**
			Paroxetine	Quinolones
			Sertraline	Macrolide antibiotics
			Methadone	Antifungals
			Doxorubicin	Amiodarone
			Vinblastine	Grapefruit juice
				HIV protease inhibitors
Inducers		Corticosteroids		**St. John's Wort**
				Barbiturates
				Phenytoin
				Corticosteroids
				Rifampin

Note: This table highlights *some* of the major known P450 drug interactions. Antidepressants are shown in bold. Appropriate, updated reference material should be consulted to establish the presence or absence of important P450 interactions. The clinical significance of these kinds of interactions are not well understood.

Table 47.6. Drug categories for management of anxiety

Benzodiazepines
Antidepressants
Neuroleptics
Antihistamines

they are effective first-line agents. These medications may cause significant sedation or trigger delirium in patients who are on other psychoactive medications (including opioids) or who are particularly frail. These drugs should be used cautiously and, when feasible, should be discontinued. The short-acting benzodiazepines lorazepam and alprazolam are used most frequently. These drugs should be dosed at 0.25–0.5 mg tid initially. For patients with panic disorder, alprazolam is effective as are several antidepressants (imipramine, sertraline, paroxetine). For patients with co-existing delirium or possible opioid toxicity, haloperidol or other neuroleptic agents are useful for symptom management while the underlying problem is addressed. Finally, antihistamines can also provide useful anxiolysis, particularly at night when insomnia is an issue.

BIBLIOGRAPHY

Sentinel articles

Chochinov HM, Wilson KG, Enns M, Lander S. Prevalence of depression in the terminally ill: effects of diagnostic criteria and symptom threshold judgments. *Am J Psychiatry* 1994;151: 537–40.

Chochinov H, Wilson K, Enns M, Lander S. "Are you depressed?" Screening for depression in the terminally ill. *Am J Psychiatry* 1997;154:674–6.

Derogatis L, Feldstein M, Morrow G et al. A survey of psychotropic drug prescriptions in an oncology population. *Cancer* 1979;44:1919–29.

Fisch MJ, Loehrer PJ, Passik SD, Kristellar JL, Jung S, Einhorn LH. Fluoxetine versus placebo in advanced cancer outpatients: a placebo-controlled, double-masked trial of the Hoosier Oncology Group. *Proc Annu Meet Am Soc Clin Oncol* 2001;20:Abstr 1530.

Lloyd-Williams M, Friedman T, Rudd N. A survey of antidepressant prescribing in the terminally ill. *Palliat Med* 1999;13:243–8.

Musselman DL, Lawson DH, Gumnick JF et al. Paroxetine for the prevention of depression induced by high dose interferon alfa. *N Engl J Med* 2001;344:961–6.

Passik SD, Dugan W, McDonald MV, Rosenfeld B, Theobald DE, Edgerton S. Oncologists' recognition of depression in their patients with cancer. *J Clin Oncol* 1998;16:1594–600.

Razavi D, Allilaire JF, Smith M et al. The effect of fluoxetine on anxiety and depression symptoms in cancer patients. *Acta Psychiatr Scand* 1996;94:205–10.

Whooley M, Avins A, Miranda J, Browner W. Case-finding instruments for depression: two questions are as good as many. *J Gen Intern Med* 1997;12:439–45.

Review articles

American Psychiatric Association. *Diagnostic and Statistical Manual of Mental Disorders* (DSM–IV) (4th edn) Washington, DC: APA, 1994.

Beliles K, Stoudemire A. Psychopharmacologic treatment of depression in the medically ill. *Psychosomatics* 1998;39:S2–19.

Bernard SA, Bruera E. Drug interactions in palliative care. *J Clin Oncol* 2000;18:1780–99.

Block SD. Assessing and managing depression in the terminally ill patient. *Ann Intern Med* 2000;132:209–18.

Holland JC. NCCN practice guidelines for the management of psychosocial distress. *Oncology* 1999;13:113–48.

Komaroff AL. Symptoms: in the head or in the brain? *Ann Intern Med* 2001;134:783–5.

Kroenke K, Harris L. Symptoms research: a fertile field. *Ann Intern Med* 2001;134(Suppl.):801–2.

Payne DK, Massie MJ. Anxiety in palliative care. In *Handbook of Psychiatry in Palliative Care*, ed. HM Chochinov, W Breitbart, pp. 63–74. Oxford: Oxford University Press, 2000.

Psychiatric aspects of excellent end-of-life care: a position statement of the Academy of Psychosomatic Medicine. *J Palliat Med* 1998;1:113–15.

Wilson KG, Chochinov HM, de Faye B, Breitbart W. Diagnosis and management of depression in palliative care. In *Handbook of Psychiatry in Palliative Care*, ed. HM Chochinov, W Breitbart, pp. 25–49. Oxford: Oxford University Press.

Internet sites

This site is sponsored by the National Cancer Institute and includes detailed supportive care statements on depression and anxiety for the health professional. There are separate statements on each topic written for patients.

http://www.cancer.gov/cancer_information/coping/

NIH State-of-the-Science Statement on Cancer Pain, Depression, Fatigue

http://www.consensus.nih.gov/ta/022/022_intro.htm

48

Delirium

Peter G. Lawlor

University of Alberta Hospital, Edmonton

Introduction

Delirium is a common and frequently distressing neuropsychiatric complication in cancer patients. It has been defined as a transient global disorder of cognition and attention. These features are highlighted in the *Diagnostic and Statistical Manual of Mental Disorders* (4th edition; DSM–IV) core diagnostic criteria for delirium (Table 48.1), which also includes perceptual disturbance, acuity of onset (hours to days), fluctuation in clinical features, and the presence of an underlying cause, such as a general medical condition, substance induced, multiple etiologies, or unknown etiology. Delirium is associated with increased morbidity and mortality, prolonged hospital stay, and especially in the elderly, an increased requirement for institutional care.

Epidemiological aspects

Delirium occurrence rates in the range of 8–88% have been reported in hospitalized cancer patients. This wide range likely represents differences in diagnostic criteria, and populations selected on the basis of admission to different settings (for example, early versus advanced disease) or referral to different consult services such as psychiatry or neurology. Prospective studies have reported delirium in 40% of advanced cancer patients on hospital admission and in almost 90% of these patients in the last hours or days prior to death. Despite its remarkable frequency as a terminal event, delirium reversal has been reported in approximately 50% of episodes.

Clinical features

Delirium is a syndrome with protean manifestations. Perceptual disturbance, one of the potential core criteria, includes misperceptions, illusions, and hallucinations.

Table 48.1. DSM–IV diagnostic criteria for delirium due to a medical condition

---

A. Disturbance of consciousness (i.e., reduced clarity of awareness of the environment) with reduced ability to focus, sustain, or shift attention.

B. A change in cognition (such as memory deficit, disorientation, language disturbance) or the development of a perceptual disturbance that is not better accounted for by a pre-existing, established, or evolving dementia.

C. The disturbance develops over a short period of time (usually hours to days) and tends to fluctuate during the day.

D. There is evidence from the history, physical examination, or laboratory findings that the disturbance is caused by the direct physiological consequences of a general medical condition.

Source: Reprinted with permission from the *Diagnostic and Statistical Manual of Mental Disorders* (4th edn). Copyright 1994 American Psychiatric Association.

Hallucinations are most commonly visual but tactile and auditory types can also occur. In addition to the core DSM–IV diagnostic criteria, disturbances of sleep–wake cycle, emotional lability, alteration in psychomotor activity, anxiety, fear, depression, delusions, apathy and disordered thoughts are recognized as associated clinical features. Alteration in psychomotor activity can involve a hyperactive or agitated state, a hypoactive or hypoalert state, or more commonly, a mixed variety with fluctuating periods of hyper- and hypoactivity.

Delirium is most frequently misdiagnosed as dementia or depression. Dementia shares many features with delirium but usually attentional capacity is relatively well preserved and the onset is gradual over months or years. The quiet hypoactive subtype of delirium is liable to be misdiagnosed as depression. Although cognitive deficit can also occur as part of a depressive pseudodementia, it is relatively uncommon. Fluctuation in symptomatology is less likely to occur in both depression and dementia.

Pathophysiology and pathogenesis

Delirium represents a neuropsychiatric manifestation of an underlying generalized disorder of cerebral metabolism and neurotransmission. Decreased cerebral cholinergic transmission or an imbalance between dopaminergic and cholinergic transmission is foremost among the studied derangements of neurotransmission in delirium.

Advanced age is recognized as one of the major risk factors for development of delirium in the general population. In advanced cancer multiple additional risk factors usually exist, for example, nutritional deficit, functional status impairment, and multiple organ impairment. Specific risk factors for opioid toxicity are likely to

Table 48.2. Precipitants associated with delirium in advanced cancer

Category	Precipitating factor
Intracranial	Primary and metastatic brain neoplasms
	Leptomeningeal metastatic disease
	Postictal
Organ failure	Cardiac
	Hepatic
	Renal
	Respiratory
Infection	Any site
Psychotropic medications	Opioids
	Benzodiazepines
	Tricyclics
	Anticholinergics
	Selective serotonin reuptake inhibitors
	Neuroleptics
	Antihistamines
Other medications	Steroids
	H_2 blockers
	Ciprofloxacin
Hematological	Anemia
	Disseminated intravascular coagulation
Metabolic	Dehydration
	Hypercalcemia
	Hyponatremia
	Hypomagnesemia
	Hypoglycemia

include those factors that are associated with a poorer prognosis for achieving good pain control: neuropathic pain, incidental pain, opioid tolerance, somatization, and a history of drug or alcohol abuse. The etiological picture is usually multifactorial with precipitant factors superimposed on a high level of baseline vulnerability. Four major causal categories have been identified: Primary intracranial disease, systemic disease affecting the brain such as metabolic disorders or infection, exogenous agents affecting the brain such as psychoactive medications, and withdrawal from substances of abuse such as alcohol or benzodiazepines. A more extensive list of causative factors is presented in Table 48.2.

Significance and impact

For the patient, delirium can result in much distress, whether associated with perceptual disturbances, paranoid delusions, disorientation, emotional lability, or agitation. For the family, there is the loss of communication at a time when it is often most precious. There is a risk of misinterpreting psychomotor agitation as pain. The family will often advocate in good faith for more analgesia. Physicians and nursing staff are at risk of adopting a reflex response to such requests, and therefore may increase the dose of opioid without conducting a disciplined clinical assessment.

Assessment

A detailed history (especially collateral) and physical examination is required. It is particularly important to inquire about the temporal onset of symptoms (acute or gradual) and the premorbid cognitive status. Physical examination of the cancer patient should include careful assessment of signs of infection, dehydration, myoclonus, asterixis, stigmata of liver disease, and neurological deficit. Baseline laboratory investigations include a complete blood count, electrolytes, creatinine, calcium, albumin, bilirubin, liver enzymes, and urinalysis. These investigations and additional ones such as chest radiology and blood cultures are dictated by the goals of care, which are determined in each individual case following discussion with the patient or more especially family members.

Delirium is frequently either not recognized or misdiagnosed. Failure to objectively assess cognition as a component of delirium, fluctuation in clinical features, and the presence of a lucid interval are commonly cited reasons for missing the diagnosis. The Mini-Mental State Examination (MMSE) is the instrument most commonly used to detect cognitive deficit, and normative data exist for age and educational level. The Confusion Assessment Method (CAM) is also used for screening and diagnosis, in association with a formal test of cognition such as the MMSE. The Memorial Delirium Rating Scale (MDAS), a severity-rating scale for delirium, allows prorating of scores for items on which the patient cannot be assessed.

Approach to management

For the clinician, management challenges and dilemmas can arise regarding a number of issues: the likelihood of an episode being reversible vis-à-vis "terminal" or irreversible; the burden–benefit ratio of specific medical interventions; the assessment of pain and other symptoms during delirium; the presence of concurrent

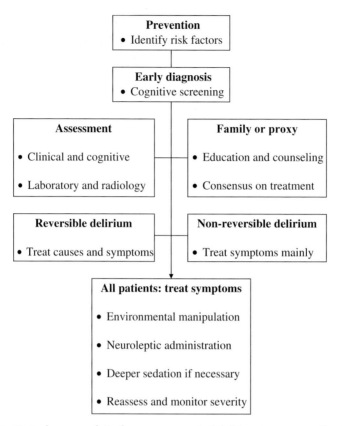

Figure 48.1 Strategic approach to the management of delirium in cancer patients.

medical problems and the patient's potential quality of life; and the prior or currently expressed wishes of the patient and family regarding medical interventions. It is essential to spend time with the family to address their concerns, to educate them regarding the nature of the delirium syndrome, and finally to establish a consensus regarding the goals of care. A management strategy is summarized in Figure 48.1.

The standard approach to treatment involves a search for underlying reversible precipitating factors. Psychoactive medications, especially opioids, benzodiazepines and anticholinergics are among the most common reversible precipitants of delirium. Opioids, especially in high doses, can give rise to a neurotoxic syndrome including delirium, hyperalgesia, allodynia, myoclonus, and even seizures. The standard approach to opioid toxicity involves either switching opioid, thereby facilitating elimination of potentially neurotoxic opioid metabolites, or alternatively, reducing the dose. The treatment of hypercalcemia with bisphosphonates, the treatment of dehydration with administration of fluid by hypodermoclysis, and an opioid switch or dose reduction are examples of relatively low burden interventions that are commonly used in the successful treatment of delirium.

Symptomatic treatment of delirium is essential, irrespective of whether investigation and treatment of reversible causes are pursued. The nonpharmacological component of treatment involves environmental manipulation such as optimizing lighting conditions, arranging for the presence of a relative or in some cases, a special nurse. The mainstay of pharmacological management is neuroleptic treatment. Haloperidol is the drug of first choice, usually given in a dose of 0.5 to 4 mg q 6–8 hourly, using oral, intravenous, subcutaneous, or if necessary, intramuscular routes. Alternatives that are more sedating include loxapine, methotrimeprazine, and chlorpromazine. Newer antipsychotics such as risperidone or olanzapine have fewer extrapyramidal side effects but currently are unavailable in parenteral formulation. Lorazepam has been shown to worsen symptoms of delirium.

Although deeper sedation can increase the risk of aspiration pneumonia, it may be required to control an agitated delirium where attempts at reversal have failed, are not possible, or are incompatible with family wishes. Midazolam, a short-acting benzodiazepine given by continuous subcutaneous infusion, is the agent most commonly used for this purpose. Careful assessment in addition to team and family discussions are essential to avoid the pitfalls of premature sedation or misunderstandings regarding the goals of care.

Box 48.1 Summary – delirium

Delirium is usually associated with a high level of symptom distress.

Death is preceded by an episode of delirium in most patients with cancer.

The reversibility of delirium can be as high as 50% in some settings.

Although delirium is multifactorial in origin, medications are among the most common
   precipitants.

BIBLIOGRAPHY

Sentinel articles

American Psychiatric Association. Practice guideline for the treatment of patients with delirium. *Am J Psychiatry* 1999;156(Suppl.):1–20.

Breitbart W, Marotta R, Platt M et al. A double-blind trial of haloperidol, chlorpromazine, and lorazepam in the treatment of delirium in hospitalized AIDS patients. *Am J Psychiatry* 1996;153:231–7.

Bruera E, Miller L, McCallion J, Macmillan K, Krefting L, Hanson J. Cognitive failure in patients with terminal cancer: a prospective study. *J Pain Symptom Manage* 1992;7:192–5.

Bruera E, Franco JJ, Maltoni M, Watanabe S, Suarez-Almazor M. Changing pattern of agitated impaired mental status in patients with advanced cancer: association with cognitive monitoring, hydration, and opioid rotation. *J Pain Symptom Manage* 1995;10:287–91.

De Stoutz ND, Bruera E, Suarez-Almazor M. Opioid rotation for toxicity reduction in terminal cancer patients. *J Pain Symptom Manage* 1995;10:378–84.

Inouye SK, van Dyck CH, Alessi CA, Balkin S, Siegal AP, Horwitz RI. Clarifying confusion: the confusion assessment method. A new method for detection of delirium. *Ann Intern Med* 1990;113:941–8.

Lawlor PG, Gagnon B, Mancini IL et al. Occurrence, causes, and outcome of delirium in advanced cancer patients: a prospective study. *Arch Intern Med* 2000;160:786–94.

Massie MJ, Holland J, Glass E. Delirium in terminally ill cancer patients. *Am J Psychiatry* 1983;140:1048–50.

Tuma R, DeAngelis LM. Altered mental status in patients with cancer. *Arch Neurol* 2000;57: 1727–31.

Review articles

Lawlor PG, Fainsinger RL, Bruera ED. Delirium at the end of life. *J Am Med Assoc* 2000;284: 2427–9.

Lipowski ZJ. Delirium in the elderly patient. *N Engl J Med* 1989;320:578–82.

Meagher DJ. Delirium: optimising management. *Br Med J* 2001;322:144–9.

Internet site

National Cancer Institute and National Institute of Health, Supportive Care PDQ section. http://www.cancer.gov/cancer_information/coping/

49

Constipation

Florian Strasser

Kantonsspital, St. Gallen, Switzerland

The moment you reach this page half of the job is done: considering the diagnosis of constipation.

How frequent is constipation in patients with advanced cancer? Epidemiology and definition

Several studies have documented the frequency of symptoms in patients with advanced cancer. However, constipation is not a symptom, such as pain or dyspnea, but a diagnosis, such as a fracture causing pain or hypoxemia causing dyspnea, respectively. Therefore only data from institutions assessing and documenting constipation routinely are reliable, but they seldom include all groups of patients with advanced cancer. Even less is known about the frequency of symptomatic constipation, i.e., which has an impact on quality of life, in contrast to asymptomatic constipation. Overall, both asymptomatic and symptomatic constipation are widely underestimated, even in specialized palliative care settings.

The range of the "normal frequency" of bowel movements, i.e., up to three bowel movements per day and more than one bowel movement every third day, illuminates the individual variation. Therefore each patient should be asked about "normal" bowel habits before the actual disease, as well as about meaningful changes both compared with "normal" and with the last few weeks or days. However, in light of the paradox of "overflow" diarrhea, or the case of diminishing stool volumes in the context of dehydration, the number of bowel movements does not reliably predict the presence of symptomatic constipation. A diagnosis of constipation (Table 49.1) has to include stool volume and quality. A "working" definition for constipation with a high sensitivity reads as follows: "A decrease in the number of bowel movements and/or of stool volume and/or of the stool water-content resulting in more difficult defecation and finally retaining hard fecal material in the intestines." However, in clinical practice stool volume is seldom measured routinely, and stool inspection or rectal examination to assess water content is underused.

Table 49.1. Diagnosis and evaluating severity of constipation

Bowels	Changes in bowel habits, irregular bowel movements, difficulty voiding, diarrhea, number of bowel movements in past weeks, bowel sounds
Stool	Volume, quality, rectal and/or colonic localization (inspection, rectal examination, flat x-ray), abdominal examination revealing distension, firmness, tenderness, or palpable fecal masses, impaction proximal (empty rectal vault) or distal (hard impacted feces). Severity estimated by "constipation score" (flat x-ray)
Laxatives	Dose and types of laxatives used in the past weeks, both oral and rectal preparations
Symptoms	Nausea, bloating, tenesmus, pain bowel movements, flatulence, sensation of incomplete evacuation, etc.

A high level of clinical suspicion is called for: do a full bowel assessment in patients with advanced cancer

Atypical symptoms may be present: nausea, abdominal distension, (overflow) diarrhea

The type and dose of the laxatives used during the past week will provide additional information. In patients with cognitive impairment or pediatric patients it is often impossible to obtain a useful history as required.

Since a definition is difficult, an estimation of fecal material retained in the colon using plain abdominal films can be very useful, or even indispensable. For each abdominal quadrant the stool content is ranked from 0–3, resulting in scores from 0–12, as reported by Bruera et al. (1994).

Associated symptoms, such as nausea, bloating or distension, abdominal pain, flatulence, sensation of incomplete evacuation or rectal fullness, anorexia, early satiety, halitosis, etc., are not specific for the diagnosis of constipation, but they can be helpful in monitoring the treatment effects. Sometimes constipation is manifest by nongastrointestinal symptoms such as urinary retention or cognitive failure.

There are no established staging systems for the severity of constipation, such as for pain or depression. Severe constipation turns into "primary" fecal impaction, which is almost always symptomatic with abdominal pain, distension or colic, spasmodic rectal pain, or vomiting, and typically presents with a change in stool quality since overflow diarrhea and fecal leakage or oozing of stool occur. "Secondary" impaction, with softer stool, can occur due to extrinsic or intrinsic blockage of the colon.

Patients with a colostomy may frequently be constipated, since normal bowel habits are bothersome as they are visualized in the bags, and the patient tries to achieve the same stool quality as via naturalis. This may be ameliorated with proper coaching.

What causes constipation? Pathogenesis and causes

Normal bowel function depends on the one hand on a subtle regulated intestinal fluid managment and on the other hand on intestinal integrity including the intestinal motility.

The intestines handle 8–9 liters of secretions and fluids per day, of which three-quarters are absorbed in the small bowels. The colon is able to absorb up to 5 liters per day, but normally only 100 ml fluids are excreted and about 150 ml fluids per day distinguish between diarrhea and constipation. However, increased water absorption has not been identified as an important factor in causing constipation, except when the stool remains for an extended time in the colon. Bile acids, prostaglandins, and bacterial toxins stimulate secretion, whereas short-chain amino acids increase absorption. Gut fluid absorption is an active process with different passive (cotransport of Na^+, glucose, and amino acids) and active (basal Na^+K^+-ATPase, mucosal cyclic-AMP-dependent Cl^- secretion) mechanisms involved in the intestinal epithelium, which are mainly regulated cholinergically and mediated through changes of intracellular calcium. This leads over to the central role of the intestinal neuro-muscular system, since both electrolyte control and muscle function are under neuronal control, particulary via the parasympathetic system. Peristalsis consists of ascending contractions (mediated by acetylcholine) and descending relaxation (mediated by vasoactive intestinal peptide). There are segmental and propulsive movements. Opioid μ-receptors are found mainly in the myenteric plexus and opioid δ-receptors in the submucosal plexus. Endogenous opioids seem to influence bowel function on many levels including increased electrolyte (and therefore water) absorption and reduced peristalsis in the whole intestine, reduction of sensitivity to colon distension, and increase of ileocecal and internal anal sphincter tonus.

Based on this understanding most causes of constipation are obvious and can be structured in four overlapping groups (Table 49.2).

1. Decreased activity (performance status) and advanced age slacken performance of many organs including the intestine. Simply the difficulty of reaching a toilet or lack of privacy can be important factors too.
2. Injured anatomic integrity of the intestine including the anal sphincters; frequent causes are tumors causing internal or external bowel obstruction or anal injuries.
3. Poor nutritional intake results in decreased intestinal fluids, the leading cause by far is dehydration, which is common in patients with decreased activity, advanced age, cognitive impairment, or depression, or is caused by diuretics.
4. Impaired intestinal neuromuscular system, caused by increased endogenous or exogenous (both oral and parenteral) opioids, hypercalcemia or high oral

Table 49.2. (Common) causes of constipation

Causes	Assessment	Management
Immobility/inactivity/age	History	Mobilization, physical therapy
Poor fluid intake/dehydration	History, clinically	Rehydration, alternative of diuretics
Opioids (no tolerance)	History	Proactive prevention, opioid rotation
Other drugs (many)[a]	History, know drugs	Proactive prevention, change drugs
Hypercalcemia or hypokalemia	Lab value	Correct electrolyte imbalance
Neural plexus/spinal cord invasion	Exam, MRI	Prokinetics, agressive managment
Autonomic neuropathy/cachexia	History, exam, EKG	Prokinetics, treat anorexia/cachexia
Tumor compression of bowel	Bowel series	Palliative surgery, stent
Severe depression	Exam, questionnaire	Counseling, antidepressants
Severe pain	Pain assessment	Pain management
Hypothyroidism	TSH, f T4, f T3	Substitute

[a] Anticholinergics, diuretics, NSAIDs, tricyclics, phenothiazines, antihistamines, iron, thalidomide, others.
MRI, magnetic resonance imaging; EKG, electrocardiogram; TSH, thyroid-stimulating hormone.

calcium intake or calcium-channel antagonists (nifedipine, verapamil), hypokalemia, drugs with anticholinergic effects (tricyclic antidepressants, phenothiazines, hyoscine, antiparkinsonian drugs), 5-HT$_3$-antagonists, sympatomimetics (clonidine), iron, autonomic failure (a paraneoplastic syndrome overlapping with the cancer cachexia syndrome), neuropathy (neurotoxic drugs, diabetes mellitus, paraneoplastic pseudo-obstruction), nerve damage (lumbosacral spinal cord, caudae equina, pelvic plexus), abdominal tumor involvment in absence of bowel obstruction, and hypothyroidism.

Many drugs which cause constipation have effects both on the mucosal fluid balance and the neuronal intestinal control.

Assessment/monitoring

The crucial step is to perform a continuous assessment towards a diagnosis of constipation or identification of patients at risk (see above). After constipation has been diagnosed the assessment relies on the different causes (Table 49.2) and laxative treatment. Monitoring treatment is based on the items used for diagnosis and auxilliary both on the daily laxative dose and symptom measurement by visual analog scales. However, there is no established instrument available to measure constipation, and a score can be misleading since the number of bowel movements can be normal in paradox diarrhea. It has to be kept in mind, that the expression of constipation by the patient is, as with any other symptom (well known for "total" pain), modulated by other symptoms, and psychosocial and spiritual distress.

Management

If it is possible to treat the underlying cause, do it first. However, since in most patients with advanced cancer constipation is a multifactorial problem induced by causes unlikely to be reversible, management of constipation is an ongoing process of assessment and treatment, with emphasis on a multiprofessional team.

Since many new drugs come on the market, it is necessary in any patient with advanced cancer to have a good understanding of the actual pharmacological treatment: justification of the actual indication, typical side effects, metabolism including excretion, influence on liver metabolism and renal function, and pharmacological interactions. So the side effect constipation will not be missed.

Constipation is an inevitable side effect of any opioid therapy, both oral and parenteral, with no development of tolerance, in contrast to tolerance to opioid-induced nausea after a few days of dose adjustments. Increasing doses of opioids correlate weakly with more severe constipation and/or higher laxative doses. Typically, constipation occurs on a lower dose than analgesia is achieved. Methadone or fentanyl are probably associated with less constipation than other opioids, but there is still a lack of good evidence from prospective double-blind controlled trials. Intrathecal opioids probably cause less constipation, however, the indication of neuraxial analgesia remains to be established in advanced cancer patients.

Patients with advanced cancer will generally need laxatives. Despite optimized management an oral-only laxative regimen can be achieved in two-thirds of patients, the other one-third will need rectal laxatives too. Patients with advanced cancer are often at risk for both constipation and dehydration, therefore bulk-forming drugs (fiber) are rarely used, since the risk of impaction is higher. The other laxatives are lubricants (liquid paraffin, mineral oil), salines (Mg, Na-phosphate, Na-sulfate), osmotic agents (lactulose, sorbitol (30–70%), mannitol), and contact laxatives (docusate, ricinoleic acid, bile salt; polyphenolics (phenolphthalein, bisacodyl, Na-picosulfate), synthetic (danthrone) and natural anthracenes (senna, cascara, casanthranol). Many other over-the-counter substances are in use.

For the choice of laxatives several pharmacological features have to be considered. The latency period from drug administration until the bowel movement, the intensity of its effects as well as typical adverse effects need to be known (Table 49.3). A common approach for mild and moderate constipation, as well as for prophylaxis, is a combination of two laxatives with stool softening (docusate, osmotic agents) as well as peristaltic stimulatory effects (anthracenes), and the titrating up (and down) of the individual doses. Osmotic laxatives often are associated with bloating. Salines usually have a cathartic effect and can deteriorate bowel obstruction. Lubricants are used for a limited time in bowel impaction (Table 49.4).

Table 49.3. Treatment of constipation

Treat cause, if possible

Start with a combination of a peristaltic stimulant and stool softener

Titrate towards effect, there are (almost) no upper limits for the most common laxatives

Add osmotic laxatives: lactulose or sorbitol every 4–6 hours, until bowel movement, but avoid long-term use
  (fluid and electrolyte imbalances)

Treat rectal with bisacodyl suppository (needs contact to the rectal mucosa), use enemas (fleet enema,
  milk-and-molasses)

Follow "rescue" enemas, required after no bowel movement for 3 days, with an increase in oral laxatives

Distal fecal impaction (digital exam) may require digital disimpaction and oil-retention enema

Proximal fecal impaction (flat x-ray) may require magnesium citrate and oral lubricants (mineral oil)

Reconsider treating cause, may rotate opioids (consider methadone, fentanyl), may use alternative analgesics,
  may use naloxone, may change other drugs

Nonpharmacological measures can add substantially to good bowel movements and consist of good location (intimacy, comfort), timing (patience, rhythm), optimal mobility and activity, as well as good hydration.

Since recommendations vary widely between different institutions, an understanding of the general principles is of more value than following strict guidelines.

Preventing is better than treating: when and how? Prophylaxis

Prevention of constipation begins as soon as a decrease in normal bowel movements is observed, or a well-known cause associated with constipation (such as spinal cord compression, opioid therapy) occurs. Any mild laxative, usually a stool softener, contact laxative, or a mild osmotic laxative is used.

It is important to explain to the patient and family the various reasons for constipation, and discuss general measures used to mitigate it. They include encouragement of adequate fluid intake, activity, avoidance of excess dietary fiber (although fruit fiber may be beneficial), compliant use of laxatives and titration of bowel regimen to effect.

What happens if? Complications

Several complications of constipation are not obvious, but impede quality of life. Severe constipation can lead to bowel obstruction or pseudo-obstruction (Ogilvie's syndrome), urinary retention, cognitive failure, dehydration, anorexia, nausea and vomiting, abdominal pain, overflow diarrhea, hemorrhoids, or anal fissures. Many of these complications are often misinterpreted in a simplistic way as normal sequelae of advanced cancer and therefore correspondingly managed,

Table 49.4. Pharmacological agents for constipation: more than "laxatives"

Bulk-forming agents

Cellulose, psyllium seed, bran

    Increase mass and water content of stool, intraluminal fluid increased after gut microflora breakdown

    Change character of effluent from a functioning stoma?

    Worsen obstruction

Lubricants

Liquid paraffin, mineral oil

    Impair absorption of fat-soluble vitamins, irritation of perianal area, risk of lipoid pneumonia when
        aspiration occurs

    Short-term use for fecal impaction

Osmotic saline cathartics

Mg-hydroxide, Mg-citrate; Na-phosphate, Na-sulfate

    Mg: most potent, sulfate more potent than phosphate

    Increase intestinal water secretion, directly stimulate peristalsis

    Rapid onset effect throughout the gut, not only in the colon

    Systemic electrolyte accumulation and volume overload; severe cramping, bloating, dehydration, bowel
        perforation; phosphates may cause hypocalcemia

Osmotic poorly absorbed sugars

Lactulose, sorbitol (30–70%), mannitol. Sorbitol cheaper than lactulose, as effective

    Bacterial degradation in colon, no effect in small intestine, slow onset of effect

    Short-chain organic acids lower intestinal pH and stimulate peristalsis, increase stool bulk by microbial
    mass

    Flatulence 20%, sweet taste, tolerance to change in bacterial flora

Polyethylene glycol

Hyperosmolar laxative, small quantities can be useful (25–500 ml)

Contact laxatives

Increase mucosal secretion and peristalsis; probably development of tolerance

Docusate

    Detergent or surfactant effect allow water and fat to mix with feces, stool softener

Castor oil

    Hydrolyzed by gut microflora to ricinoleic acid

    Abundant mucosal secretions in the small bowel, cramping and diarrhea, malabsorption

Diphenylmethane derivates or polyphenolics

    Phenolphthalein, bisacodyl, Na-picosulfate

    Effect mainly in the colon, slow onset (12–24 hours)

    Abdominal cramps, hypokalemia, allergies

Synthetic (danthrone) or natural anthracenes/anthraquinone derivates

    Senna, cascara, casanthranol. Senna in form of glycosides, have to be converted to active aglycone form by
        colonic bacteria

continued

Table 49.4. (*cont.*)

Directly stimulate myenteric plexus, inhibition of NaK-ATPase, stimulation of cyclic AMP, mucosal electrolyte transport and motility

Effect mainly in the colon, slow onset (12–24 hours)

Pink urine can occur

Prokinetics

Cisapride

Substituted benzamine, related to metoclopramide, has no dopamine-blocking activity, and no anti-emetic effects. It is a 5-HT$_4$ agonist, and 5-HT$_3$ antagonist. Seems to increase endorphine, motiline, PP, but decrease CCK, Substance-P

Stimulates motility also in lower gastrointestinal tract. Clinical trials show effect in constipation

Used infrequently, since cardiac side effects

Metoclopramide

Dopamine antagonist in both central and peripheral levels, in addition it is a cholinergic 5-HT$_4$ agonist and weak antagonist for 5-HT$_3$

Increase tone and strength of gastroduodenal contractions. Less prokinetic in jejunum, ileum, and colon. No stimulation of gastric, pancreatic, enteric, biliary secretions

Combined action chemoreceptor-trigger zone and intestinal motility

Can cause drowsiness, lassitude, anxiety, extrapyramidal side effects (EPS)

Careful in combination with tricyclics and EPS phenothiazines

Domperidone

Peripherally acting dopamine-2 receptor antagonist, which does not cross blood–brain barrier

Effect limited to stomach

Can cause dry skin, rash, itch, diarrhea

Macrolid antibiotics, erythromycin

Mimic effect of motilin, improve gastrointestinal motility in colonic pseudo-obstruction

Enemas and suppositories

Short latency of action

Stimulation of anocolonic reflex

Phospha soda

Sodium phosphate suppository/sodium phosphate or citrate enema

Releases bound water from feces, may stimulate peristalsis in lower bowel (rectal or colonic)

May cause hypocalcemia, hyperphosphatemia

Oil retention

Arachis oil, olive oil

Softens hard, impacted stool

Glycerin suppository

Softens stool by osmosis, as well as a lubricant. Can cause mechanic stimulation

Sorbitol enema

Sodium docusate, sodium lauryl sulfoacetate, sodiulm alkyl sulfacetate

Used as microenemas, promotes water influx in rectum and penetration of hard stool

Table 49.4. (*cont.*)

Milk and molasses
   Stimulates lower bowel, sugar is an irritant, can produce gas, which distends bowel
Tap water
   Induces peristalis
Soap suds
   Stimulates lower bowel, promotes evacuation
Saline
   Stimulates lower bowel, promotes evacuation
   Rectal lavage 8 liters warm water
Harris flush (up and down)
   Promotes expulsion of flatus postoperatively
Polyphenol
   Bisacodyl suppository
   Induces colonic peristalis after 15–60 min. Bisacodyl is superior to glycerine

Opioid antagonist
Naloxone, or methylnaltrexate
   Modulate excitatory and inhibitory neurotransmission
   Act both on cholinergic and nonadrenergic/noncholinergic neurons
   Accelerate colon transit without increasing the number of bowel movements

Octreotide
Inhibit release and activity of gastrointestinal hormones
Reduce gastric acid secretion, decrease bile flow, increase mucus production, reduce splanchnic blood flow.
   Increase enteric action potentials and frequency of migrating myoelectric complexes
Increase amplitude of lower esophageal sphincter tone, enhance speed of esophageal contractions
Stimulate motility in rectosigmoid
Good tolerability, expensive

by insertion of a Foley catheter (impeding autonomy and comfort), treatment with benzodiazepines for agitated delirium, opioids for abdominal cramps, or 5-HT$_3$ antagonists for nausea/vomiting, among others.

Another common mistake is to believe that constipation is being adequately managed since a relevant amount of different laxatives per mouth and rectal are applied, rendering constipation as a cause of the above-mentioned complications unlikely. A careful continuing assessment and suspicion remains crucial.

Future directions

Since the problem of constipation is underestimated in patients with advanced cancer, an important area of future research is to establish the symptomatic and pharmacoeconomic price of neglecting it.

Table 49.5. A practical approach to constipation

Monitoring	Assessment and action
High level of suspicion	Consider constipation (almost) always: "progressive disease," cognitive impairment (delirium), loss of bladder function (urinary retention), decrease in performance status, diarrhea, bowel obstruction, etc.
	High risk: opioid-treatment, immobility, inadequate fluid intake, peritoneal carcinomatosis, colostomy
Do a good assessment	Is the stool soft/hard? Is the rectum full? Is there an impaction?
	Are the bowels moving (paralytic ileus? obstruction?)?
	Symptomatic manifestation? Impact on function, socialization?
Standard treatment	Give laxatives around-the-clock, titrate them up, use (for) breakthrough, use a combination of a mild contact-laxans and stool-softener
Is the rectum full?	Use a local contact-laxans (bisacodyl-supp) and a mild enema
Is the colon full?	Hydrate. Titrate laxatives up. Combine with osmotic laxatives. For hard stool use for a few days mineral oil p.o.
Is there an impaction?	Manual impaction, if hard stool mineral oil retention enemas, then mild enemas, soap enemas only short time
Prevention	Prevention not emergencies: do laxative orders "on hold, if," not "prn." Educate patient/caregivers. Hydrate. Toilet habits and comfort, privacy

The diagnosis of constipation needs to be improved, mainly by a better awareness and understanding of continuous symptom assessment. There is not a lack of a "good" assessment instrument, rather than the need for a persuasive use of established, simple, guidelines (Table 49.1).

The growing understanding of the neurohormonal enteral regulation, involving substance P, neurokinins, tachykinins, 5-HT$_4$ receptors, among others, will lead to the development of new laxatives. 5-HT$_4$ agonists, such as prucalopride, are under evaluation in human phase II/(III) trials, involving patients with chronic opioid-associated constipation. The value of NK1-receptor antagonists remains to be established.

The oral administration of opioid-antagonists can alleviate constipation, but the therapeutic window towards opioid-withdrawal is very narrow. Methyl-naltrexone is the first quaternary ammonium opioid-receptor antagonist, that does not cross the blood–brain barrier in humans. Preliminary human data with intravenous as well as oral methyl-naltrexone suggest a dose-dependent increase in the numbers of bowel movements with a good volume and decrease of the oral–cecal transit time, with mild side effects of abdominal cramping.

In addition to new (and probably expensive) drugs, traditionally used remedies, such as "Fresh Baker's yeast" merit systematic evaluation.

Summary

Constipation is often under-recognized or misunderstood as a symptom. It requires a practical approach on all levels of prevention, assessment, and multimodal treatment (Table 49.5).

The moment you leave this page the challenge continues: prevent, assess, treat multimodally

Acknowledgement

Florian Strasser is supported by a grant from Swiss Cancer Research (BIL grant KFS 950-09-1999).

BIBLIOGRAPHY

Sentinel articles

Bruera E, Suarez-Almazor M, Velasco A, Bertolino M, MacDonald SM, Hanson J. The assessment of constipation in terminal cancer patients admitted to a palliative care unit: a retrospective review. *J Pain Symptom Manage* 1994;9:515–19.

Yuan CS, Foss JF, O'Connor M et al. Methylnaltrexone for reversal of constipation due to chronic methadone use: a randomized controlled trial. *J Am Med Assoc* 2000;283:367–72.

Review articles

Derby S, Portenoy R. Assessment and managment of opioid-induced constipation. In *Topics in Palliative Care*, Vol. 1, ed. R Portenoy, E Bruera, pp. 95–112. Oxford: Oxford University Press, 1997.

Mancini I, Bruera E. Constipation in advanced cancer patients. *Support Care Cancer* 1998;6:356–64.

Ripamonti C, Rodriguez C. Gastrointestinal motility disorders in patients with advanced cancer. In *Topics in Palliative Care*, Vol. 1, ed. R Portenoy, E Bruera, pp. 61–94. Oxford: Oxford University Press, 1997.

Sykes N. Constipation and diarrhea. In *Oxford Textbook of Palliative Medicine*, 2nd edn, ed. D Doyle, G Hanks, N MacDonald, pp. 513–26. Oxford: Oxford University Press, 1998.

Internet sites

A wonderful site about the symptom constipation and research. But more than research, it is helpful for practical tips too.

http://www.symptomresearch.org/chapter_3/index.htm

A comprehensive site about palliative care, with practical tips for assessing and managing constipation.

http://www.palliative.org/PC/ClinicalInfo/PCareTips/ConstipationInTheCancerPatient.html

50

Palliation of fever and sweats: the heat is on!

Donna S. Zhukovsky

U.T. M.D. Anderson Cancer Center, Houston

Introduction

Almost all have experienced fever and the associated chills and sweats. Sweating also occurs independently of fever in various disease states, in normal situations like exercise and in common nondisease states such as menopause. Like other symptoms in advanced cancer, fever and sweats may be multifactorial, with different etiologies predominating at different points in the disease trajectory. Optimal management is predicated on an understanding of the contributing causes and pathophysiologic mechanisms, as well as knowledge of patient goals relative to the disease course.

Fever

Pathophysiology

In normal individuals, core body temperature is maintained within a tightly controlled range by a dynamic balance of heat production, heat conservation, and heat loss. There are three phases of fever. In the initiation phase, endogenous or exogenous pyrogens elevate the thermoregulatory set point above normal. Cutaneous vasoconstriction promotes heat retention and shivering produces additional heat. Behaviorally, the individual feels cold and seeks warmer clothing. When steady state fever is achieved, heat production balances heat loss and shivering ceases. During defervesence, the set point decreases to the normal core temperature and heat loss prevails. Heat loss occurs as a consequence of cutaneous vasodilation and sweating, with radiant and evaporative heat loss to the environment, respectively. There is a paucity of data describing the symptom complex associated with fever in the cancer patient.

Definition

Most oncologists consider a temperature in excess of 38.5 °C or 38 °C on three occasions at least 1 hour apart as clinically significant. The classic definition of

Table 50.1. Causes of fever in cancer patients

Infection

Tumor

Drugs

   Cytotoxic, BRMs, amphotericin, other

Drug withdrawal

   Opioids, benzodiazepines

Obstruction of a hollow viscus

Blood product transfusion

Tumor embolization (i.e., hepatic)

Graft versus host disease

Other medical comorbidities

   Thrombosis, connective tissue disorders, CNS bleed/stroke

Note: BRM, biologic response modifiers; CNS, central nervous system.

fever of unknown origin (FUO) includes an illness of more than 3 weeks' duration, fever higher than 101 °F (38.3 °C) on several occasions and uncertain diagnosis after 1 week's investigation in hospital.

Prevalence

Cancer as a cause of FUO occurs in 7–19% of cancer patients. Many authors have evaluated fever in patients with cancer diagnoses. Infection as a cause of fever occurs in less than 15–57% of cancer patients and paraneoplastic fever ranges from 5–56%. The wide variation in fever frequency and its causes likely relates to differences in definition of fever, the population studied, primary tumor site, and medical advances over the period studied. Paraneoplastic fever is considered to be more common in malignancies such as renal cell cancer or lymphomas, but available data suggest that it occurs in diverse primaries.

Etiology

Causes of fever are numerous (Table 50.1). The differentiation of infection from other causes of fever may be difficult. From a palliative perspective, differentiation is important, as the specific fever diagnosis impacts management, comfort, and prognosis. This is especially true in neutropenic fever, which is associated with a high risk of medical complications and death.

Treatment interventions
Primary interventions

Treatment of fever consists of therapy directed at the underlying cause, combined with nonspecific therapies to lower fever. For patients with infections, antibiotics palliate by controlling fever and associated constitutional symptoms, as well as site-specific symptoms (i.e., cough, pain related to abscess formation). Febrile neutropenia requires urgent broad-spectrum antibiotic treatment to minimize associated morbidity and mortality. Antibiotic use is guided by knowledge of the treating institution's antimicrobial spectrum and antibiotic resistance pattern. Further treatment is guided by individual patient risk factors (i.e., presence of a central line, prior use of steroids, history of injection drug use) and response to initial treatment. Models predicting risk groups of febrile neutropenia have been developed, with implications for management. The reader is directed to specialized sources for specific management recommendations.

Response to antineoplastic therapy results in control of paraneoplastic fever. Drug-associated fever responds to discontinuation of the offending agent, if possible. Drug fever is often a diagnosis of exclusion, although its occurrence is predictable with many cytotoxic agents and biologic response modifiers (BRMs). Fever due to BRM administration is type, dose, route, and schedule dependent. These parameters may sometimes be modified for fever control without sacrificing antineoplastic efficacy. Similar findings are noted with fever related to some cytotoxic chemotherapy and to antimicrobials (i.e., amphotericin). Premedication with acetaminophen, nonsteroidal anti-inflammatories (NSAIDs) and steroids is often of benefit. Amphotericin-associated chills may be diminished by slowing the rate of infusion and by premedication with meperidine. The frequency of fever with blood product transfusion is diminished by use of leukocyte-depleted products.

Nonspecific interventions

Palliative fever control measures combine antipyretic administration with physical methods. Acetaminophen and non-aspirin NSAIDs have largely replaced the use of aspirin for fever control in children due to the risk of Reye's syndrome with aspirin use. Naproxen and indometacin may preferentially control paraneoplastic fever relative to other NSAIDs or acetaminophen. Response to an adequate dose of naproxen has been proposed as diagnostic of tumor fever. However, efficacy of naproxen and other NSAIDs for infection-related fever is a common clinical observation. When tumor fever controlled by NSAID use relapses, rotation to an NSAID with a different chemical structure can yield additional fever control.

Sponging with various solutions lowers fever. Sponging combined with acetaminophen results in more rapid fever control than use of either modality alone. In a placebo-controlled, randomized trial, ratings of comfort were greatest in patients receiving either placebo or sponging alone, followed by those that received acetaminophen combined with tepid water sponging. Acetaminophen combined with ice water or isopropyl alcohol sponging resulted in the best fever control, but the most discomfort. These results bear further study, as they have implications for comfort in the management of fever. Carefully designed studies evaluating the impact of pharmacotherapy, sponging, and other interventions on symptoms associated with fever in cancer patients are indicated.

Sweats

Definition

Sweating is a form of body temperature regulation that results in evaporative heat loss via the skin. It is associated with fever, and occurs with exercise, warm environments, and the hormonal changes of menopause. Sweating is part of the hot flash symptom complex that accompanies the vasomotor instability of menopause. Qualitative definitions of hot flashes consist of somatic, behavioral, emotional, and temporal components. As hot flash severity increases from mild to very severe, the sensation of increased heat and associated diaphoresis intensifies and becomes more generalized; emotional perceptions including anxiety and embarrassment become more prominent, symptoms last longer and the individual feels a greater need to modify behavior by actions such as fanning, uncovering, and opening windows.

Prevalence

Limited data suggest that sweating occurs in approximately 14–16% of cancer patients receiving palliative care and is frequently nocturnal. Severity is typically moderate or severe. In 1635 cancer patients referred to an anesthesiology-based pain service, sweating was reported by 28%. Tumor stage was III or IV in 72% of the 1244 patients for whom stage was available. Sweating occurred in 40% of a convenience sample of 25 patients receiving treatment for prostate cancer at a comprehensive cancer center.

Hot flashes occur in approximately 65% of postmenopausal women with a breast cancer history, include night sweats in 44% and are typically moderate to very severe in intensity. There are no comparable data available for women with metastatic breast cancer. Approximately 75% of men with locally advanced or metastatic prostate cancer treated with bilateral orchiectomy report hot flashes. Intensity is moderate to severe in 76%.

Etiology

Sweats in the cancer patient may be associated with the tumor, its treatment, or unrelated disorders, including primary disorders of sweating. A major distinction exists between sweats associated with fever and those that occur independently. The latter are often hormonally mediated (Table 50.2). In postmenopausal women with a history of breast cancer, a high-school education or less, younger age at diagnosis and tamoxifen use have been associated with the presence of hot flashes. Predictors

Table 50.2. Causes of sweats in cancer patients

Fever
Menopause (female)[a]
Natural
Surgical
Chemical
Cytotoxic
Radiation
Androgens
Castration (male)[a]
Orchiectomy
Gonadotropin-releasing hormones
Estrogens
Drugs
Tamoxifen (females)
Opioids
Tricyclic antidepressants
Steroids
Neuroendocrine tumors[a]
Carcinoid
Hypothalamic disturbances
Idiopathic[a]

[a] Hot flashes may accompany sweats.

of hot flash severity include higher body mass index, younger age at diagnosis, and tamoxifen use. Unlike for other postmenopausal women, hot flash prevalence does not decrease with time in breast cancer survivors.

Treatment interventions

Sweats

Treatment directed at the underlying cause, when possible, combined with palliative (nonspecific) management interventions forms the basis of the treatment plan. Notwithstanding, since sweats are associated with defervescence and not steady-state fever, more needs to be known about its epidemiology to improve nonspecific management techniques of fever-associated sweats. Low dose thioridazine has been used for the management of sweats in advanced cancer, but is no longer recommended in view of a recent drug warning circulated by the US Food and Drug Administration reporting an association with torsade de pointes type of arrhythmias and sudden death. Clinical experience suggests a role for the H_2 blocker cimetidine in the management of malignancy-associated sweating. Recent reports suggest that low dose

Table 50.3. Pharmacologic treatment interventions for hot flushes in cancer patients

Estrogens
Systemic
Topical
Androgens
Cyproterone acetate
Progestational agents
Megesterol acetate
SSRIs
Alpha adrenergic agonists
Methyl dopa
Transdermal clonidine
Beta blockers
Propranolol
Veralipride (antidopaminergic)
Vitamin E

thalidomide may play a role in the management of sweats associated with terminal malignancy. Somatostatin analogs are a primary treatment for flushing and sweats associated with some neuroendocrine tumors. Given the vascular actions of 5-HT, these agents may have a role to play in nonspecific sweat management. Further study of these agents and others is warranted.

Hot flashes

Estrogen replacement is well documented as efficacious for the management of hot flashes in postmenopausal women. However, many women have relative or absolute contraindications to estrogen replacement therapy. Other agents with reported efficacy are noted in Table 50.3. Inferior efficacy and associated side effects limit use of many of these agents.

A series of double-blind, placebo-controlled studies have been carried out in women with a history of breast cancer and men with prostate cancer who have undergone androgen-deprivation therapy and experience distressing hot flashes. Low-dose megesterol acetate use (20 mg by mouth twice daily) is the most effective agent in diminishing hot flash frequency and intensity in both men and women, decreasing both hot flash frequency and intensity in 79%. In women receiving concomitant tamoxifen therapy, an initial flare of hot flash activity occurs during the first few days. Maximal efficacy was achieved after 2–3 weeks of treatment. Of study participants, 45% continued to use megesterol acetate over the ensuing

3 years with benefit. Those that discontinued use cited reported lack of efficacy in 23%, resolution of hot flashes in 16% and side effects in 48% as the reason. It is uncertain what effect low-dose progestational agents have on breast cancer pathophysiology or on the outcome of tamoxifen treatment. Similar concerns exist with the use of soy phytoestrogens, weak estrogen-like substances found in soybean that demonstrate a mixture of estrogen agonist and/or antagonist effects. However, they have no demonstrated efficacy in the alleviation of hot flashes.

Recent studies of selective serotonin reuptake inhibitor antidepressants (SSRIs) suggest activity in the treatment of hot flashes in breast cancer survivors, and men treated with androgen deprivation. Response for venlafaxine is dose-related, and plateaus at a daily dose of 75 mg. Frequency of some side effects (dry mouth, decreased appetite, nausea, and constipation) is also dose related. Responses occur within days rather than the weeks associated with response to megesterol acetate. As clinically significant responses occur at low doses, the investigators suggest starting at 37.5 mg per day and increasing to 75 mg per day at 1 week, if necessary. Minimal to modest efficacy has been noted for vitamin E and transdermal clonidine, respectively, in hot flash management.

Many affected breast cancer survivors use or are interested in learning more about a variety of complementary and alternative interventions for palliation. Relaxation response training in healthy, postmenopausal women is associated with decreased hot flash intensity, anxiety, and depression. Further evaluation of behavioral methods as a primary or adjunctive modality for management of hot flashes in the cancer population may prove beneficial. Benefits of these techniques may generalize to other symptoms.

Clinical decision making in the management of fever and sweats

The differential diagnosis of fever and sweats is extensive. Relatively little is known about symptom epidemiology, and contributing pathophysiologies in advanced cancer patients. Further work is needed to develop improved management strategies.

Despite current limitations, much can be gained from careful history taking and physical examination. Information thus gained is used to develop a plan for diagnostic evaluation. Which tests are performed and treatment interventions utilized ultimately depend on where the patient is in the disease spectrum, his/her personal goals of care and quality-of-life factors. Quality-of-life factors include symptom burden, potential diagnostic interventions, and treatment modalities. For example, investigation of neutropenic fever with daily blood counts, frequent blood cultures and diagnostic imaging may be consistent with goals of care in a patient newly diagnosed with acute leukemia. In the patient with progressive disease, the value of repeated phlebotomies and hospitalization for empirical antibiotic treatment must be weighed against the value of avoiding the associated discomfort and remaining at home. For some individuals, improved quality of life supersedes potential survival benefits. The relative value of competing therapeutic goals (quantity versus quality) varies throughout the disease trajectory and is perceived differently by each patient. Optimal management, therefore, is contingent on medical expertise in the setting of good physician–patient communication.

BIBLIOGRAPHY

Sentinel articles

Boggs DR, Frei E. Clinical studies of fever and infection in cancer. *Cancer* 1960;13:1240–53.

Briggs LH. The occurrence of fever in malignant disease. *Am J Med Sci* 1923;166:846–53.

Klastersky J, Weerts D, Hensgens C, Debusscher L. Fever of unexplained origin in patients with cancer. *Eur J Cancer* 1973;9:649–56.

Loprinzi CL, Michalak JC, Quella SK et al. Megestrol acetate for the prevention of hot flashes. *N Engl J Med* 1994;331:347–52.

Loprinzi CL, Kugler JW, Sloan JA et al. Venlafaxine in management of hot flashes in survivors of breast cancer: a randomised controlled trial. *Lancet* 2000;356:2059–63.

Quigley CS, Baines M. Descriptive epidemiology of sweating in a hospice population. *J Palliat Care* 1997;13:22–6.

Steele RW, Tanaka PT, Lara RP, Bass JW. Evaluation of sponging and of oral antipyretic therapy to reduce fever. *J Pediatr* 1970;77:824–9.

Tsavaris N, Zinelis A, Karabelis A et al. A randomized trial of the effect of three non-steroid anti-inflammatory agents in ameliorating cancer-induced fever. *J Intern Med* 1990;228: 451–5.

Review articles

Boulant JA. Thermoregulation. In *Fever: Basic Mechanisms and Management*, ed. P Mackowiak, pp. 1–22. New York: Raven Press, 1991.

Clark WG. Antipyretics. In *Fever: Basic Mechanics and Management*, ed. P Mackowiak, pp. 297–340. New York: Raven Press, 1991.

Cleary JF. Fever and sweats: including the immunocompromised hosts. In *Principles and Practice of Supportive Oncology*, ed. A Berger, RK Portenoy, DE Weissman, pp. 119–31. Philadelphia: Lippincott-Raven, 1998.

Quesada JR, Talpaz M, Rios A, Kurzrock R, Gutterman JU. Clinical toxicity of interferons in cancer patients: a review. *J Clin Oncol* 1986;4:234–43.

Internet site

http://www.cancer.gov/cancerinfo/pdq/supportivecare/fever

51

Bleeding in advanced cancer patients

Isabelle Mancini and J. J. Body

Institut Jules Bordet, Université Libre de Bruxelles, Brussels

Bleeding is a common presenting problem at the time of initial diagnosis in several types of cancers. It is less frequent in the palliative care setting and has been estimated to affect 6–10% of patients. Although they are less frequent, these bleeding events can be frightening and dramatic for the patients, their families, and healthcare professionals, especially if the hemorrhaging is massive.

Clinical approach

In the palliative care setting, management of bleeding requires consideration of many factors. The clinician has not only to consider the underlying cause, the clinical presentation, and the severity of the event, but he also needs to take into account other salient factors such as the setting of care, the availability of various resources, the overall disease burden, the life expectancy, the patient's overall quality of life, and the wishes of the patient and family.

Malignancies involving the upper and lower gastrointestinal tracts, lungs, kidneys, bladder, and female genital tract can produce massive bleeds that present as hematemesis, hematochezia, melena, hemoptysis, hematuria, and vaginal bleeding, respectively.

These hemorrhages can result in catastrophic events that may cause hypovolemic shock and are immmediately life threatening. They can also give rise to chronic, low-volume bleeding or occasional hemorrhages of low to medium intensity.

Systemic disorders such as coagulation and platelet abnormalities, and disseminated intravascular coagulation may cause hemorrhages or increase their risk. Clotting and fibrinolysis abnormalities are thus detectable in up to 50% of palliative care patients.

General measures

The first step when approaching the problem of hemorrhaging in patients with advanced cancer is to identify those patients who are at increased risk of massive external bleeding. Risk factors include large, fungating head and neck or lung tumors that are close to large blood vessels; recurrent episodes of mild hemoptysis, hematemesis, or hematuria; and large intra-abdominal tumors. Patients with liver failure, bone marrow suppression, or hematological diseases may also be at increased risk.

The next step in the management of patients at increased risk of significant bleeding is to inform caring family members. Given the potentially distressing nature of the topic, great sensitivity is required when discussing the risk with the patient or the family. Dark towels and dark-colored bassinets need to be at hand to make the blood loss less evident than it would be with white or light-colored utensils and bed sheets. The availability of a sedating drug such as midazolam, that can be administered rapidly and acts quickly, may be useful under these circumstances.

Local interventions

Local measures include local packing and wound dressing. Packing can be used with or without pressure to assure hemostasis, particularly in the case of bleeding from organs such as the rectum, nose, or vagina. In some cases, surgical swabs can be coated with various chemicals to facilitate hemostasis. Some hemostatic dressings, such as the compressed pack form of purified gelatin solution (Gelfoam®) or mesh impregnated with bovine collagen (Colagen®) or thromboplastin (Thrombostat®) are useful in managing oozing blood from capillaries and small venules in accessible sites.

The palliative role of radiotherapy in controlling bleeding, particularly of lung, vaginal, bladder, or rectal origin, has been well documented and should always be considered early.

Endoscopic techniques may be considered in selected cases, particularly in upper gastrointestinal and bladder-related bleeding and, to a lesser extent, in bleeding from the lower gastrointestinal tract and the lungs.

Transcatheter arterial embolization is a well-recognized radiological technique that has been used for many years. Embolization has been successfully used in the management of hemorrhaging due to head and neck tumors, pelvic malignancies, and lung cancers. Limiting factors include the availability of radiologists with the appropriate expertise and skills and the presence of a systemic bleeding disorder.

Systemic interventions

Systemic measures include the use of vitamin K, somatostatin analogues, antifibrinolytic agents, and transfusion of blood products.

Vitamin K is necessary for hepatic production of several clotting factors, including factors II, VII, IX, and X. Metastatic liver involvement can lead to deficiencies in the above-mentioned clotting factors. Often other signs of liver involvement, such as jaundice or encephalopathy, are present. Coagulation screening studies will reveal prolonged prothrombin time (PT) and partial thromboplastin time (PTT), with normal thrombin time (TT), fibrinogen, and fibrin–fibrinogen degradation products (FDP). Parenteral administration (intravenous or subcutaneous) of 5–10 mg vitamin K once or twice a week could potentially prevent some hemorrhagic complications.

Octreotide, an analogue of somatostatin, can play a role in the systemic management of upper gastrointestinal bleeds. However, most of the data related to its use in bleeding problems come from noncancer patients and one can only speculate on its possible role in palliative care. The benefit of somatostatin probably derives from its effect on mesenteric blood flow and pressure, and possibly its concomitant cytoprotective effects and suppression of gastric secretion. A starting dose of 50–100 μg twice daily is generally recommended. The dose should be increased according to the clinical response but seldom needs to exceed 600 μg/day.

Tranexamic acid (TA) and aminocaproic acid are synthetic antifibrinolytic agents that act by blocking the lysine binding sites of plasminogen, thereby inhibiting the conversion of plasminogen into plasmin by tissue plasminogen activator. The end result is a decreased lysis of fibrin clots. Various therapeutic schemes have been used and we suggest an intravenous dose of 10 mg/kg three or four times a day.

In advanced cancer patients, platelet transfusions should be considered only when symptoms such as mucosal bleeding or epistaxis are distressing, or when the patient suffers from painful hematomas or continuous bleeding through the gastrointestinal, gynecological, or urinary systems.

The use of packed red cell transfusions has to be limited to the patients with chronic bleeding resulting in symptomatic anemia. In palliative care, its use for resuscitation of patients in hypovolemic shock is generally not appropriate.

Conclusions

Bleeding, although relatively uncommon in patients with advanced cancer, is stressful for both patients and caregivers. These episodes require an individualized approach based on the specific needs of the patient and family, including the level of distress, the stage of disease, and the available expertise. A multidisciplinary approach using various treatment modalities may be required. Treatments range from simple hemostatic techniques to more invasive endoscopic and embolization techniques. Minimal management requires identification of the patients at risk of massive hemorrhage and to take appropriate preparatory measures to empower caregivers to deal appropriately with the situation if and when it arises.

BIBLIOGRAPHY

Sentinel article

Gagnon B, Mancini I, Pereira J et al. Palliative management of bleeding events in advanced cancer patients. *J Palliat Care* 1998;14:50–4.

Review articles

Hoskin P, Makin W (ed.) *Oncology for Palliative Medicine,* pp. 229–234. Oxford: Oxford University Press, 1998.

Pereira J, Bruera E. Miscellaneous aspects of decision making in palliative care. In *The Edmonton Aid to Palliative Care*, ed. J Pereira, E Bruera, pp. 3–6. Edmonton: University of Alberta Press, 1996.

Pereira J, Mancini I, Bruera E. The management of bleeding in advanced cancer patients. In *Topics in Palliative Care*, ed. R Portenoy, E Bruera, pp. 163–83. Oxford: Oxford University Press, 2000.

52

Thrombosis

Lukas Radbruch

University of Cologne, Cologne

It is not easy to determine whether the use of anticoagulants in patients with far advanced and incurable disease is good palliative care or not. Most palliative care specialists will follow standard procedures in their units for the handling of thrombosis or pulmonary embolism. However, when the subject comes to discussion in international meetings, vast differences are found. Some palliative care professionals will reject the use of anticoagulants as life-prolonging but otherwise useless measures, and consider death from pulmonary embolism as part of the natural course of the malignant disease. Others will hold that anticoagulant therapy is necessary to relieve symptoms such as pain and swelling from deep vein thrombosis or prevent dyspnea from pulmonary embolism. In our palliative care unit in the University of Cologne, standard procedures for bedridden patients include regular application of low molecular-weight heparin.

Prevalence

There is no doubt that the incidence of deep vein thrombosis is high among cancer patients. Thromboembolic episodes were reported for approximately 15% of cancer patients. The incidence seems to be higher for pancreatic and gastric cancer and especially high for patients with lung cancer with an incidence of up to 30%. Pulmonary embolism and deep vein thrombosis have been found in even higher incidences in a large series of necropsies, and again cancer of the peritoneal cavity was correlated with particularly high incidences. Impediment of venous drainage from the lower limbs by these cancers has been proposed as the reason for these high incidences. Venous and arterial thromboembolic episodes are also termed Trousseau's syndrome following the author of the first description, Armand Trousseau, who described high incidences of venous thrombosis in gastric cancer patients in 1865. Apart from deep vein thrombosis, a variety of other locations such as mesenterial, hepatic, or portal veins has been reported. Arterial embolism may be caused by

Table 52.1. Activated clotting system and venous thromboembolism in cancer patients (reviewed in Schmitt et al. 1999)

Tumor	Activation of clotting system
	Stimulation of mononuclear cells
Therapy	Chemotherapy
	Hormonal therapy
	Surgery
Others	Prolonged bed rest
	Dehydration
	Infection
	Long-term catheters

nonbacterial thrombotic endocarditis, and intravasal tumor growth may be associated with pulmonary tumor embolization. Thrombophlebitis migrans and saltans is a rare form with short but recurrent thrombosis of superficial veins which may be very painful.

Pathophysiology

The thrombophilic state in cancer patients has multiple causes. The tumor cells can activate the clotting system directly or by stimulation of mononuclear cells (Table 52.1). This leads to the release of thromboplastin or the cancer procoagulant factor, a specific cysteine protease directly activating factor X. In some patients with genetically based deficiencies the risk for thrombosis may also be increased by antithrombin deficiency or resistance to activated protein C. Cancer cells not only activate the clotting system, but also reinforce fibrinolysis with the expression of plasminogen-activator receptors and the production of urokinase-like plasminogen-activator and plasminogen-activator inhibitors. However, these fibrinolytic activities do not revoke the prothrombotic state in cancer patients. Elevated fibrinogen levels, thrombocytosis, infections or dehydration further increase the incidence of thromboembolic episodes.

Antineoplastic therapies also may be associated with thrombosis. The hepatic veno-occlusive disease is a complication of allogenic and autogenic stem cell transplantations, and has recently also been described following monoclonal antibody therapy. Chemotherapeutic agents such as mitomycin C, cisplatin, bleomycin, or fluorouracil can damage the endothelial cells or induce allergic reactions with circulating immunocomplex proteins. Venous and sometimes also arterial thromboembolism may be a complication of hormonal therapy with tamoxifen, probably related to reduced levels of antithrombin or protein C. With newer substances for hormonal therapy such as toremifene the incidences of thrombo-embolic complications may be lower. Patients undergoing surgical procedures have a higher risk of thromboembolism in the perioperative phase. Not only in the peri-operative phase, but also in patients with far advanced disease, prolonged bed rest or the need to insert central venous lines may further increase the risk.

Thromboembolic episodes are also not uncommon in noncancer patients requir-ing palliative care. Patients with amyotrophic lateral sclerosis or geriatric patients may be bedridden or requiring infusion therapy with central venous lines for pro-longed periods of time. The risk for deep vein thrombosis is increased in patients with HIV infection, probably correlated with reduced heparin cofactor II and free protein S levels. Drug interactions between warfarin and protease inhibitors may reduce the anticoagulant effects in these patients.

Diagnosis

Clinical investigation and laboratory findings are helpful in the diagnosis of venous thromboembolism. Painful swelling in the legs, differences in the circumference between the legs and alleviation of pain with elevation of the leg are clinical signs of deep vein thrombosis. Sudden onset of dyspnea in combination with signs of deep vein thrombosis lead to the diagnosis of pulmonary embolism.

The plasma concentration of D-dimer, a degradation product of fibrin, is almost always raised after a thromboembolic event. Lower limb venous compression ultra-sonography detects deep vein thrombosis with high sensitivity and specificity, especially in the proximal veins. As the sensitivity is lower for thrombosis in the distal veins, it has been recommended to repeat negative investigations after some days to detect eventual proximal extensions of distal thrombosis. A diagnostic strat-egy with a combination of clinical assessment, D-dimer measurement, lower limb venous ultrasonography and lung scan was used for noninvasive diagnosis in out-patients with good results. With adequate use of noninvasive diagnostic procedures phlebography or angiography are indicated only rarely in palliative care patients.

Prophylaxis and treatment

Options for prophylaxis of deep vein thrombosis include pharmacological and non-pharmacological approaches. Mechanical methods such as intermittent pneumatic calf compression or compression stockings may be used perioperatively, but effec-tiveness is limited in high-risk cancer surgery patients. Mechanical methods also are not practical for long-term use or home treatment.

Pharmacological treatment with anticoagulants is used most commonly (Table 52.2). For shorter periods of time unfractionated heparin or low molecular-weight heparin are used. Administration of 5000 IU unfractionated heparin

Table 52.2. Effectiveness of anticoagulant therapies in cancer patients in different settings (reviewed in Kakkar and Williamson 1998)

	Method	Control group %	Treatment group %	Number needed to treat
Perioperatively	Intermittent pneumatic calf compression	20	13	14.3
	Unfractioned heparin	30	13	5.9
	Unfractioned heparin (pulmonary embolism)	1.6	0.4	83.3
Chemotherapy	Warfarin	4.4	0.7	27.0
Central venous line	Warfarin	37	10	3.7
	Low molecular-weight heparin	62	6	1.8

preoperatively and 2–3 times daily for 7–10 days after the operation has reduced the rates of thrombosis significantly. Low molecular-weight heparin also has been used in perioperative prophylaxis with good effect.

Low molecular-weight heparin has to be given only once daily with doses of 2500–5000 IU. This makes it practical also for the prevention of chemotherapy-associated thrombosis or for inpatients with increased risk of thrombosis, for example, bedridden patients or patients with central venous catheters. For long-term prophylaxis, oral treatment with warfarin is the drug of choice. Monitoring of the international normalized ratio (INR) is used to titrate the dosage. However, cancer patients have a higher risk of bleeding with warfarin, and archiving steady-state INR levels may be more difficult. Administration of vitamin K or even of factor concentrates may be necessary to stop bleeding in palliative care patients. Close monitoring of INR therefore is required.

If thromboembolic complications are diagnosed, treatment with unfractionated or low molecular-weight heparin is initiated or continued. Higher doses than for prophylaxis may be necessary. In severe cases of veno-occlusive disease fibrinolytic regimens with tissue plasminogen activator or defibrotide have been used with limited effect, but these substances should not be used in palliative care patients.

Surgical procedures have been used in the treatment of recurrent thrombo-embolic episodes in cancer patients. However, procedures such as arterio-venous shunts, intravenous stent implantation or vena caval filters usually are not indicated for palliative care patients.

Problems with anticoagulant therapy

The use of anticoagulant drugs in palliative care patients has not been subjected to much research. However, there are some ethical and medical problems arising with the use of these drugs. In advanced progressive disease, deep-vein thrombosis may lead to lower extremity edema, induce pulmonary embolism and should be treated. In a postal survey most of 131 palliative physicians reported that they would anticoagulate outpatients and inpatients sometimes or always, and only 2% never would use anticoagulants. On the other hand, patients may have an increased risk of bleeding, especially if they develop complications such as gastric ulcers in the course of the disease, and staff and relatives therefore may reject anticoagulants. In other patients treatment with anticoagulants may have been initiated before admission to the palliative care ward, and the staff will want to discuss discontinuation of these drugs with the patient and his family. Anticoagulant therapy may be part of the standing order for bedridden patients in the hospital, but the question can be raised whether this is appropriate for patients on the palliative care ward. Appropriateness of the therapy was named as one of the major problems associated with anticoagulation in the postal survey. Patients with a history of heart operations may have been treated with anticoagulants for long periods of time before the cancer was diagnosed. Though usually anticoagulant medication will be continued for these patients, it may be impossible to continue the oral medication due to cancer progression. The switch to subcutaneous anticoagulant injections may be questioned by patient, relatives, and staff.

These problems will have even more impact on patients with nonmalignant disease and longer life expectancy. Neurologic patients with amyotrophic lateral sclerosis requiring palliative care may be bedridden early in the course of their disease, and anticoagulant medication for prophylaxis of venous thrombosis and pulmonary embolism may be necessary for years.

CASE   A 68-year-old woman suffered from lung cancer diagnosed only 4 months before, and was treated with chemotherapy with monthly courses. A metastasis in the left suprarenal gland was suspected. In the medical history venous thrombosis on the left side due to varicose veins 5 years ago was reported. She was admitted to the palliative care ward because of pain and restlessness. With admission to the palliative care unit, symptoms resolved almost spontaneously and the patient reported that most of her previous distress had been related to psychosocial problems with the family. In the unit she felt extremely well. Oral application of tramadol drops 125 mg per day resulted in complete pain relief. Low-dose acetylsalicylic acid had been part of her previous regimen and was continued throughout her inpatient treatment.

However, after 7 days she complained of slight pain in the left leg, and noticed a swelling of the ankle joint. Ultrasonography showed a thrombosis from the upper thigh to the calf, with no signs of thrombosis in the proximal or the lower abdominal veins.

The patients started wearing her own compression stockings, and anticoagulant treatment with 0.6 ml low molecular-weight heparin twice daily was initiated. Though the patient had only minimal pain and no other symptoms, bed rest was kept for 1 week to prevent pulmonary embolism. Coagulation parameters were in the normal range, but the nurses reported that the patient bled easily after the heparin injections, leading to painful hematomas at the injection sites in both upper thighs. Control ultrasonography after 1 week showed recanalization of the thrombus and no proximal extension. The patient was discharged 6 days later.

The case report shows that symptoms from deep venous thrombosis were treated effectively and pulmonary embolism was prevented. However, anticoagulant treatment was not without side effects and resulted in painful hematomas.

An individualized approach to anticoagulation is necessary to consider advantages and disadvantages in the specific setting and for the individual patient.

BIBLIOGRAPHY

Sentinel articles

Johnson MJ. Problems of anticoagulation within a palliative care setting: an audit of hospice patients taking warfarin. *Palliat Med* 1997;11:306–12.

Johnson MJ, Sherry K. How do palliative physicians manage venous thromboembolism? *Palliat Med* 1997;11:462–8.

Kakkar AK, Williamson RC. Thromboprophylaxis in the cancer patient. *Haemostasis* 1998;3:61–5.

Perrier A, Desmarais S, Miron M et al. Non-invasive diagnosis of venous thromboembolism in outpatients. *Lancet* 1999;353:190–5.

Schmitt M, Kuhn W, Harbeck N, Graeff H. Thrombophilic state in breast cancer. *Semin Thromb Hemost* 1999;25:157–66.

Internet sites

Guide to anticoagulant therapy of the American Heart Association
   www.americanheart.org/

Consensus guidelines for warfarin therapy from the Australasian Society of Thrombosis and Haemostasis
   www.mja.com.au/public/issues/172_12_190600/gallus/gallus.html

Patient regulated or monitored oral anticoagulant therapy
   www.promoat.org

Information about coumadin
   www.coumadin.com/hcp/hcp.shtm

53

Hypercalcemia of malignancy

Paul W. Walker

U.T. M.D. Anderson Cancer Center, Houston

Introduction

Hypercalcemia of malignancy and tumor-induced hypercalcemia are the two terms used to describe this common and life-threatening complication of cancer. This paraneoplastic syndrome produces a metabolic emergency. It occurs in 10–20% of patients with cancer.

Etiology

A common misconception of the student is that metastases to bone is required to produce hypercalcemia. Although this "local osteolytic hypercalcemia" does occur, particularly in breast cancer and multiple myeloma, a more important cause overall is that termed "humoral hypercalcemia of malignancy." This is the paraneoplastic process where humoral and paracrine factors produced by tumor cells stimulate osteoclast activity and proliferation resulting in bone resorption, liberating calcium into the circulation. Even in situations of tumor involving bone, such as in breast cancer and multiple myeloma, this humoral process has been demonstrated. Although many substances have been implicated in this role, it is not surprising that the agent deemed most responsible for this syndrome is a protein produced by the cancer that mimics normal parathyroid hormone (PTH). This peptide, termed parathyroid hormone-related protein (PTHrP), shows considerable homology with the natural PTH at the N-terminal, with 8 of the first 13 amino acids being identical. This protein has been found to interact with the PTH receptor with equal affinity to natural PTH. Therefore it has the same effect as PTH, which causes increased bone resorption by osteoclasts and renal calcium reabsorption. The clinician's level of suspicion for hypercalcemia should be raised in cancers where it occurs commonly (Table 53.1).

Table 53.1. Hypercalcemia of malignancy

Common in:
    Multiple myeloma
    Breast cancer
    Squamous cell lung cancer
    Squamous cell head and neck cancer
    Genitourinary neoplasms
Rare in:
    Small cell lung cancer
    Prostate cancer
    Adenocarcinoma of colon and stomach

Clinical manifestations

This condition typically has a sudden onset in advanced cancer patients. Less frequently a patient will present with symptoms due to hypercalcemia together with weight loss and is then found to have cancer on further investigations. This can be contrasted to individuals with primary hyperparathyroidism who typically present with no or vague symptoms of a chronic nature. These patients are relatively well when they are found to be hypercalcemic on routine laboratory screening. As the two clinical presentations are markedly different, it is usually not difficult to differentiate between these two most common causes of hypercalcemia. If necessary, an elevated PTH level can confirm primary hyperparathyroidism.

Even though hypercalcemia of malignancy is common, the diagnosis may be delayed due to the nonspecific nature of the symptoms produced. These symptoms do not closely correlate with the calcium level in the individual. Rather, it is believed that the rate of increase in the serum calcium level is a more significant factor in symptom development. Anorexia, nausea, and vomiting commonly result. Constipation is usually seen and may progress to the status of ileus in severe situations. Due to the acute nature of the elevation in serum calcium, cramping abdominal pains, acute pancreatitis and peptic ulceration, that may be seen with the more chronically elevated calcium levels of primary hyperthyroidism, are exceedingly rare. Renal concentrating ability is impaired by the toxic effects of high calcium levels on the renal tubules, with polyuria resulting. Together with the gastrointestinal effects which produce decreased fluid intake or vomiting, severe volume depletion results. Muscle weakness and lethargy are common. Impairment in mental status occurs producing confusion, which progresses to coma (Table 53.2).

The clinician must entertain the diagnosis of hypercalcemia or the diagnosis will be missed. Until a serum calcium level is drawn, the patient may erroneously

Table 53.2. Clinical findings in hypercalcemia of malignancy

Anorexia
Nausea and vomiting
Constipation or ileus
Polyuria
Dehydration
Fatigue and weakness
Confusion
Coma

Table 53.3. "Corrected" serum calcium

Ca (corrected) = Ca (measured) + [0.02 (40-serum albumin)]
SI units (e.g., mmol/l)
Ca (corrected) = Ca (measured) + [0.8 × (4-serum albumin)]
Conventional units (e.g., mg/dl)

be believed to have nausea attributed to chemotherapy, chronic nausea of cancer, anorexia secondary to the cachexia syndrome, simple constipation, ileus, or delirium secondary to a number of possible causes. It is therefore important to obtain an indication of the serum calcium level in cancer patients with any of these symptoms.

Determining hypercalcemia

Serum calcium is highly protein bound. Approximately 45% of the total plasma calcium is bound to albumin and 10% is complexed with bicarbonate and citrate. The remaining 45% is ionized calcium, which is the physiologically active form of interest to the clinician. As the measurement of total serum calcium will fluctuate with changes in the serum protein concentration, this measurement does not represent a value useful for clinical purposes. Measurement of the ionized calcium is available in many institutions and directly measures the physiologically active component. This is much preferable to using the total serum calcium level. If the ionized calcium measurement is unavailable, then a formula may be used to "correct" the total serum calcium for the usually reduced serum albumin concentration found in advanced cancer patients (Table 53.3). Measurement of the ionized calcium directly or calculation of the corrected calcium level, are required for correct diagnosis and management.

Treatment

In situations where antineoplastic therapy is effective, that treatment can resolve the hypercalcemia. Frequently, however, this complication occurs in the advanced cancer patient where these options are unavailable. In this setting it is important to have clear goals. Although the prognosis for advanced cancer patients who developed hypercalcemia has not been extensively evaluated, most studies report a median survival of approximately 1 month. Sometimes a view is expressed by clinicians that the patient may be better served by not treating the hypercalcemia. This may be true in situations where, prior to the development of hypercalcemia, the patient's quality of life was deemed unacceptable secondary to pain or other issues. Alternatively, treatment that corrects the hypercalcemia can resolve the nausea, vomiting, anorexia, constipation, and delirium. The complete reversal of this devastating symptom complex is often greeted with appreciation from the patient and family. Even if the patient's life may be in the order of a short number of weeks, this intervention allows meaningful interaction with loved ones, and may provide significant time to complete unfinished business.

The first step in treatment is to address the severe volume depletion by administering parenteral fluid (i.v. or hypodermoclysis). Normal saline is the preferred solution and the rate of administration is dependent on the patient's cardiac status and ability to handle a rapid volume increase. Young individuals with a previously good performance status may tolerate 3 liters per day or more while an elderly advanced cancer patient with a previous cardiac disorder may safely tolerate only 1–2 liters per day. Fluid administration should continue until the calcium level is normalized through the use of therapeutic agents. In cases of mild hypercalcemia, hydration alone may be enough to produce normocalcemia. Little role exists for furosemide except to manage overzealous hydration. Use of furosemide early in management, before rehydration is adequate, may exacerbate the condition.

Together with hydration, the administration of a bisphosphonate has become the treatment of choice. These drugs are potent inhibitors of osteoclast-mediated bone resorption and are the most efficacious agents to date. Fortunately they have almost no side effects and are well tolerated. Their oral bio-availability is poor. This, together with the urgency of the patient's condition, necessitates parenteral administration. Table 53.4 indicates the bisphosphonates currently recommended. Clodronate produces normocalcemia in approximately 80% of patients within 3 days of administration. It has the added advantage in the palliative setting that it may be administered via a subcutaneous infusion thereby obviating the need for initiation and maintenance of an i.v. site. This agent is available in Canada and Europe. Pamidronate is an amino bisphosphonate. It produces normocalcemia in approximately 90% of patients and is administered intravenously. It produces

Table 53.4. Hypercalcemia: treatment modalities

Parenteral fluid rehydration (i.v. or s.c.)
with normal saline 1–3 L/day or more
Bisphosphonates
Clodronate 1500 mg i.v. or s.c. over 2 hours
Pamidronate 90 mg i.v. over 2 hours
Ibandronate 4 mg i.v. over 2 hours
Zoledronate 4 mg i.v. over 15 minutes
Corticosteroids
Dexamethasone 6–16 mg/day
Prednisone 40–100 mg/day
Calcitonin 4 IU/kg s.c. q 12 hour–8 IU/kg s.c. q 6 hr (approx. 300–600 IU per dose)

Note: i.v., intravenously; s.c., subcutaneously.

normocalcemia in the same time frame as clodronate but its duration of activity is longer (median 28 days) than clodronate (median 14 days). Ibadronate is a newer amino bisphosphonate that produces normocalcemia in approximately 75% of patients and has been used in Europe. Intravenous infusion of these agents has been reduced to 2 hours duration in order to facilitate outpatient administration. The development of newer, more potent bisphosphonates have held the hope that shorter and more effective treatment would be available. The latest and most potent of these drugs is zoledronate. This agent may become the drug of choice. It has been administered over an infusion time as short as 5 minutes intravenously and has a success rate of approximately 90%. The amino bisphosphonates have the small complication of causing an acute-phase reaction on initial administration. This produces a transient elevation in temperature as well as myalgias and leukopenia. It is important to recognize, so as not to misattribute this reaction to another cause, such as a neutropenic sepsis. It may be possible to avoid this phenomenon by administration of 500–650 mg of acetominophen orally prior to pamidronate infusion. All biphosphonates may produce a transient elevation in the serum creatinine level, especially if prehydration has not been adequate. Symptomatic hypocalcemia occurs rarely.

Treatment with a bisphosphonate should occur whenever the patient is symptomatic with hypercalcemia. In the absence of overt symptoms, hypercalcemia requiring bisphosphonate treatment occurs at a corrected calcium of 3.0 mmol/L (12 mg/dl), whereas clinical judgement is required at less elevated levels. In urgent situations, where the hypercalcemia is deemed to be life threatening, it is prudent to co-administer calcitonin with the bisphosphonate, to achieve its more rapid effect, while waiting for the bisphosphonates to be effective. Calcitonin is a less efficacious agent in reducing serum calcium levels and unfortunately is subject to tachyphylaxis, which develops in 2–3 days, due to downregulation of calcitonin receptors. Plicamycin and gallium nitrate unfortunately are less effective and have greater toxicity than the biphosphonates. The use of corticosteroids such as dexamethasone or prednisone are indicated in steroid-responsive hematological malignancies such as myeloma and lymphoma. Medications that may contribute to hypercalcemia such as vitamin D and thiazide diuretics should be discontinued.

Concerns about limiting dietary calcium intake (milk, etc.) are not warranted as levels of $1,25\text{-}[OH]_2D_3$ are low in most cases of hypercalcemia of malignancy, and gastrointestinal calcium absorption is not a significant factor. Monitoring of the serum calcium level should be performed every 1–2 days until normocalcemia has returned. Determination of electrolyte and magnesium levels are prudent due to volume expansion. Thereafter, serum calcium determinations approximately weekly may be performed to monitor for recurrence of hypercalcemia. Each individual's response to the bisphosphonate treatment is unpredictable and patients may relapse much sooner or later than the median duration stated for the effectiveness of the respective agent. It is important to remember that this treatment does not provide a cure but temporarily reduces the calcium level through inhibition of bone resorption. Repeat treatments are frequently required. Approximately 10–20% of patients will be resistant to management with a bisphosphonate. In these situations, humoral hypercalcemia of malignancy is the primary mechanism and renal re-absorption of calcium limits biphosphonate effectiveness. Unfortunately there are no agents to directly antagonize the effect of PTHrP on the kidney. In these situations switching to a different or more potent bisphosphanate may be attempted.

Summary

Hypercalcemia of malignancy is a common complication of advanced cancer and requires a high level of clinical suspicion on the part of the practitioner, but it is easily diagnosed with the appropriate laboratory tests. It produces marked symptom distress, which can usually be alleviated safely with volume repletion and bisphosphonate administration. In the majority of cases it is a gratifying condition to manage by improving the quality of life for patients in their last remaining weeks of life.

BIBLIOGRAPHY

Body JJ. Current and future directions in medical therapy: hypercalcemia. *Cancer* 2000;88:3054–8.

Body JJ, Bartl R, Burckhardt P et al. Current use of bisphosphonates in oncology. *J Clin Oncol* 1998;16:3890–9.

Major P, Lortholary A, Hon J et al. Zoledronic acid is superior to pamidronate in the treatment of hypercalcemia of malignancy: a pooled analysis of two randomized, controlled clinical trials. *J Clin Oncol* 2001;19:558–67.

Morton AR, Ritch PS. Hypercalcemia. In *Principles and Practice of Supportive Oncology*, ed. A Berger, RK Portenoy, DE Weissman, pp. 411–25. Philadelphia: Lippincott-Raven, 1998.

Walker P, Watanabe S, Lawlor P, Hanson J, Pereira J, Bruera E. Subcutaneous clodronate: a study evaluating efficacy in hypercalcemia of malignancy and local toxicity. *Ann Oncol* 1997;8: 915–16.

Warrell RP. Metabolic emergencies: hypercalcemia. In *Cancer: Principles and Practices of Oncology*, 5th edn, ed. VT Devita Jr, S Hellman, SA Rosenberg, pp. 2486–500. Philadelphia: Lippincott-Raven, 1997.

54

Lymphedema

Mabel Caban

Baylor College of Medicine, Houston

Introduction and natural history

Lymphedema occurs when there is an imbalance of the lymphatic load in relation to the transport capability of the lymphatics. Lymphedema presents as swelling of any tissue but typically it manifests with swelling of a limb. Lymph flow is impaired and cannot return back to the circulation, resulting in formation of edema, chronic inflammation, and fibrosis of the tissue.

A normal lymphatic system can manage an increased protein and water load without leading to edema. However, other factors that increase the capillary filtration or impair lymphatic drainage can alter the equilibrium causing clinical edema. The increase in capillary filtration is known as high-output lymph failure. It occurs when the lymph flow is increased and incapable of keeping up with the microcirculatory demand, such as portal hypertension secondary to cirrhosis. The impaired lymph flow caused by blockage of lymph flow is low-output lymph failure, that presents as lymph stasis.

Lymphedema is classified as primary or secondary. Primary causes are usually congenital or hereditary from abnormalities of the lymphatic vessels. Secondary lymphedema is typically the result of blockage from tumor compression, or dissection of the lymph nodes or infections (filariasis). In the US the most common cause of secondary lymphedema is cancer and cancer treatment, but filariasis is the most common cause of lymphedema worldwide.

Clinical manifestation

The most common symptoms of lymphedema are presented in Table 54.1. These are mostly subjective symptoms that should be closely monitored. The differential diagnoses include deep venous thrombosis and soft tissue infections. A careful history and physical exam (see Table 54.2) are needed to diagnose lymphedema.

Table 54.1. Signs and symptoms of early lymphedema

Heaviness
Tightness
Hardness
Numbness
Stiffness
Erythema
Pain
Weakness
Seroma
Limitation of motion

Table 54.2. Details of the physical exam

Detectable enlargement of the limb or trunk
Number of skin folds at the axilla, along the limb, digits
Skin color
Skin texture (soft, hard, shiny, taut)
Asymmetric increase in the adiposity of the subcutaneous tissue
Pitting edema 1–4, or no pitting edema
Pulses
Range of motion
Neurological exam
Measurement of the limb

Previously, the concept of assessing the size of the extremity to find asymmetry was essential for the diagnosis. For example, a difference of 2 cm is no longer required to make the diagnosis of lymphedema. Current thinking emphasizes qualitative signs of the physical examination, particularly skin texture, which can be important in the early stages as well as advanced lymphedema. Initially, the edema may be pitting, with some fullness palpable. In later stages, hardness and fibrosis of the skin are predominant. A lymphedema symptom assessment sheet is recommended (see Figure 54.1) to note changes in the subjective symptoms. Both subjective symptoms and measurement of the limb are recommended in the evaluation of the patients with lymphedema to ensure success or failure of therapies. Symptoms in the history that may alert to the presence of recurrent cancer are the presence of neuropathic pain (radiating, lancinating), burning, allodynia, the presence of weakness or inability to move the limb. Physical signs such as new or unusual lesions of the skin, lymphadenopathy, weakness or sensory loss related to radicular or plexus

Table 54.3. Alert symptoms and signs for malignant lymphedema

Inability to move the limb
Neuropathic pain
Radicular or plexus-like lesions
Weakness
Unusual skin lesions
Violaceous skin discoloration
Lymphadenopathy

Lymphedema Symptom Assessment

1. Do you experience tension of the swollen arm or leg or chest?
0 ————————————————————— 10 (cm)
No tension   Tension as bad as it
                                    could possibly be

2. Do you experience heaviness?
0 ————————————————————— 10 (cm)
No heaviness   Heaviness as bad as it
                                    could possibly be

3. Do you experience pain?
0 ————————————————————— 10 (cm)
No pain   Pain as bad as it
                                    could possibly be

4. Do you experience abnormal sensations of the swollen arm or leg?
0 ————————————————————— 10 (cm)
No abnormal sensation   Abnormal sensation as bad as it
                                    could possibly be

5. Do you experience hardness of the skin in the arm, leg, or the chest?
0 ————————————————————— 10 (cm)
No hardness   Hardness as bad as it
                                    could possibly be

Figure 54.1   Visual analog scale proposed for the evaluation of subjective symptoms of lymphedema.

involvement suggest recurrent cancer and require further diagnostic imaging and contact with the oncologist or surgeon. Swelling caused by tumor cells infiltrating the lymph nodes or by tumor bulk compressing the lymphatics is known as malignant lymphedema. Table 54.3 depicts the alerting signs and symptoms associated with malignant lymphedema. Sustained reduction of the swelling is rare in spite of treatment efforts, some authors recommend the use of diuretics with this severity of malignant swelling plus the concomitant use of cancer treatments.

The patient with lymphedema faces a higher risk of soft tissue infections. The most common are:

1. Cellulitis – acute inflammation of the deep subcutaneous tissues and muscle associated with edema.

2. Erysipelas – acute, superficial form of cellulitis involving the dermal papillae. It is characterized by hot, bright red, edematous, well-defined margins with a raised indurated border. Pain, fever, and intense red color are present; resolution follows initiation of antibiotic.

3. Lymphangitis – inflammation of a lymphatic vessel characterized by a painful, subcutaneous red streak along the lymphatic vessel.

Potential life-threatening infections may ensue. Prompt attention with antibiotics is necessary. The most common organism is group A Streptococcus, so a penicillin, such as dicloxacillin 500 mg orally every 6 hours, is a good choice for treatment. Massage or the use of a low-stretch compression bandage should be deferred until response to antibiotics occurs.

Prevention

Prevention is the best way to treat lymphedema. Newer surgical techniques are trying to spare the lymph nodes from removal if at all possible. Other ways to prevent the onset or recurrence of lymphedema are:

1. Avoid cuts or needle sticks on the affected arm or leg.
2. Avoid blood pressure check-up on the affected limb.
3. Avoid burns or sunburn on the affected limb.
4. If air travel is necessary, wear a compression sleeve or hose.
5. Prompt treatment of infections.

Treatment

Decongestive lymphatic therapy is widely acceptable (previously known as complex physical therapy). It consists of manual lymph drainage, exercises and low-stretch compression bandaging. Manual lymph drainage is a specialized superficial massage technique; the mechanism of action proposed is that it stimulates the motoricity of the lymphatic system. In combination with exercises and low-stretch compression bandaging it is very effective for most cases of nonmalignant lymphedema. It requires daily treatments for 2–3 weeks until the swelling reduces, progressing into a maintenance program of daily exercises and the use of a daytime elastic compression hose or sleeve. Recent literature comparing manual lymph drainage with standard therapy of compression garment and exercises find that both are effective in reducing limb volume. Much controversy exists about the use of manual lymph drainage in patients with malignant lymphedema because some practitioners fear the spread of tumor. However, manual lymph drainage is acceptable as palliation in addition to treatment with radiation or chemotherapy. The mobilization of tumor cells by manual lymph drainage is considered unfounded. The exception would be in cases of diffuse carcinomatous infiltrates when mobilization of tumor cells can occur by mechanical massage, but in those cases the prognosis is already poor so that palliation with manual lymph drainage is indicated.

Other treatment available is the use of the pneumatic pump in combination with exercises for proximal decongestion. Low pressures of about 30 mm Hg for the arms or about 40 mmHg for the legs appear safe and successful when using pneumatic compression pumps. High pressures of 70–100 mm Hg are not recommended because this can damage the lymphatic vessels. Both the massage and the compression should use low pressure.

Medications have not been successful in the treatment of lymphedema. Diuretics are indicated at times, particularly in the presence of malignant lymphedema. Careful follow-up of the patient's electrolytes is recommended when initiating diuretics. The use of benzopyrones to stimulate breakdown of protein, therefore the absorption of protein, has not proved to benefit patients in the short term. Benzopyrones are associated to liver damage so they are banned from use in many countries of the world, including the US. Initial reports using micronized purified flavonoid fraction (MPFF) that stimulates macrophages appear to reduce effectively the swelling in lymphedema. MPFF is not available for clinical use but initial clinical trials appear promising to treat lymphedema.

Surgical options are few. They are mostly used for debulking in cases of lymphedema of the genitalia or when there is elephantiasis. Liposuction is controversial because there is resection of the superficial lymphatics, but recent reports with the use of compression hose or sleeves after liposuction advocate excellent results. Microsurgery for lymph vessel transplantation or the use of lymph–venous and lymph–nodal shunts is promising in selected cases.

BIBLIOGRAPHY

Sentinel articles

Andersen L, Hojris I, Erlandsen M, Andersen J. Treatment of breast-cancer-related lymphedema with or without manual lymphatic drainage – a randomized study. *Acta Oncol* 2000;39:399–405.

Badger CM, Peacock JL, Mortimer PS. A randomized, controlled, parallel-group clinical trial comparing multilayer bandaging followed by hosiery versus hosiery alone in the treatment of patients with lymphedema of the limb. *Cancer* 2000;88:2832–7.

Brennan MJ, Miller LT. Overview of treatment options and review of the current role and use of compression garments, intermittent pumps, and exercise in the management of lymphedema. *Cancer* 1998;83:2821–7.

Brorson H. Liposuction gives complete reduction of chronic large arm lymphedema after breast cancer. *Acta Oncol* 2000;39:407–20.

Eliska O, Eliskova M. Are peripheral lymphatics damaged by high-pressure manual massage? *Lymphology* 1995;28:21–30.

Johansson K, Lie E, Ekdahl C, Lindfeldt J. A randomized study comparing manual lymph drainage with sequential compression for treatment of postoperative arm lymphedema. *Lymphology* 1998;31:56–64.

Kocak Z, Overgaard J. Risk factors of arm lymphedema in breast cancer patients. *Acta Oncol* 2000;39:389–92.

Olszweski W. Clinical efficacy of micronized purified flavonoid fraction (MPFF) in edema. *Angiology* 2000;51:25–9.

Swedborg I. Effects of treatment with an elastic sleeve and intermittent pneumatic compression in post-mastectomy patients with lymphoedema of the arm. *Scand J Rehab Med* 1984;16:35–41.

Review articles

Consensus Document of the International Society of Lymphology Executive Committee. The diagnosis and treatment of peripheral lymphedema. *Lymphology* 1995;28:113–17.

Erickson VS, Pearson ML, Ganz PA, Adams J, Kahn KL. Arm edema in breast cancer patients. *J Natl Cancer Inst* 2001;93:96–111.

O'Brien P. Lymphedema. *Principles Pract Support Oncol Updates* 1999;2:1–11.

Olszewski WL. Clinical picture of lymphedema. In *Lymph Stasis: Pathophysiology, Diagnosis and Treatment*, ed. WL Olszewski, p. 348. Boca Raton: CRC Press, 1991.

Szuba A, Rockson S. Lymphedema: anatomy, physiology and pathogenesis. *Vasc Med* 1997;2: 321–6.

Szuba A, Rockson S. Lymphedema: classification, diagnosis and therapy. *Vasc Med* 1998;3:145–56.

Internet sites

National Lymphedema Network
   www.lymphnet.org
Cancernet
   http://www.cancer.gov
International Society of Lymphology
   www.u.arizona.edu/~witte/ISL.htm

55

Wound care of the advanced cancer patient

Kathryn G. Froiland
U.T. M.D. Anderson Cancer Center, Houston

Introduction

Pressure ulcers, surgical wounds, malignant cutaneous wounds, radiation therapy-induced skin alterations, and incontinence-induced wounds are commonly experienced by cancer patients.

Assessment

Wound assessment and documentation should include the following findings:
- Degree of tissue layer destruction or color.
- Anatomic location.
- Length, width, depth, and tunneling using consistent units of measure.
- Appearance of the wound bed and surrounding skin.
- Drainage, specifying amount, color, and consistency.
- Pain or tenderness.
- Temperature (Hess 1999).

These parameters were developed to assess pressure ulcers, but they are useful guidelines for assessing other types of wounds.

The skin surrounding the wound must be assessed for color, temperature, and swelling. The wound's epithelial edge is assessed for continuity and integrity. Excessive dryness or moisture or the presence of nonviable tissue or exudate may delay re-epithelialization once granulation occurs. Finally, assess the wound for the presence of foreign objects such as sutures, staples, or environmental debris (Hess 1999).

Urinary or fecal incontinence

Skin-related damage may appear as an irritant contact dermatitis, involving erythema, edema, and vesicle formation. Failure to remove the irritant (urine or stool) will result in progressive inflammation of the skin, resulting in blistering, erosion of epidermis, weeping, and pain. Itching and burning occur with mild inflammation, whereas severe inflammation is associated with epidermal loss and exposure of dermal nerve endings, causing pain. *Candida albicans* yeast infection commonly causes a rash in these patients.

Prognosis and treatment

Topical wound management is designed to keep the wound moist, clean, warm, and protected from trauma and secondary infection. A limited number of examples of wound care products are included here. The reader is referred to wound care texts (Hess 1999; Bryant 2000) and to manufacturers' packaging information for greater detail. Consultation with a nurse certified in wound, ostomy, and continence care is also advised.

- Alginates, derived from seaweed, absorb up to 20 times their weight. The formed gel maintains a moist wound environment and is easy to apply and remove (Bard AlgiDERM; Smith & Nephew AlgiSite M; Coloplast Comfeel SeaSorb).
- Hydrocolloids, occlusive or semi-occlusive dressings are composed of gelatin, pectin, or carboxymethylcellulose. Creation of a moist environment allows clean wounds to granulate and necrotic wounds to debride autolytically. They are self-adhesive and mold well. The edges may curl and injure fragile skin when removed. When placed along the edges of surgical wounds, they will protect periwound skin from moisture and dermal stripping due to traumatic tape removal (ConvaTec DuoDERM; Coloplast Comfeel; 3M Tegasorb).
- Hydrofiber dressing. AQUACEL (ConvaTec) is a nonwoven dressing made from sodium carboxymethylcellulose fibers. It is highly absorbent for managing exudating wounds. As absorption occurs, gel forms, providing a moist environment that promotes debridement.
- Hydrogels are water- or glycerin-based amorphous gels, impregnated gauze, or sheet dressings. They maintain a moist environment, promote granulation and epithelialization, and facilitate autolytic debridement. They are soothing and may reduce pain. They provide minimal to moderate absorption, dehydrate if not covered with a secondary dressing, and may cause periwound breakdown if the hydrogel is allowed to contact intact skin (Carrington Carrasyn Gel; ConvaTec SAF-Gel; Bard Vigilon).

Selected other products

- Cream or emulsion dressings. BIAFINE Radiodermatitis Emulsion dressing (Medix Pharmaceuticals Americas, Inc.) recruits macrophages to promote granulation, debrides autolytically, creates a moist environment, absorbs exudate, and decreases odor.
- Debriding agent. ACCUZYME Papain-Urea Debriding Ointment (Healthpoint) contains a proteolytic enzyme that digests nonviable protein matter without

harming healthy tissue. It is indicated to debride necrotic tissue and to liquefy slough in pressure ulcers, burns, surgical wounds, vascular wounds, and infected wounds. Collagenase SANTYL Ointment (Smith & Nephew) is a collagen-specific proteolytic enzyme that debrides necrotic tissue without harming healthy tissue. Debridement of chronic dermal ulcers and burned areas is its indicated usage.

- Skin sealants provide a transparent waterproof barrier that protects skin from excess moisture. Several manufacturers make such barriers as wipes, sprays, or gels. Those containing a minimal amount of alcohol or none at all are most comfortable.

- Vacuum-assisted closure/negative pressure wound therapy (Kinetic Concepts, Inc.). This mechanical treatment evacuates wound fluid, reduces localized edema, stimulates granulation tissue formation, and reduces bacterial colonization counts. Therapy is applied until closure is achieved or until the wound has granulated sufficiently for surgical closure.

Care of irradiated skin

Cleaning with tepid water is advisable. The skin should be patted dry with a soft towel, or may be dried with a hair dryer set on a low/cool setting. Applications of heat or cold, perfume, deodorant, makeup, scented soaps, adhesives, and tight-fitting clothes should not be used in the treatment area.

Itching is often due to dryness. The use of moisturizers should be approved by the radiation oncologist so as not to interfere with treatment. Hydrogels, wafers, and sheets may be applied to provide comfort to inflamed areas.

Nonadherent absorptive dressings can be applied to moist skin. Non-binding elastic mesh garments can secure them to intact, nonirradiated skin. The patient must be supported with adequate pain medication. Symptom management should be continued following completion of radiation therapy, as reactions continue for several weeks or months following treatment.

Care of malignant cutaneous wounds

If the wound is painful, nonadherent dressings offering long wear times (i.e., changed no more often than every 2–3 days), should be considered. Hydrocolloid dressings applied to fragile skin will decrease trauma. Nontraumatic tapes and mesh netting can be used to affix dressings and ease dressing removal.

Hemostatic dressings, nonadherent gauze, alginates, and silver nitrate can be used to control minor bleeding. Appropriate precautions must be taken when sharply debriding these wounds, as vascular structures are often difficult to identify and bleeding may be difficult to control.

Necrotic tissue, infection, or saturated dressings are sources of odor. Ionic irrigants or wound cleansers can mechanically remove odorous necrotic tissue.

Absorbent dressings, polysaccharide beads (Healthpoint IODOSORB), sodium-impregnated gauze (Molnlycke MESALT), and alginates absorb odorous wound fluid. Charcoal-impregnated dressings (ConvaTec CARBOFLEX and LYOFOAM C; Johnson & Johnson ACTISORB PLUS), used as the outermost layer of the dressing, suppress odor until saturated.

Conservative autolytic or enzymatic debridement can soften and remove necrotic tissue. Surgical debridement may be appropriate but is used less commonly because of the risk of bleeding.

Antimicrobial creams, dressings with antibacterial properties, antibiotic solutions, and sodium-impregnated gauze may reduce bacterial load and thereby reduce odor. Metronidazole (gel or crushed tablets in normal saline solution) applied one to two times daily to the wound bed suppress odor (not an FDA-approved indication; Bryant 2000). Biologic odor-eliminating sprays can aid in controlling environmental odors. Spray deodorizers, vanilla extract or orange oil, although readily available and less costly, only mask odor, not eliminate it. It is advisable to change odorous dressings when strikethrough of drainage occurs.

The volume of exudate varies and determines the type of dressing required to contain it. Alginates and foam dressings contain moderate to large amounts of exudate. Heavily exudative wounds need superabsorbent pads as well as an alginate or hydrofiber dressing, or absorptive powder, beads, or wound-filler products.

Wound drainage pouches should be considered when dressings require frequent changing, when odor is uncontrolled, or when the periwound skin shows signs of impending breakdown. Pouching may facilitate the patient's ability to ambulate without concern for dislodging bulky dressing material.

Cutaneous lesions associated with mycosis fungoids may appear as blisters or bullae that vary in size and number. These lesions drain watery fluid, can be painful, and cause heat loss as drainage evaporates. Surrounding skin may be friable. The skin may be dry, cracked, and inelastic. Itching is usually remedied with application of a heavy petrolatum-based moisturizer (Beiersdorf AQUAPHOR) after bathing and as needed. Antibiotic ointment applied to open areas protects against infection. Whirlpool treatments may be comforting and can debride nonviable tissue. Absorbent, nonadhering dressings secured with roll gauze collect drainage between treatments.

Care of skin affected by urinary and/or fecal incontinence

Mild cleansers provide cleaning action, require no rinsing, and leave a protective barrier on the skin. These products minimize patient discomfort and shorten caregiver's cleaning time.

Use of a moisture barrier cream or ointment is advised for both prevention and treatment of skin breakdown. Petrolatum, dimethicone, and zinc oxide are common ingredients in these products. An antifungal agent may be added to the ointment and is effective in treating yeast-induced rashes.

Devices for managing urinary incontinence for men include external condom catheters and adhesive urinary pouches. Both types of devices are attached to collection bags that can measure volume and contain urine. External collection pouches for women are available, but only useful for short-term urine collection in the bedfast patient.

Indwelling catheters may be the best option for managing urinary incontinence in the terminally ill patient. The perineum and the catheter should be cleansed daily. A closed drainage system should be maintained and changed as a unit.

Rectal tubes are not advised, as an inflated anchoring balloon can cause local tissue necrosis in the rectum. An appropriately applied fecal incontinence collector is an alternative management device. Denuded skin can be prepared with moisture-absorbing powder and skin sealants or thin hydrocolloid dressings to provide a dry surface for pouching.

Absorbent pads and garments are available in many sizes and designs and are either disposable or reusable. Those containing polymer products wick urine away from the skin and contain it in gel. Unfortunately, absorbent pads and garments for containment of stool and control of its odor are not as readily available.

REFERENCES

Bryant RA (ed.) *Acute and Chronic Wounds: Nursing Management*, 2nd edn. St. Louis: Mosby, 2000.

Hess CT. *Clinical Guide: Wound Care*, 3rd edn. Springhouse: Springhouse Corporation, 1999.

Internet sites

Wound, Ostomy, and Continence Nurses Society
www.wocn.org

56

Infections in patients with advanced cancer

Rudolph M. Navari

Walther Cancer Research Center, University of Notre Dame, Notre Dame, IN

Introduction

Patients with advanced or terminal cancer are at high risk for infections as a result of the underlying disease, a poor nutritional state, and/or a direct suppression of the hematological system due to chemotherapy or radiation treatments. An infectious complication may occur due to an alteration in the phagocytic, cellular, or humoral immunity, an alteration or breach of their skin or mucosal defense barriers, indwelling catheters, or a splenectomy. A high index of suspicion, a consideration of the empirical institution of antimicrobials, an awareness of the possibility of unusual infectious agents, and a constant surveillance of the hematological status of the patients are necessary in order to provide optimal management of infections in this patient population.

This review will consider the initial evaluation of fever, the use of antimicrobial agents, the predominant organisms associated with infection, and the management of infectious complications in this specific patient population. Special consideration and discussion will be given to patients receiving hospice and palliative care.

Evaluation of fever

In patients with advanced cancer, fever is very common and it may or may not have an infectious etiology. It must be noted that fever may be the only manifestation of an infection in an immunocompromised patient and there is no pattern of fever that can be used to definitively rule out an infectious etiology. Fever may also be modified by the use of specific medications such as corticosteroids or nonsteroidal anti-inflammatory agents.

Fever in patients with advanced or terminal cancer must be evaluated in terms of the underlying disease, the specific risk for a local or systemic infection, the urgency for empirical antimicrobial therapy, the presence or absence of neutropenia, and any signs or symptoms which may suggest a site of infection. Attention should be directed to the most common sites of infection such as the oral cavity, lungs, perirectal area, urinary tract, skin, and soft tissues. In patients with fever and neutropenia, the initial evaluation does not identify a site of infection in the majority of patients.

Depending on the status of the patient at the time of the fever, in addition to the history and physical examination, an initial evaluation may include a hematologic profile, cultures of nose and throat, urine, blood, stool, and cerebrospinal fluid, and radiological evaluations of the chest and sinuses. Whether or not antimicrobials are begun at the time of the initial fever, patients should be carefully re-evaluated at least every 24 hours. It must be remembered that in patients with profound and prolonged neutropenia, multiple sites of infection and multiple organisms may be present.

Empirical treatment – febrile neutropenia

Empirical treatment with broad-spectrum antimicrobial therapy is justified in patients with advanced cancer with febrile neutropenia due to the high frequency of severe infections. As previously noted, signs and symptoms of infection in these patients are often minimal, and life-threatening septicemia may be present. Empirical initiation of antimicrobials is indicated without waiting for microbiological and/or clinical documentation.

Prognostic factors recently have been identified for patients with febrile neutropenia. Approximately 25–30% of patients with febrile neutropenia have a low risk of complications and death. These low-risk patients are those who develop febrile neutropenia outside the hospital, whose neoplasms are under reasonable control, and who do not have serious cofactors. These cofactors include the degree and duration of neutropenia, post chemotherapy or radiotherapy breaches of physical defense barriers such as oral and gastrointestinal mucositis, absence of dehydration or hypotension, absence of chronic obstructive pulmonary disease, and/or splenectomy. Recent studies have suggested that these low-risk patients may be considered for treatment as outpatients with oral amoxicillin–clavulanate plus ciprofloxacin or intravenous once-daily ceftriaxone plus amikacin. Current clinical trials are underway to further define the safety and efficacy of this approach.

Patients with febrile neutropenia not in the low-risk group should be hospitalized and treated with a single broad spectrum antibiotic (monotherapy) which covers both gram-positive and gram-negative organisms if the neutropenia is moderate and expected to be short-lived. Agents such as cefepime, ceftazidime, meropenem, and piperacillin–tazobactam appear to be adequate. None of these antibiotics cover methicillin-resistant coagulase-negative staphlococci which are very common in patients with febrile neutropenia. The low pathogenicity of these organisms, however, allows a delay of specific therapy with a glycopeptide (vancomycin or teicoplanin) until a specific microbiological diagnosis is made.

In patients presenting with clinical signs of gram-negative sepsis, such as high fever and hypotension, or with an unexpected high degree and long duration of neutropenia and/or the presence of serious cofactors, combination therapy (multiple antibiotics) with consideration of an aminoglycoside should be utilized. If a serious gram-positive infection is suspected such as in a patient with an infected intravenous line or severe mucositis, the addition of a glycopeptide may be warranted. Vancomycin is the drug of choice for methicillin-resistant strains of coagulase negative and coagulase positive staphylococcus infections. Because of emerging resistance in enterococci and staphylococci, vancomycin should be used for very specific indications. Quinupristin/dalfopristin, a streptogramin antibiotic, and linezolid, an oxazolidinone, may be useful for some strains of gram-positive bacteria that are resistant to vancomycin.

After a 2–3 day period, antimicrobial therapy should be re-evaluated and modified if necessary based on microbiological data, in order to limit toxicity and cost. Antimicrobials should be discontinued after 5–6 afebrile days and/or when the neutropenia resolves, to avoid superinfection with resistant organisms.

There is limited information on the efficacy of using colony-stimulating factors as an addition to empirical antibiotics for the treatment of patients with febrile neutropenia. The current recommendations of the American Society of Clinical Oncology suggest that growth factors be considered only for high-risk patients with neutropenia, mainly those with severe sepsis or organ involvement such as renal failure or pulmonary infiltrates. The guidelines suggest that low-risk patients may not need treatment with growth factors.

In patients who continue to have fever and negative cultures after the initiation of empirical combination antibiotics, empirical antifungal therapy is indicated, particularly if the duration of neutropenia is expected to be prolonged. Amphotericin B and the azoles, fluconazole and itraconazole, have been used in this setting, but drug toxicities and resistant organisms have limited the efficacy of these agents. A new semisynthetic antifungal, caspofungin acetate, is in phase III clinical trials and may be approved in 2002. It is reported to have a broad spectrum, to be fungicidal, and have few side effects.

Predominant organism

The most probable offending organisms in patients with advanced cancer are dependent on the degree and duration of the immunosuppression, the type of immune defect, the chemotherapy or radiotherapy treatment regimen, as well as where the patient resides and receives care.

Bacteria represent the most immediate threat to the immunocompromised, and over the past 20 years, there has been a significant change in the predominant organisms responsible for infections in patients with neutropenia. Gram-positive organisms, particularly the coagulase-negative staphylococci, have been the leading cause of acute bacterial infections in patients with febrile neutropenia in the US and Western Europe. This may be due at least partially to the increased use of indwelling intravenous access devices.

In addition to the coagulase-negative staphylococci, *Staphylococcus aureus*, streptococci, and enterococcus are the predominant gram-positive isolates representing the majority of the infections in this patient population. These organisms have replaced the gram-negative organisms (*Pseudomonas aeruginosa*, *E. coli*, and *Klebsiella* sp.) which were the common organisms in the US and Europe 30–40 years ago and which are still the common organisms in the developing countries.

Infections and antibiotic use in palliative care

Patients with advanced cancer who are receiving palliative care or hospice care have a lower frequency of febrile neutropenia mainly due to the limited use of chemotherapy and radiotherapy. The frequency of infections, however, remains high due to the underlying disease, the generally poor functional status of the patients characterized by impaired cognition and immobility, as well as the use of indwelling urinary catheters and vascular access devices.

Recent studies have suggested that during a stay of 30 days or less on an inpatient palliative care unit, 36–55% of patients had at least one or more infections, which were considered for antimicrobial treatment. The most common clinical conditions were urinary tract infections, respiratory tract infections, skin and subcutaneous tissue infections, and a small number of positive blood cultures. The most common organisms were *E. coli*, *Staphylococcus aureus*, and enterococcus.

Studies suggest that antimicrobials are initiated in the overwhelming majority (70–90%) of patients receiving palliative care when they have fever or a suspected or documented infection. The response rate to antibiotics appears to be at least 50%, and although symptoms appear to be improved, survival does not appear to be affected. A small number of catastrophic fatal events may be secondary to infections, but it is unlikely that the institution of antibiotics would affect the outcome.

The decision-making process in the use of antimicrobials in patients receiving palliative care is highly complex. In most situations, the approach should be individualized for each patient based on the desires of the patient, the control of symptoms, and quality-of-life issues. Issues to be considered include the potential benefit of the use of antimicrobials compared with the potential toxicities that may result from the extent of the investigation of a suspected infection, the number of diagnostic tests to be employed, and the means to be employed to treat a suspected or documented infection. It may be appropriate to treat a fever with an antipyretic alone in a patient whose death is imminent rather than proceed with an extensive laboratory work-up and the initiation of antimicrobials. Alternatively, the pain resulting from a symptomatic, localized skin or soft tissue infection may be treated more successfully with both antibiotics and pain medications.

For patients receiving hospice care at home or in an institution such as a hospital palliative care unit or a chronic care facility, consideration should be given to initiating oral or parenteral antibiotics based only on clinical indications without the use of laboratory or imaging criteria. Mobilization of the patients for diagnostic interventions may be associated with significant discomfort.

For community-acquired bacterial pneumonia, an oral macrolide (erythromycin, azithromycin, or clarithromycin), doxycycline, or a fluoroquinolone with good antipneumococcal activity (levofloxacin, gatifloxacin, or moxifloxacin) is recommended. For patients who require parenteral antibiotics, cefotaxime or ceftriaxone may be reasonable first choices. An antipneumococcal fluoroquinolone may be added to cover *Legionella*, *Mycoplasma*, and *Chlamydia*. These agents would not require monitoring of blood levels.

Patients with uncomplicated cystitis can be effectively and inexpensively treated with a 3-day course of oral trimethoprim-sulfamethoxazole or a fluoroquinolone. Acute uncomplicated pyelonephritis can often be managed with a 7-day course of an oral fluoroquinolone.

The issues that patients, families, and physicians consider when making decisions concerning the use of a respirator, cardiac resuscitation, dialysis, etc. should, in general, also apply to the use of antimicrobials. Antimicrobial use in patients receiving palliative care may be a part of symptomatic care, may or may not result in life prolongation, and/or may be associated with symptom-producing interventions such as laboratory testing, venous access, and direct antimicrobial toxicities. The goal of antimicrobial therapy in palliative care is symptom control, in contrast to the goal of decreased morbidity and mortality in acute medical or surgical situations.

In order to develop guidelines for these choices, a recent study reported that antimicrobial options were discussed with patients at the time they began palliative care. During a 6-month period, in a community-based hospice and palliative care program, over 300 consecutive patients were asked to elect one of three options: full antimicrobial use for suspected or established infections, antimicrobial use for symptomatic treatment only, or no antimicrobial use. More than half of the patients elected symptomatic treatment only, and one-third of the patients elected no antibiotics. There were no differences in overall survival among the three groups, and antimicrobial use did not affect survival. The number of deaths attributable directly to infection was small and not different among the three groups.

The study suggests that when asked about the use of antimicrobials, patients in a palliative care program choose antimicrobial use for the control of symptoms and reject antimicrobial use for decreased mortality. A discussion of antimicrobial use with patients who elect hospice and palliative care may contribute to effective symptom control and enhanced quality of life.

BIBLIOGRAPHY

Ahronheim JC, Morrison RS, Baskin SA et al. Treatment of the dying in the acute care hospital. *Arch Intern Med* 1996;156:2094–100.

Bruera E. Intractable pain in patients with advanced head and neck tumors: a possible role of local infection. *Cancer Treat Rep* 1986;70:691–2.

Finberg RW, Talcott JA. Fever and neutropenia – how to use a new treatment strategy. *N Engl J Med* 1999;341:362–3.

Klastersky J. Empirical treatment of sepsis in neutropenic patients. *Int J Antimicrob Agents* 2000;16:131–3.

Klastersky J, Paesmans M, Rubenstein EB et al. The multinational association for supportive care in cancer risk index: a multinational scoring system for identifying low-risk febrile neutropenia cancer patients. *J Clin Oncol* 2000;18:3038–51.

Navari RM, Daskal F. Antibiotic use in advanced cancer patients receiving end of life palliative care. *ASCO* 2001;20:1554.

Pereira J, Watanabe S, Wolch G. A retrospective review of the frequency of infections and patterns of antibiotic utilization on a palliative care unit. *J Pain Symptom Manage* 1998;16:374–81.

Pizzo PA. Fever in immunocompromised patients. *N Engl J Med* 1999;341:893–900.

Steinberg JP, Clark CC, Hackman BO. Nosocomial and community-acquired *Staphylococcus aureus* bacteremias from 1980 to 1993: impact of intravascular devices and methicillin resistance. *Clin Infect Dis* 1996;23:255–9.

The choice of antibacterial drugs. *Med Letter* 2001;43:69–78.

Vazquez JA, Lynch M, Boikov D, Sobel JD. In vitro activity of a new pneumocardin antifungal, L-743,872, against azole-susceptible and resistant Candida species. *Antimicrob Agents Chemother* 1997;41:1612–14.

Vitetta L, Kenner D, Sali A. Bacterial infections in terminally ill hospice patients. *J Pain Symptom Manage* 2000;20:326–34.

Walsh TJ, Finberg RW, Arndt C et al. Liposomal amphotericin B for empirical therapy in patients with persistent fever and neutropenia. *N Engl J Med* 1999;340:764–71.

57

Urogenital complications

Romano T. DeMarco and Richard S. Foster

Indiana University Medical Center, Indianapolis

Introduction

Genitourinary and other primary malignancies cause frequent and common urogenital complications. Healthcare providers need to be cognizant of these unique problems inherent in treating cancer patients. In this chapter, we will discuss the most common urogenital complications of patients with cancer.

Ureteral obstruction

Primary malignancies can spread from their original location to the retroperitoneum and lead to ureteral obstruction. The obstruction typically occurs from either direct extension from the tumor itself or metastases to the retroperitoneal lymph nodes. Malignancies originating from the genitourinary system are the most common cause of ureteral obstruction in patients with cancer. However, other malignant tumors can be culprits (Table 57.1). Additionally, other therapies such as radiation therapy can result in ureteral obstruction.

Patients with ureteral obstruction typically present with flank pain, oliguria, or azotemia. Renal sonography, abdominal-pelvic computed tomography (CT) scan, or intravenous pyelogram (IVP) usually demonstrate unilateral or bilateral hydronephrosis in patients with significant ureteral obstruction.

Internal double-J stents, placed in a retrograde fashion through the bladder and into the renal pelvis, usually relieve the obstruction. Occasionally, significant retroperitoneal disease precludes the placement of internal stents. In these situations, percutaneous nephrostomy tubes placed into the kidneys relieve the obstruction.

Patients may exhibit a marked polyuria following the relief of bilateral ureteral obstruction. This postobstructive diuresis is usually physiologic and self-limited. If the polyuria is persistent and associated with elevation of serum creatinine and blood

Table 57.1. Common malignancies associated with ureteral obstruction

Prostate
Bladder
Cervical
Colon
Uterine
Ovarian
Breast

urea nitrogen (BUN), the patient needs aggressive monitoring of urine output, blood pressure, intravenous fluids, and serum electrolytes.

Gross hematuria

Transitional cell carcinoma of the bladder commonly causes gross hematuria. Patients with prostate cancer, renal cell carcinoma, and transitional cell carcinoma of the ureter or renal pelvis can also present with gross hematuria. Patients undergoing radiation therapy for genitourinary or other pelvic malignancies, and those patients receiving cyclophosphamide, which can cause hemorrhagic cystitis, are at risk for significant hematuria.

If gross hematuria occurs, a patient may present with an inability to void because of large obstructing clots, known as clot retention. In this situation, a large urethral catheter can evacuate the clots. Additionally, a three-way Foley catheter with continuous bladder irrigation using saline or sterile water keeps the catheter patent and draining.

Bladder irrigation with 1% alum can control persistent bleeding. The consulting urologist may use other agents, such as silver nitrate or formalin, to control the hematuria. Occasionally, cystoscopy with fulguration of the bleeding areas, removal of the bladder tumor, or in rare cases, cystectomy, are interventions used to control bleeding.

Urinary incontinence

Urinary incontinence is a particularly disturbing genitourinary complication. Prostate cancer patients undergoing radical retropubic prostatectomy may sustain injury to their external urinary sphincter causing either limited or persistent problems with urinary incontinence. Radiation therapy for prostate cancer may also cause urinary incontinence. Vesicovaginal or ureterovaginal fistulae can occur after surgical extirpation or radiation therapy for pelvic malignancies causing continual incontinence.

Initial management of incontinence includes conservative measures such as urinary pads or diapers. Indwelling urinary catheters can be useful for short periods. An artificial urinary sphincter for men incontinent after radical retropubic prostatectomy is an option. Surgical takedown of the fistula corrects the incontinence for patients with incontinence secondary to urinary fistulae.

Urinary retention

In direct contrast to urinary incontinence, urinary retention can be a significant problem for the cancer patient. Urinary retention is commonly caused by prostatic obstruction from a large tumor, clot retention from active bleeding, or less frequently, from urethral stricture disease from previous trauma during therapies for the prostate or bladder cancer. Radiation or operative therapies to the pelvis occasionally cause a noncontractile (neurogenic) bladder. Vertebral involvement of tumors may cause spinal cord compression and result in urinary retention. Finally, medications such as opioids and anticholinergic agents are sometimes the cause of urinary retention in older adults with cancer.

Anchoring an indwelling Foley catheter is the first step. Clean intermittent urinary catheterizations to empty the bladder work well in motivated and dexterous patients. If obstruction by a large prostate tumor is the cause, a transurethral resection of the prostate may relieve the obstruction and allow the patient to void normally. In patients with refractory retention, occasional placement of a suprapubic catheter is necessary.

Erectile dysfunction

A common complaint among men undergoing surgery or radiation therapy for prostate cancer is erectile dysfunction. The nerves controlling potency are at significant risk of injury from either surgery or radiation therapy. Although newer nerve-sparing techniques during surgery have increased the chance of maintaining potency, it is still a frequent cause of patient and partner distress.

Oral medications such as Viagra (sildenafil citrate) are the first line of therapy. Patients with cardiac disease or who fail Viagra are candidates for other modalities. These include penile injection therapy, the vacuum pump, or surgical insertion of a penile prosthesis.

Conclusion

The urogenital complications of patients with cancer span a spectrum from mild to life threatening. Potential morbidity can be lessened or negated, by recognition and appropriate intervention in patients with urogenital complications from their primary malignancy.

BIBLIOGRAPHY

Chiou RK, Chang WY, Horan JJ. Ureteral obstruction associated with prostate cancer: the outcome after percutaneous nephrostomy. *J Urol* 1990;143:959–9.

Harris J. The prevalence of impotence after radical prostatectomy. *Urol Nurs* 1997;17: 142–5.

McIntyre JF, Eifel PJ, Levenback C, Oswald MJ. Ureteral stricture as a late complication of radiotherapy for stage IB carcinoma of the uterine cervix. *Cancer* 1995;75:836–43.

Sise JG, Crichlow RW. Obstruction due to malignant tumors. *Semin Oncol* 1978;5:213–24.

Smith DB. Urinary continence issues in oncology. *Clin J Oncol Nurs* 1999;3:161–7.

Teloken C. Management of erectile dysfunction secondary to treatment for localized prostate cancer. *Cancer Contr* 2001;8:540–5.

Wahle GR. Urinary incontinence after radical prostatectomy. *Semin Urol Oncol* 2000;18:66–70.

58

Brain metastases

Doreen Oneschuk

Grey Nuns Hospital and Community Health Center, Edmonton

Introduction

Brain metastases are the most common intracranial tumors among adults, with a reported incidence of 20–40% in patients with cancer. In descending order, lung, breast, malignant melanoma, renal, and gastrointestinal are the most common tumors giving rise to brain metastases. Metastases can be single, solitary, or multiple. "Single" metastases refers to the presence of only one brain metastasis and implies nothing about the extent of cancer that may or may not be present elsewhere; "solitary" refers to a single metastasis that is the only known site of metastatic cancer in the body; and "multiple" refers to the presence of more than one metastasis and makes no distinction regarding the presence of systemic cancer. Approximately two-thirds to three-quarters of patients with brain metastases have multiple lesions. Single metastasis is more common with breast, renal, and colon cancer. Multiple lesions are more commonly seen with malignant melanoma and lung cancer.

This chapter will address the pathophysiology, clinical features, radiographic diagnosis, and treatment of brain metastases.

Pathophysiology

Intracranial metastases may involve the brain parenchyma, the blood vessels (including the dural sinus), the cranial nerves, the dura, the leptomeninges, and the inner table of the skull (Figure 58.1). Most brain metastases are the result of hematogenous spread, usually through the arterial circulation, and are distributed throughout the brain in proportion to the cerebral blood flow, with approximately 80% being located in the cerebral hemispheres, 15% in the cerebellum, and 5% in the brain stem. Metastases are commonly located in the region directly below the grey–white junction, where narrowed vessels act as a trap for emboli. Cerebral edema secondary to brain metastases is primarily vasogenic in origin implying that

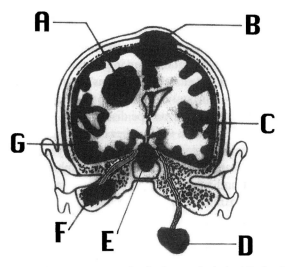

Figure 58.1   Sites of metastases to the brain can include (A) the brain parenchyma; (B) the calvar-
ium compressing the sagittal sinus and raising intracranial pressure; (C) leptomeningeal
metastases invading the brain; (D) tumor growth from the face or ear growing within the
parenchyma of the cranial nerves to secondarily invade the brain; (E) extracerebral structures such as the pineal or pituitary gland that secondarily compress the brain; (F) base of
the skull involving exiting cranial nerves; (G) subdural metastases secondarily compressing the brain. Source: Posner JB. Brain metastases: 1995. A brief review. *J Neuro-Oncology*
1996;27:287. Figure 1, with kind permission from Kluwer Academic Publishers.

the edema is localized in the extracellular space of mainly the white matter and is
caused by changes in the blood–brain barrier.

Clinical features

More than two-thirds of patients with brain metastases experience some neurological symptoms during their illness trajectory. The clinical presentation is primarily
dependent on the location of the brain metastases within the brain and is similar
to that of other mass lesions in the brain. The four most common symptoms are
headaches, focal weakness, cognitive dysfunction, and seizures. Headaches occur
in approximately 50% of patients and are more common in patients with multiple
metastases and with metastases in the posterior fossa. Focal weakness is the presenting symptom in 20–40% of patients, and is usually mild or moderate and gradual in
onset. Cognitive dysfunction, as detected by standard tests of mental status, may be
present in as many as 75% of patients. One-third of patients report general memory problems and mood or personality disturbances. Focal or generalized seizures
occur in approximately 10% of patients as the first sign of metastases. However, as
many as 40% of patients will develop seizures during the course of their disease.

Use of anticonvulsants

Any patient with brain metastases who has experienced a seizure should be treated with a standard anticonvulsant, although which anticonvulsant is the most effective is not known. The most commonly used anticonvulsant is phenytoin, although other options for use include carbamazepine, phenobarbital, and valproic acid. No study has compared the effectiveness of these anticonvulsants. A meta-analysis of randomized clinical trials addressing the issue of prophylactic anticonvulsants concluded that there is no statistical evidence showing a significant benefit of prophylactic anticonvulsants. Prophylactic use is not supported by any studies except in two situations: in patients with brain metastases from melanoma because of the high incidence of seizures; and in tumors located in an area of high epileptogenicity, such as the motor cortex. When prescribing anticonvulsants, the risk for intrinsic side effects and potential for drug–drug interactions must be heeded.

Radiographic diagnosis

The diagnosis of brain metastases can be established by a contrast-enhanced computed tomography (CT) scan or magnetic resonance imaging (MRI). The MRI with gadolinium contrast enhancement is the most sensitive diagnostic tool in the general detection of brain metastases and appears to be superior to double-dose delayed contrast CT scan for detection, anatomical localization, and differentiation of solitary versus multiple brain metastases. Delayed-contrast CT has been shown to have a higher (by as much as 67%) sensitivity for detecting metastases than immediate CT scanning. Brain metastases should be distinguished from primary brain tumors, abscesses, demyelination, cerebral infarctions or hemorrhages, progressive multifocal leukoencephalopathy, and the effects of treatment including radiation necrosis.

Treatment

The main purposes of treatment are to reverse the patient's neurological deficits and to prolong life. Systemic cancer rather than neurologic disease usually limits life expectancy. Patients with a better prognosis include those with a solitary lesion, a good performance status, young age (less than 60 years), a primary tumor that is in remission, and metastases confined to the brain. The available treatments include the use of corticosteroids, radiotherapy, surgery/radiosurgery, and chemotherapy. The median survival of patients who are untreated is 1 month. The addition of corticosteroids increases survival to 2 months, while whole brain radiotherapy (WBRT) improves survival to 3–6 months.

Corticosteroids

Corticosteroids are often the first therapeutic intervention initiated for the management of brain metastases. Exactly how corticosteroids achieve their effect in the management of brain metastases remains unknown. Dexamethasone appears to be the preferred corticosteroid owing to its lower mineralocorticoid activity and the convenience of twice-a-day dosing. The effect of corticosteroids is often rapid and dramatic. Clinical effects are noticeable within 6–24 hours following the first dose and reach their maximum effect in 3–7 days, although neurological improvements have been noted within a few hours after administration. Significant clinical improvement occurs in approximately 70–80% of patients. Divided doses of 16 mg per day of dexamethasone have been recommended on the basis of empirical clinical observations. However, other studies suggest that patients not responsive to this dosage may benefit from doses up to 100 mg per day. Corticosteroids are administered to radiotherapy patients 48–72 hours before initiating treatment and during radiation to lessen the chance of symptomatic deterioration resulting from radiation-induced edema. Corticosteroids should be tapered and discontinued in most patients once radiotherapy is completed or reduced to the minimal effective dose that prevents or reduces symptoms associated with the metastases. A small percentage of patients may require the use of corticosteroids indefinitely to control symptoms. Potential side effects of corticosteroids include infections (immunosuppression), insomnia, hyperglycemia, systemic edema, cushingoid appearance, dyspepsia, easy bruisability, weight gain, myopathy, osteoporosis, avascular necrosis, and neuropsychiatric symptoms.

Radiation therapy

Whole brain radiotherapy has been the mainstay of treatment for single or multiple brain metastases for over 40 years. The combination of WBRT and corticosteroids is effective palliative treatment for brain metastases providing symptomatic relief in 70–90% of patients. There is currently no consensus on the optimal radiation schedule for patients with brain metastases. Late complications of WBRT can be debilitating and include leukoencephalopathy, brain atrophy, brain necrosis, and communicating hydrocephalus. Regarding reirradiation, there is no consensus as to which dose-fractionation schedule is most appropriate or the optimal interval between the initial course and reirradiation.

Surgery

For patients who are candidates for surgery, the most important factor to consider is the extent of extracranial disease. For single brain metastases, several studies support the use of surgery in addition to WBRT in patients with stable disease. The studies for surgical treatment of multiple brain metastases are conflicting, making it difficult to draw firm conclusions regarding the value of surgical resection. For recurrent brain metastases, several studies support surgical resection in selected patients with symptomatic lesions. Stereotactic radiosurgery is a technique of external irradiation that utilizes multiple convergent beams to deliver a high single dose of radiation to a radiographically discrete treatment volume. Radiosurgery can be performed with high-energy x-rays produced by linear accelerators, with gamma rays from the gamma knife, and less frequently, with charged particles, such as protons produced by cyclotrons. Young patients with good performance status, limited extracranial disease, and fewer than three lesions are particularly suited to radiosurgery. Radiosurgery can be used alone or in combination with WBRT, and several studies suggest a trend for superior local control when radiosurgery is used in conjunction with WBRT. Radiosurgery also has an important role in patients who experience a recurrence of brain metastases following WBRT. The morbidity of radiosurgery is low. The most serious side effects are radiation necrosis and cranial nerve damage, which occur in relatively small percentages of patients.

Chemotherapy

Chemotherapy has limited value in the treatment of brain metastases. Although the results of chemotherapy for brain metastases have been disappointing, a number of uncontrolled studies have demonstrated favorable response rates for chemosensitive tumors such as breast cancer, small-cell lung cancer, and germ cell tumors.

Conclusions

Not an uncommon complication of advanced cancer, brain metastases can cause neurological impairment that contributes to a decreased quality of life. Left untreated, patients with brain metastases survive approximately 1 month. Goals of treatment include life prolongation and improvement of neurological deficits. Treatment options include the use of corticosteroids, radiation therapy, surgery, and chemotherapy. Radiosurgery is gaining in popularity for the treatment of brain metastases.

Box 58.1 Summary – brain metastases

Brain metastases are more common than primary brain tumors.

Cerebral edema from brain metastases is primarily vasogenic in origin.

The four most common neurological symptoms from brain metastases are headaches, focal weakness, cognitive dysfunction, and seizures.

In general, prophylactic anticonvulsants are not recommended.

Corticosteroids are the first therapeutic intervention advised upon identification of brain metastases.

Other treatment options include radiation, surgery, and radiosurgery.

BIBLIOGRAPHY

Sentinel articles

Cho KH, Hall WA, Gerbi BJ, Higgins PD, Bohen M, Clark HB. Patient selection criteria for the treatment of brain metastases with stereotactic radiosurgery. *J Neuro-Oncol* 1998;40:73–86.

Delattre JY, Krol G, Thaler HT, Posner J. Distribution of brain metastases. *Arch Neurol* 1988;45:741–4.

Lagerwaard FJ, Levendag PC, Nowak PJCM, Eijkenboom WMH, Hanssens PEJ, Schmitz PIM. Identification of prognostic factors in patients with brain metastases: a review of 1292 patients. *Int J Radiat Oncol Biol Phys* 1999;43:795–803.

Maor MH, Dubey P, Tucker SL et al. Stereotactic radiosurgery for brain metastases: results and prognostic factors. *Int J Cancer (Radiat Oncol Invest)* 2000;90:157–62.

Patchell RA, Tibbs PA, Walsh JW et al. A randomized trial of surgery in the treatment of single metastases to the brain. *N Engl J Med* 1990;322:494–500.

Patchell RA, Tibbs PA, Regine WF et al. Postoperative radiotherapy in the treatment of single metastases to the brain. A randomized trial. *J Am Med Assoc* 1998;280:1485–9.

Walker AE, Robins M, Weinfeld FD. Epidemiology of brain tumors: The national survey of intracranial neoplasms. *Neurology* 1985;35:219–26.

Review articles

Boyd TS, Mehta MP. Stereotactic radiosurgery for brain metastases. *Oncology* 1999;13:1397–409.

DeAngelis LM. Mangement of brain metastases. *Cancer Invest* 1994;12:156–65.

Oneschuk D, Bruera E. Palliative management of brain metastases. *Support Care Cancer* 1998;6:365–72.

Patchell RA. The treatment of brain metastases. *Cancer Invest* 1996;14:169–77.

Posner JB. Management of brain metastases. *Rev Neurol (Paris)* 1992;148:477–87.

Posner JB. Brain metastases: 1995. A brief review. *J Neuro-Oncol* 1996;27:287–93.

Rude M. Selected neurologic complications in the patient with cancer. Brain metastases and spinal cord compression. *Crit Care Nurs Clin N Am* 2000;12:269–79.

Wen PY, Loeffler JS. Management of brain metastases. *Oncology* 1999;13:941–61.

59

Bowel obstruction

Carla Ripamonti

National Cancer Institute of Milan, Milan

Introduction

Bowel obstruction is defined as any process preventing the movement of bowel contents, thus leading to the partial or complete blocking of feces and gas through the intestinal passage. Malignant bowel obstruction (MBO) is a distressing outcome in patients with abdominal and pelvic primary cancer or metastases. MBO may be the first manifestation of the abdominal disease or the consequence of advanced disease due to failure of anticancer treatments.

The exact frequency of MBO in cancer patients is not known. In highly selected groups of patients, retrospective and autopsy studies have estimated that MBO occurs in 4–28.4% of patients with gastrointestinal cancer and in 5–51% of patients with gynecological disease, in particular with ovarian cancer, where it is a major cause of death (Feuer et al. 1999*a*; Ripamonti et al. 2001).

Multifactorial and often coexisting malignant and benign pathophysiologic mechanisms may be involved in the onset of and worsening of MBO (Box 59.1) (Ripamonti et al. 2001).

The obstruction can be partial or complete, single or multiple. The small bowel is more commonly involved than the large bowel (61% versus 33%) and both are involved in over 20% of the patients (Ripamonti et al. 2001).

Some reports suggest a benign cause is responsible in about 50% of the patients with colorectal cancer as compared with only 6% of patients with gynecological cancers (Ripamonti et al. 2001). Other causes such as inflammatory edema, fecal impaction, constipating drugs (such as opioids, anticholinergics, etc.), and dehydration, are likely to contribute to the development of bowel obstruction or to worsen the clinical picture.

> **Box 59.1** Pathophysiological mechanisms of malignant bowel obstruction
>
> Mechanical obstruction is caused by:
>
> 1. Extrinsic occlusion of the lumen due to an enlargement of the primary tumor or recurrence, mesenteric and omental masses, abdominal or pelvic adhesions (caused either by the tumor or secondary to surgery), postirradiation fibrosis.
> 2. Intraluminal occlusion of the lumen due to neoplastic mass or annular tumoral dissemination.
> 3. Intramural occlusion of the lumen due to intestinal linitis plastica.
>
> Functional obstruction (or adynamic ileus) is caused by intestinal motility disorders consequent to:
>
> 1. Tumor infiltration of the mesentery or bowel muscle and nerves (carcinomatosis), malignant involvement of the celiac plexus.
> 2. Paraneoplastic neuropathy in patients with lung cancer.
> 3. Chronic intestinal pseudo-obstruction (CIP) mainly due to diabetes mellitus, previous gastric surgery and other neurological disorders.
> 4. Paraneoplastic pseudo-obstruction.

Clinical features

As a consequence of the partial or complete occlusion of the lumen, the accumulation of the unabsorbed secretions produce nausea, vomiting, pain and colicky activity (not present in functional obstruction) to surmount the obstacle that causes intermittent colicky pain (Figure 59.1). Abdominal distension may be absent in high obstruction, i.e., of the duodenum or proximal jejunum, and when the bowel is "plastered" down by extensive mesenteric spread.

Table 59.1 shows the most frequent symptoms of bowel obstruction in cancer patients according to the site of obstruction.

Differential diagnosis and symptom assessment

When a cancer patient presents suspected bowel obstruction, all the possible causes of constipation (see Chapter 49) and nausea and vomiting (Follon 1998; Pisters et al. 1998; Ripamonti et al. 2002; Twycross et al. 1998) have to be ruled out. The possible metabolic alterations, the type and dosages of drugs taken as well as the state of hydration and nutrition must be assessed. The patient must be investigated regarding a relapse or a disease progression, bowel movements, and the presence of overflow diarrhea which could lead to underestimating of the problem.

Abdominal examination can show the presence of abdominal cancer or fecal masses, distension to all the abdomen or above the obstacle, the eventual presence of ascites as well as painful sites. Rectal exploration can show the absence or presence of feces in the rectal ampulla. The symptoms referred to by the patient should be

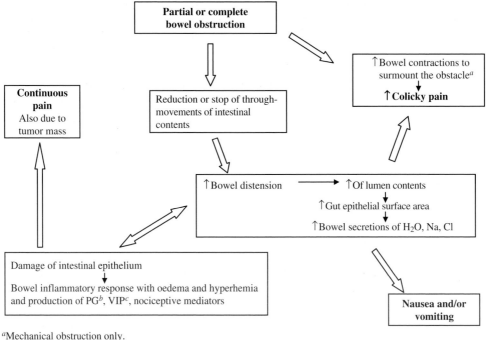

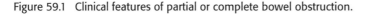

[a]Mechanical obstruction only.
[b]Prostaglandins.
[c]Vasoactive intestinal polypeptide.

Figure 59.1 Clinical features of partial or complete bowel obstruction.

monitored daily. Vomiting can be evaluated in terms of quantity, quality, and number of daily episodes. Other symptoms such as nausea, pain, dry mouth, drowsiness, dyspnea, hunger, thirst, etc. can be assessed by numerical or verbal scales.

An abdominal x-ray taken in a supine or standing position is the first investigation in patients with suspected small bowel obstruction to document the dilated loops of bowel, air–fluid interfaces, or both. Contrast radiography can help to evaluate dysmotility, partial obstruction, and to define the site and extent of the obstruction. Retrograde transrectal radiographic contrast studies should be used to rule out or to diagnose isolated or concomitant obstruction of the large bowel.

An abdominal computed tomography (CT) scan is useful for evaluating the global extent of disease, to perform staging, and to assist in the choice of surgical, endoscopic, or simple pharmacological palliative intervention for the management of the obstruction.

Prognosis and treatment

Because the obstruction of the lumen develops slowly and often remains partial, MBO in advanced cancer patients is rarely an emergency event and intestinal

Table 59.1. Common symptoms in cancer patients with malignant bowel obstruction

Vomiting	Intermittent or continuous	It develops early and in great amounts in gastric, duodenum and small bowel obstruction and develops later in large bowel obstruction	Biliary vomiting is almost odorless and indicates an obstruction in the upper part of the abdomen. The presence of bad smelling and fecaloid vomiting can be the first sign of a ileal or colic obstruction
Nausea	Intermittent or continuous		
Colicky pain	Variable intensity and localization due to distension proximal to the obstruction; secondary to gas and fluid accumulation most of which are produced by the gut	If it is intense, periumbilical and occurring at brief intervals, may be an indication of an obstruction at the jejunum–ileal level. In large bowel obstruction the pain is less intense, deeper, occurring at longer intervals and spreads toward the colon wall	An overall acute pain which begins intensely and becomes stronger, or a pain which is specifically localized, may be a symptom of a perforation or an ileal or colic strangulation. A pain which increases with palpation may be due to peritoneal irritation or the beginning of a perforation
Continuous pain	Variable intensity and localization	It is due to abdominal distension, tumor mass and/or hepatomegaly	
Dry mouth		It is due to severe dehydration, metabolic alterations, but above all it is due to the use of drugs with anticholinergic properties and poor mouth care	
Constipation	Intermittent or complete	In case of complete obstruction there is no evacuation of feces and no flatus	In case of partial obstruction the symptom is intermittent
Overflow diarrhea		It is the result of bacterial liquefaction of the fecal material	

strangulation is uncommon, thus there is time to evaluate the most suitable thera-peutic intervention for each patient.

Curative or palliative surgical intervention

Surgical intervention should be considered in all patients with bowel obstruction. However, it is important to consider whether palliative surgery is technically feasible and whether the patient is likely to benefit from surgery (Feuer et al. 1999*b*; Ripamonti et al. 2001). According to the literature contraindication factors to surgery include: (1) a previous laparotomy/surgery which showed diffuse metastatic cancer thus considered unfit for surgery; (2) multiple partial bowel obstructions; (3) severe motility problems due to intraperitoneal carcinomatosis; (4) massive ascites which rapidly recur after drainage; (5) extra-abdominal metastases produc-ing symptoms difficult to control such as severe dyspnea (Ripamonti et al. 2001).

Seeing that not all the advanced cancer patients can be operated on, the physician has to deal with a patient suffering from nausea, vomiting, and pain, with a short life expectancy, who can only be treated with self-expanding metallic stents or with pharmacological palliative therapies.

Self-expanding metallic stents

Stents are an option in malignant obstruction of the gastric outlet, proximal small bowel, and colon. The stents may be useful in the management of patients who are at surgical risk or in those presenting large bowel obstruction in which decompression by a stent allows treatment of coexisting medical complications to enable surgery to be carried out at a later date, after staging of the disease and an optimal colonic preparation (Wallis et al. 1998). However, their usefulness in patients with end-stage cancer has not yet been formally evaluated.

Venting procedures

Nasogastric suction is the usual hospital treatment to reduce secretions, vomiting, pain, and abdominal distension. However, long-term use of a nasogastric tube is very uncomfortable and should only be considered when drugs are ineffective for symptom control or when a venting gastrostomy cannot be performed. Operative or percutaneous endoscopic gastrostomy are much more acceptable methods for longer-term decompression of an obstructed gastrointestinal tract, rather than a nasogastric tube (Ripamonti et al. 2001).

Pharmacological palliative treatment

Drug therapy comprising analgesics, antisecretory drugs, and anti-emetics, without using a nasogastric tube was first described by Baines et al. (1985). Several authors have confirmed the efficacy of this approach (Ripamonti et al. 2001). Medications should be tailored to each patient regarding both the drugs to be administered, the

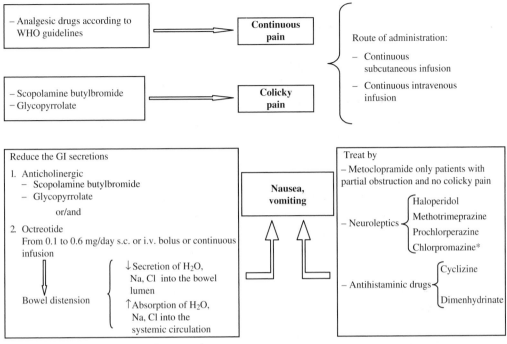

* Skin irritation when administered subcutaneously

Figure 59.2   Symptomatic pharmacological approach in bowel-obstructed patients (Ripamonti et al. 2001).

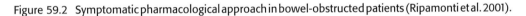

dosages, the drug associations and the route of their administration (Figure 59.2) (Ripamonti et al. 2001). In most bowel-obstructed patients, oral administration is not suitable and alternatives routes have to be considered. Most of the recommended drugs can be administered in association via parenteral continuous infusion.

To relieve continuous abdominal pain, opioid analgesics via continuous subcutaneous or intravenous infusion are necessary in most of the patients. The dosage has to be titrated for each patient until pain relief is achieved. Anticholinergics may be administered in association with opioids to control colicky pain (Mercadante 1995).

Vomiting can be managed using two different pharmacological approaches: (1) drugs such as anticholinergics and/or octreotide, which reduce gastrointestinal secretions; (2) anti-emetics acting on the central nervous system, alone or in association with drugs to reduce gastrointestinal secretions.

Vomiting should be reduced to an acceptable level for the patient (e.g., 1–2 times/day). Among the anti-emetics, parenteral metoclopramide is the drug of choice in patients with functional bowel obstruction. Octreotide inhibits the release of several gastrointestinal hormones, reduces gastrointestinal secretions, reduces the secretion going into the bowel lumen and increases the absorption into the systemic circulation of H_2O, Na, Cl (Fallon 1994). Two randomized controlled studies have been carried out comparing the antisecretory effects of octreotide and scopolamine butylbromide in patients with inoperable MBO (Mercadante et al. 2000;

Ripamonti et al. 2000). Octreotide was significantly more effective and faster than scopolamine butylbromide in reducing the amount of gastrointestinal secretions, the intensity of nausea and the number of vomiting episodes. Octreotide was also effective in patients with upper abdominal obstruction where scopolamine butylbromide had failed.

The role of corticosteroids in treating bowel obstruction is still controversial (Feuer et al. 1999*a*).

Parenteral nutrition and hydration

The role of total parenteral nutrition in patients with malignant bowel obstruction should not be considered a routine part of a terminal care regimen but should be used in selected patients who may die of starvation rather than from tumor spread (Bozzetti et al. 1996; Cozzaglio et al. 1997). A favorable criterion for selecting these patients is a Karnofsky performance status > 50 (Cozzaglio et al. 1997).

The need to treat dehydration in terminally ill patients remains a controversial issue (MacDonald 2002; Fainsinger 2002). The intensity of dry mouth and thirst are independent of the quantity of parenteral hydration, whereas the intensity of nausea and drowsiness is significantly lower in inoperable obstructed patients treated with more than 1 liter/day of parenteral fluids (Ventafridda et al. 1998; Mercadante et al. 2000; Ripamonti et al. 2000). As a high level of hydration may increase the GI secretions, it is necessary to keep a balance between the efficacy of the treatment and the adverse effects.

Intravenous hydration can be difficult and uncomfortable for terminal cancer patients who have not had a central venous catheter previously inserted. Hypodermoclysis (Fainsinger et al. 1994) is a valid alternative with few problems and several potential advantages over the intravenous route. It is a simple and inexpensive way of managing patients both at hospital and at home, and can be started by any staff member able to give a subcutaneous injection.

Box 59.2 Summary – bowel obstruction

Bowel obstruction is a distressing outcome, above all in patients with abdominal and pelvic cancer in the advanced and terminal stage of disease.

Surgery should not routinely be undertaken in patients with poor prognostic criteria such as intra-abdominal carcinomatosis, poor performance status, and massive ascites.

Medical measures such as analgesics, antisecretory drugs, and anti-emetics administered alone or in combination should be used to relieve symptoms.

A nasogastric tube should be used only as a temporary measure and a venting gastrostomy should be considered if drugs fail in reducing vomiting to an acceptable level.

Total parenteral nutrition should be considered only for patients who may die of starvation rather than from tumor spread. Parenteral hydration is sometimes indicated to correct nausea and regular mouth care is the treatment of choice for dry mouth.

A collaborative approach by surgeons and physicians can offer patients an individualized and appropriate symptom management plan.

BIBLIOGRAPHY

Sentinel articles

Baines M, Oliver DJ, Carter RL. Medical management of intestinal obstruction in patients with advanced malignant disease. A clinical and pathological study. *Lancet* 1985;Nov 2:990–3.

Cozzaglio L, Balzola F, Cosentino F et al. Outcome of cancer patients receiving home parenteral nutrition. *J Parenteral Enteral Nutrition* 1997;21:339–42.

Davis MP, Furste A. Glycopyrrolate: a useful drug in the palliation of mechanical bowel obstruction. *J Pain Symptom Manage* 1999;18:153–4.

De Conno F, Caraceni A, Zecca E, Spoldi E, Ventafridda V. Continuous subcutaneous infusion of hyoscine butylbromide reduces secretions in patients with gastrointestinal obstruction. *J Pain Symptom Manage* 1991;6/8:484–6.

Fainsinger RL, MacEachern T, Miller MJ et al. The use of hypodermoclysis for rehydration in terminally ill cancer patients. *J Pain Symptom Manage* 1994;9:298–302.

Fainsinger RL, Spachynski K, Hanson J, Bruera E. Symptom control in terminally ill patients with malignant bowel obstruction (MBO). *J Pain Symptom Manage* 1994;9/1:12–18.

Mercadante S, Ripamonti C, Casuccio A, Zecca E, Groff L. Comparison of octreotide and hyoscine butylbromide in controlling gastrointestinal symptoms due to malignant inoperable bowel obstruction. *Support Care Cancer* 2000;8:188–91.

Ripamonti C, Mercadante S, Groff L, Zecca E, De Conno F, Casuccio A. Role of octreotide and scopolamine butylbromide, and hydration in symptom control of patients with inoperable bowel obstruction and nasogastric tubes: a prospective randomized trial. *J Pain Symptom Manage* 2000;19:23–34.

Ventafridda V, Ripamonti C, Caraceni A, Spoldi E, Messina L, De Conno F. The management of inoperable gastrointestinal obstruction in terminal cancer patients. *Tumori* 1990;76:389–93.

Wallis F, Campbell KL, Eremin O, Hussey JK. Self-expanding metal stents in the management of colorectal carcinoma – a preliminary report (see comments). *Clin Radiol* 1998;53:251–4.

Review articles

Baines MJ. Nausea, vomiting and intestinal obstruction. In *ABC of Palliative Care*, ed. M Fallon, B O'Neill, pp. 16–18. London: BMJ Books, 1998.

Baines MJ. The pathophysiology and management of malignant intestinal obstruction. In *Oxford Textbook of Palliative Medicine*, ed. D Doyle, GWC Hanks, N MacDonald, pp. 526–34. Oxford: Oxford University Press, 1998.

Bozzetti F, Amadori D, Bruera E et al. Guidelines on artificial nutrition versus hydration in terminal cancer patients. *Nutrition* 1996;12:163–7.

Fainsinger R. Hydration. In *Gastrointestinal Symptoms in Advanced Cancer Patients*, ed. C Ripamonti, E Bruera, pp. 395–410. Oxford: Oxford University Press, 2002.

Fallon MT. The physiology of somatostatin and its synthetic analogue, octreotide. *Eur J Palliat Care* 1994;1:20–2.

Feuer DJ, Broadley KE with members of the Systematic Review Steering Committee. Systematic review and meta-analysis of corticosteroids for the resolution of malignant bowel obstruction in advanced gynaecological and gastrointestinal cancers. *Ann Oncol* 1999a;10:1035–41.

Feuer DJ, Broadley KE, Shepherd JH, Barton DPJ. Systematic review of surgery in malignant bowel obstruction in advanced gynecological and gastrointestinal cancer. *Gynecol Oncol* 1999*b*;75:313–22.

Follon BG. Nausea and vomiting unrelated to cancer treatment. In *Principles and Practice of Supportive Oncology*, Vol. 12, ed. A Berger, RK Portenoy, DW Weissman, pp. 179–90. Philadelphia: Lippincott-Raven, 1998.

MacDonald N. Ethical considerations in feeding or hydrating advanced cancer patients. In *Gastrointestinal Symptoms in Advanced Cancer Patients*, ed. C Ripamonti, E Bruera, pp. 411–23. Oxford: Oxford University Press, 2002.

Mercadante S. Pain in inoperable bowel obstruction. *Pain Digest* 1995;5:9–13.

Pisters KMS, Kris MG. Treatment-related nausea and vomiting. In *Principles and Practice of Supportive Oncology*, Vol. 11, ed. A Berger, RK Portenoy, DW Weissman, pp. 165–77. Philadelphia: Lippincott-Raven, 1998.

Ripamonti C. Bowel obstruction. In *Principle and Practice of Supportive Oncology*, ed. A Berger, RK Portenoy, DW Weissman, pp. 207–16. Philadelphia: Lippincott-Raven, 1998.

Ripamonti C, Bruera E. Chronic nausea and vomiting. In *Gastrointestinal Symptoms in Advanced Cancer Patients*, ed. C Ripamonti, E Bruera, pp. 169–92. Oxford: Oxford University Press, 2002.

Ripamonti C, Twycross R, Baines M et al. Clinical-practice recommendations for the management of bowel obstruction in patients with end-stage cancer. Working group of the European Association for Palliative Care. *Support Care Cancer* 2001;9:223–33.

Rousseau P. Management of malignant bowel obstruction in advanced cancer: a brief review. *J Palliat Med* 1998;1:65–72.

Twycross R, Back I, et al. Nausea and vomiting in advanced cancer. *Eur J Palliat Care* 1998;5:39–45.

Ventafridda V, Ripamonti C, Sbanotto A, De Conno F. Mouth care. In *Oxford Textbook of Palliative Medicine*, ed. D Doyle, GWC Hanks, N MacDonald, pp. 691–707. Oxford: Oxford University Press, 1998.

60

Bone metastases

Carlos Centeno[1] and Alvaro Sanz[2]

[1] Hospital Los Montalvos, Salamanca, Spain
[2] Hospital Universitario de Valladolid, Spain

Introduction

The tumors that most frequently develop bone metastases are those from the breast, prostate, thyroid, lung, and kidney. The most common sites of bone metastases include vertebrae (70%), pelvis (40%), femur, and ribs.

Bone metastases are due to the hematogenous dissemination of neoplastic cells from the primary tumor. Metastatic cells settle in the bone marrow before affecting the cortex. Around those cells a release of factors takes place activating the osteoclasts and increasing bone resorption. As a reaction, the osteoblasts increase bone formation. Thus, lytic and blastic components coexist in bone metastases. X-ray imaging not only shows the tumor occupying bone volume, but a complex of neoplastic tissue and bone reaction both lytic and blastic.

Although many bone metastases are asymptomatic, the main clinical features (Table 60.1), where present, are usually localized pain, fractures, and collapses, with their functional (instability), neurological (spinal cord compression) or metabolic (hypercalcemia) complications. The alkaline phosphatase that indicates osteoblastic activity rises in 70% of the patients diagnosed with bone metastases. X-ray, computer-assisted tomography (CAT) and magnetic resonance imaging (MRI) show bone metastases as an increase or decrease of density in relation to the adjacent bone. Bone scintigraphy is more sensitive than conventional radiographs, and it shows the blastic activity around the metastases. MRI is even more sensitive and can be used to confirm early metastases shown by bone scan but not by conventional x-rays.

Bone metastases are not life threatening in themselves, but their presence means that there is a hematogenous tumor dissemination. However, there are patients who can survive a long time with bone metastases, especially if it is of small extent and the primary tumor responds to systemic treatment, as in the case of breast and prostate

Table 60.1. Clinical findings in patients with bone metastases

Symptom or syndrome
Pain
Continuous bone pain
Incidental pain
Pain with mixed bone and neuropathic component
Neuropathic pain
Impaired mobility
Anemia or marrow depression
Deterioration in performance status
Bone fractures
Vertebral collapses
Nerve root compression
Spinal cord compression
Hypercalcemia

cancers, where the median survival is about 24–36 months. Nevertheless, bone pain and complications can affect the patient's mobility and general well-being.

Bone pain

Two out of three patients with bone metastases suffer pain; usually of the somatic nociceptive kind. It is thought that the pain results from the release of nociceptive chemical transmitters and from the stimulation of nerve endings in the periosteum and the mechanoreceptors in the bone marrow. Other causes of pain are the effects on nerve structures, microfractures, and reactive muscular spasms.

The pain is usually described as aching, persistent, intense, and localized. Weight carrying, movement, and pressure on the affected area increase it, and rest lessens it. Pain is often localized in an area where there is a selective zone of hyperalgesia over the bone level. There may not be any relation between the intensity of the pain and the radiological appearance of the lesion.

Analgesic drugs

To deal with bone pain it is necessary to use analgesic drugs before and during any other analgesic treatment; but if analgesics are used simultaneously with other treatments such as radiotherapy, then the doses must be adjusted to avoid toxicity when the pain changes in intensity.

Bone pain is normally responsive to opioids but extra dosage may be required if the pain is intensified by movement. The occurrence of this incidental factor is an indication of bad pain-control prognosis in the control of pain. In addition, the presence of a neuropathic component worsens the prognosis.

NSAIDs are effective for mild or medium oncological pain. COX-2 selective inhibitors are preferable. However, the effect of adding them to the opioids is doubtful and their systematic use as an adjuvant for bone pain is unjustified. It is likely that a higher analgesia is obtained by increasing the doses of opioids, than by using an NSAID, while at the same time avoiding polypharmacy and adverse side effects.

Corticoids are adjuvants for bone pain. Short-term improvements can be dramatic and may be observed in 1 or 2 days. If after 5 days of treatment there is no relief, they should be stopped. The effect is transitory and rarely lasts more than a month.

Chemotherapy and hormone therapy

Chemotherapy provides symptom relief for patients in an advanced stage of cancer. Therapeutic benefit depends on patients' sensitivity to treatment and on their general condition. For chemosensitive tumors and those with a tendency to dissemination, like breast cancer or myeloma, chemotherapy is an essential part of palliative treatment. In general, there is no ideal regimen; therefore, the least toxic one is applied which does not jeopardize efficacy. Hormone therapy treatments have low toxicity and are effective for hormone-dependent cancers like those of the breast or the prostate (Table 60.2).

Radiation therapy

External radiation therapy is commonly used to provide pain relief for localized painful bone metastases due to its high efficacy and excellent tolerance. Different fractionation schedule trials (5–10 fractions; 3–5 Gy per fraction) and single fractionation trials (8–9 Gy) have yielded similar results. Both techniques achieve some pain relief in 2–3 weeks in more than 70% of the patients, with the effect lasting nearly 3 months. One year after treatment, half of the patients are still pain-free. If pain recurs, it is advisable to reirradiate the affected area.

Hemibody irradiation is a special technique for pain control in multiple bone metastases patients; 6 to 8 Gy are administered in a single dose, with pain-relieving results similar to those of more localized irradiation. Because of its high degree of toxicity, both digestive and hematogenous, this therapy is not recommended for patients with reduced blood cell counts, poor general condition, or with a very short life expectancy.

Radiopharmaceuticals

Strontium (Sr89) is a beta-particle-emitting calcium analogue. It is administered by intravenous injection and selectively retained at sites of osteoblastic lesions. It achieves palliation of the pain produced by multiple metastases sites, in 40–90%

Table 60.2. Hormonal treatment in breast and prostate cancer

	Premenopausal breast cancer	Postmenopausal breast cancer	Prostate cancer
First-line	Ovarian ablation LH–RH analogue (Gosereline or leuprolide) Radiotherapy Oopherectomy	Anti-estrogen Tamoxifen Toremifene	Complete androgenic block LH–RH analogue (Gosereline or leuprolide) + anti-androgen (Flutamide or bicalutamide) Orchiectomy
Second-line	Anti-estrogen Tamoxifen Toremifene	Aromatase inactivator Formestane Anastrozole Letrozol Exemestane	Anti-androgen withdrawal
Third-line	Progestogen Megestrol Medroxyprogesterone	Progestogen Megestrol Medroxyprogesterone	Estrogen / ketoconazole

Note: The first- and second-line treatment efficacy is similar for premenopausal and postmenopausal breast cancer patients.

of patients; the dose may be readministered for certain patients. Its analgesic effect is not immediate and it may take weeks to appear, although it may then last several months. Treatment with Sr89 should be considered for patients suffering from refractory pain, especially multifocal, caused by osteoblastic lesions. It is not recommended as a treatment on its own for patients suffering from severe cancer pain because its analgesic effects are not immediate.

Bisphosphonates

Bisphosphonates, which inhibit bone resorption, reduce the intensity of the pain and the incidence of skeletal complications in patients suffering from bone metastases. Pamidronate seems to be the most efficient bisphosphonate for the prevention of bone complications, and probably for its analgesic effects too. Pamidronate provides partial pain relief in nearly 50% of patients (Table 60.3). Its effect increases during the 2 weeks following the treatment and lasts up to 4–8 weeks. After this period of time, the dose may be readministered. For patients who wish to remain at home, 2-hour infusions of subcutaneous clodronate seem to be effective. Also, zolendronate is a new bisphosphonate more potent than others that has been used to treat bone pain.

Table 60.3. Analgesic regimens with bisphosphonates, as recommended by the Association for Palliative Medicine of Great Britain and Ireland for Palliative Care

Pamidronate	90–120 mg in 500–1000 ml of saline solution 2 hours intravenous infusion
Clodronate	600–1500 mg in 500 ml of saline solution 4 hours intravenous infusion

Pathologic fractures

Pathologic fractures occur after a minimal trauma caused to an abnormal bone and they appear in 5–10% of patients with bone metastases. Although they are usually associated with a sudden increase in pain and/or functional disability, they often initially go unnoticed.

There are few (less than 5%) pathologic fractures that mend only with immobility, since lytic activity impairs the regeneration. Therefore, orthopedic stabilization is recommended. Besides, it relieves the pain earlier, provides earlier mobility, and facilitates patient care. Fixation of lytic lesions at risk for fracture is furthermore advisable, especially if they are situated in weight-bearing bones, are big, or impair the cortical bone. For long bones, internal fixation by intramedullary pin is recommended; it is a technique with low morbidity. If the lesion is situated near a joint (head or femoral neck), prosthetic replacement is the most appropiate technique.

After orthopedic stabilization, radiotherapy is applied for its effectiveness in reducing pain and possible further fractures. There is no adverse effect from irradiating metal or plastic prostheses or fixations. Patients who are not suitable for a surgical fixation due to their poor general condition or poor prognosis can obtain some pain relief with immobility and traction, apart from the application of radiotherapy.

Vertebral collapse and instability

Vertebral collapses are common in patients with bone metastases. These can be silent or can appear as a pain in the back and/or neurologic impairment. The vertebral instability syndrome secondary to collapses is the equivalent of the unstable long bones fractures involving the axial skeleton, although x-ray only detects collapses, not fracture lines. It is characterized by severe pain whenever there is any movement. Slight pain is palliated with an orthopedic corset (or a surgical collar, if it is cervical pain). In extreme cases, relief is only obtained with total immobility in decubitus position. Since no movement is allowed, the only possible treatment is fixation of the injured vertebra. Radiotherapy only produces moderate improvement as the pain has a mechanical origin.

Spinal cord compression

Spinal cord compression syndrome appears in 5% of patients suffering from cancer and requires urgent diagnosis and treatment to avoid irreparable sequelae. It presents in the following order of frequency: in the thoracic vertebral column (60–70%), where the medullary cavity is narrower, in the lumbar spine (10%), and in the cervical spine (10–20%).

The first symptom is almost always a progressive pain, either axial or radicular, which increases with movements and is palliated by sedation. Subsequently three patients in four develop weakness or loss of strength in their legs, sensory disturbance and autonomic dysfunction such as loss of bladder control, hesitancy or urinary retention, and constipation. Finally, if it progresses, the pain diminishes and a complete paraplegia develops.

When this clinical picture is suspected (due to pain or neurologic symptoms), an urgent MRI must be performed to determine whether the compression is present and its level.

The prognosis improves if the treatment is given inmediately, especially within the first 24 hours from the beginning of the clinical picture, and if the patient keeps a good functional level. If the patient only suffers from radicular pain or paraparesis, functional recovery is achieved in 80% of cases; but when there is paraplegia, mobility is only recovered in 10%. Before confirming the diagnosis, the first step is to administer corticoids (dexamethasone 8–10 mg, tid). Decompressive surgery is recommended in vertebral instability, relapse in a previously radiated area, cervical injuries, childhood tumors, and absence of histologic confirmation of malignancy. After the laminectomy, radiotherapy is recommended. In other situations, external radiotherapy alone achieves the same results especially when combined with surgery.

Hypercalcemia

Around 10–40% of patients with advanced cancer develop hypercalcemia. In a few cases hypercalcemia is due to the bone's massive destruction by metastatic disease. For a more detailed discussion, see Chapter 53.

Conclusion

Pain is the most frequent symptom in bone metastases. Bone pain always needs a multidisciplinary and individualized therapeutic treatment. Treatment options include analgesics and coanalgesics, specific palliative oncologic treatments and bisphosphonates. When dealing with a localized phenomenon, single doses of radiotherapy can bring complete relief. Pathologic fractures must be treated with orthopedic surgery and radiotherapy. Spinal cord compression is a medical emergency and the patient's functional prognosis depends on its quick and appropriate treatment.

Box 60.1 Summary – bone metastases

The presence of an incidental or neuropathic component indicates a bad prognosis in the control of bone pain.

The additive effect of NSAIDs is doubtful and their systematic use as adjuvant analgesic drugs for bone pain is not justified.

Corticoids are good adjuvants for bone pain. Their effect is rapid and can usually be observed in 24–48 hours.

External radiation therapy is the treatment of choice to provide pain relief for localized painful bone metastases due to its high efficacy and excellent tolerance. It can be administered in only a single fraction.

Reirradiation can be performed if pain recurs, as can other techniques for multiple metastases.

Pamidronate seems to be the most efficient bisphosphonate for analgesic effect and provides partial pain relief in nearly 50% of patients.

Hormonal therapy is indicated in breast cancer and prostate bone metastases. In addition, for these tumors, as for myeloma and microcytic lung tumors, chemotherapy can be used.

Pathologic fractures do not mend with immobilization alone. They are treated with orthopedic stabilization and postradiation therapy. Fixation of lytic lesions at risk for fracture is advisable.

Spinal cord compression syndrome requires urgent diagnosis and treatment to avoid irreparable sequelae.

When spinal cord compression is suspected, due to pain or the neurologic clinical picture, an urgent MRI must always be performed.

BIBLIOGRAPHY

Sentinel articles

Eisenberg E, Berkey CS, Carr DB et al. Efficacy and safety of nonsteroidal anti-inflammatory drugs for cancer pain: a meta-analysis. *J Clin Oncol* 1994;12:2756–65.

Helweg-Larsen S, Sorensen PS. Symptoms and signs in metastasic spinal cord compression: a study of progression from first symptoms until diagnosis in 153 patients. *Eur J Cancer* 1994;30: 396–8.

Mannix K, Ahmedzai SH, Anderson H, Bennett M, Lloyd-Williams M, Wilcock A. Using bisphosphonates to control the pain of bone metastases: evidence-based guidelines for palliative care. *Palliat Med* 2000;14:455–61.

Price P, Hoskin PJ, Eaton D, Austin D, Palmer SG, Yarnold JR. Prospective randomised trial of single and multifraction radiotherapy schedules in the treatment of painful bone metastases. *Radiother Oncol* 1986;6:247.

Walker P, Watanabe S, Lawlor P, Hanson J, Pereira J, Bruera E. Subcutaneous clodronate: a study evaluating efficacy in hypercalcemia of malignancy and local toxicity. *Ann Oncol* 1997;8:915–16.

Yarnold JR, on behalf of the Bone Pain Trial Group. Bone Pain Trial: a prospective randomised trial comparing a single dose of 8 Gy and a multifraction radiotherapy schedule in the treatment of metastasic bone pain. *Br J Cancer* 1998;78(Suppl. 2):6.

Review articles

Abrahm JL. Management of pain and spinal cord compression in patients with advanced cancer. *Ann Intern Med* 1999;131:37–46.

Fulfaro F, Casuccio A, Ticozzi C, Ripamonti C. The role of bisphosphonates in the treatment of painful metastatic bone disease: a review of phase III trials. *Pain* 1998;78:157–69.

Jenkins CA, Bruera E. Nonsteroidal anti-inflammatory drugs as adjuvant analgesics in cancer patients. *Palliat Med* 1999;12:183–96.

McQuay HJ, Collins SL, Carroll D, Moore RA. Radiotherapy for the palliation of painful bone metastases (Cochrane Review). In *The Cochrane Library 1*. Oxford: Update Software, 2001.

Mercadante S. Malignant bone pain: pathophysiology and treatment. *Pain* 1997;69:1–18.

Pereira J. Management of bone pain. *Topics Palliat Care* 1998;2:79–116.

Ripamonti C, Fulfaro F. Malignant bone pain: pathophysiology and treatments. *Curr Rev Pain* 2000;4:187–96.

Sabo D, Bernd L. Surgical management of skeletal metastases of the extremities. *J Am Acad Orthop Surg* 2000;8:56–65.

Internet sites

Managing bone complications of advanced breast cancer and multiple myeloma.
    http://www.zometa.com

Center Watch: Clinical Trials in Bone Metastases.
    http://www.centerwatch.com/patient/studies/cat348.html

61

Meningeal cancer

Neil A. Hagen

University of Calgary, Calgary

Cancer can spread to the cerebral spinal fluid (CSF) and meninges, and rarely, can originate there. When cancer involves the meninges, it causes cancerous meningitis. It has clinical similarities to infectious meningitis in that it commonly causes confusion, drowsiness, a stiff neck, and other meningeal signs, and if untreated, causes death. It is different from infectious meningitis in that the time course is somewhat slower (many days or weeks) and it more commonly tends to cause focal neurological deficits. Meningeal cancer is a devastating clinical situation; it causes severe neurological impairment, and carries a grim prognosis despite treatment. Fortunately, distressing symptoms can respond to intervention.

Meningeal cancer is fairly common. About 5% of patients with metastatic cancer will develop clinically significant cancerous meningitis, although autopsy surveys show a higher prevalence, indicating it can be asymptomatic particularly in patients who are otherwise quite ill. A peculiar feature of the epidemiology of meningeal cancer is that some kinds of malignancies have a striking predilection to metastasize to the leptomeninges, such as melanoma. About 90% of patients who die from metastatic melanoma have central nervous system metastases, and this commonly includes the meninges. Other kinds of cancer are much less likely to metastasize to the leptomeninges, such as bladder or prostate cancer. However, it can occur in any kind of cancer. About 5% of patients who die from a malignant supratentorial glioma have meningeal spread of glioma at autopsy, but only rarely is gliomatous meningitis of any clinical significance.

Pathophysiologically, the process is characterized by invasion of meninges and adjacent neural tissue by cancer cells. Grossly, at autopsy the meninges have the appearance of being coated with icing sugar. In addition however, there can be areas of bulky tumor growth with a cobblestone-type appearance. Commonly this will occur at the bottom of the thecal sac, as cancer cells literally settle downward by gravity in the CSF. Cancer cells invade through the meninges into adjacent neural tissue and thereby cause symptoms. Brain involvement by meningeal cancer can result in convulsions and confusion. Brain stem invasion can result in drowsiness and difficulty in breathing. Cranial nerve dysfunction can be manifest by dysphagia, diplopia, and other consequences of focal cranial nerve palsies. Spinal cord compression from bulky meningeal spread can result in myelopathy. Peripheral nerve invasion can result in lower motor neuron type weakness, numbness, bladder failure, and constipation. The arachnoid villi can be literally plugged with cancer cells, interfering with reabsorption of cerebral spinal fluid. This can result in a syndrome of communicating hydrocephalus and raised intracranial pressure. The raised intracranial pressure can itself be life threatening.

In order to assess a patient in whom you are considering a diagnosis of meningeal cancer, the history, general physical exam, and neurological exam will often be essentially diagnostic. On history, the clinical tempo of meningeal cancer usually unfolds more quickly than the activity of the cancer elsewhere in the body; as described above, typically, neurological symptoms unfold over several days or a few weeks. The clinical features of meningeal cancer are quite varied. Often there are focal neurological symptoms, with or without achy pain. Focal symptoms can include weakness, numbness, double vision, and so on. While meningeal cancer is often painful, painless lower motor neuron weakness at multiple sites of the neuraxis is strongly suggestive of the diagnosis. On physical examination, there may be evidence of neck stiffness (meningismus). A familiar clinical pattern of meningeal cancer is that there are usually more neurological signs than there are symptoms, the neurologic signs are found at multiple levels of the neuraxis, and signs are often asymmetrical. On history and physical exam there will commonly be evidence of advanced cancer, so one would need to look for evidence of liver enlargement, adenopathy, or bone metastases.

A computed tomography (CT) scan of the head may be normal, may show a picture consistent with communicating hydrocephalus, or may show meningeal enhancement. The magnetic resonance imaging (MRI) findings are likewise quite varied. An MRI scan of the brain or spine without gadolinium enhancement can be falsely normal. Typically, a gadolinium-enhanced MRI is abnormal and can be considered diagnostic of an active meningeal process; it does not rule out infection, however. An MRI scan may also surprisingly show evidence of an intramedullary tumor (a metastasis of cancer directly into the spinal cord itself). Most patients who develop intramedullary metastasis have meningeal cancer as the underlying mechanism. After a history and physical examination, patients will generally need to have a scan of their brain in order to be sure that it is safe to perform a spinal puncture. A spinal fluid examination is the most definitive test for meningeal cancer but can be falsely negative. Up to six spinal lumbar punctures may need to be done in order to make a cytological diagnosis, although usually something is abnormal within the spinal fluid on even the first tap, such as raised protein or elevated white blood cell counts. An MRI scan with gadolinium without a spinal tap can be considered diagnostic if the clinical setting is appropriate.

The differential diagnosis of leptomeningeal cancer is essentially the differential diagnosis of focal or multifocal neurological disease in a cancer patient. One would look for disease elsewhere in the neuraxis such as metastases to the brain, brain stem, spinal cord, the epidural space (epidural cord compression or nerve root compression), plexus, or peripheral nerve. If a patient presents with diffuse problems such as diffuse achiness, one would consider diffuse bone metastasis. A presenting complaint of confusion would raise the possibility of multiple brain metastases, a metabolic abnormality such as hypercalcemia or disseminated intravascular coagulation.

Rarely, meningeal cancer is curable, such as the clinical scenario of lymphoma that has meningeal spread at the time of initial presentation. Breast cancer and other tumors can be responsive to radiation therapy or intrathecal chemotherapy and prognosis is usually several months. Usually however, meningeal cancer is not curable and typically results in death within 4–6 weeks from initial diagnosis, particularly when a solid tumor such as lung or renal cancer is the site of origin. Some patients elect not to receive any direct oncologic treatment of meningeal cancer. A conservative approach would be to offer interventions to help manage distressing symptoms: dexamethasone and analgesics for headache, regular monitoring for bladder failure, antinauseants for dizziness, and so on. Patients who have potentially chemosensitive meningeal tumors such as lymphoma, leukemia, or breast cancer can receive systemic chemotherapy or intrathecal chemotherapy through a lumbar puncture or through placement of an Ommaya reservoir into a lateral ventricle. Symptomatic areas within the neuraxis, with documented bulky disease, can respond well to focal radiation therapy. Occasional patients with severe headache from raised intracranial pressure and communicating hydrocephalus will have very good relief of symptoms with repeated palliative spinal taps.

Meningeal cancer is a devastating clinical occurrence and typically heralds the terminal phase of a malignancy. It can be of prognostic value for patients and their families to be made aware of the diagnosis, and many symptoms of meningeal cancer can be well controlled with aggressive supportive care.

Box 61.1 Meningeal involvement by cancer

Causes symptoms and signs at multiple levels of the neuraxis.

Has some clinical features in common with infectious meningitis.

Is rarely curable, and only sometimes treatable, but distressing symptoms can often be controlled.

Progressive neurologic decline and death usually occur over weeks or a few months.

BIBLIOGRAPHY

Sentinel articles

Olsen ME, Chernik NL, Posner JB. Infiltration of the leptomeninges by systemic cancer; a clinical and pathologic study. *Arch Neurol* 1974;30:122–37.

Posner JB, Chernik NL, Intracranial metastases from systemic cancer. *Adv Neurol* 1978;19: 575–87.

Wasserstrom WR. Leptomeningeal metastases. In *Neurological Complications of Cancer*, ed. RG Wiley. New York: Marcel Dekker, 1995.

Wasserstrom W, Glass JP, Posner JB. Diagnosis and treatment of leptomeningeal metastases from solid tumors; experience with 90 patients. *Cancer* 1982;49:759–72.

Internet sites

Meningeal carcinomatosis in breast cancer. This web site shows typical MRI scan findings in meningeal carcinomatosis, published in the *New England Journal of Medicine.*
  http://www.content.nejm.org/cgi/content/short/342/15/1093

Metastatic tumors to the brain and spine.
  http://medhlp.netusa.net/lib/mets.htm

The Nature of Cancer.
  http://www.carelife.com/cancer/med_onc/nature_cancer.html

Active Therapies for CNS Tumors.
  http://www.brain.mgh.harvard.edu/therapies.htm

62

Pleural and pericardial effusions

Michael J. Boyer

Royal Prince Alfred Hospital, Camperdown

Introduction

Pleural and pericardial effusions may occur in patients with advanced malignancy, or may be the presenting manifestation of malignancy. The symptoms caused by effusions can be the cause of substantial morbidity, and may limit the quality of life for patients with advanced cancer. With appropriate management, these symptoms can be minimized or eliminated. This chapter is concerned predominantly with the management of effusions in patients with pre-existing malignancy, rather than the approach to patients presenting with an undiagnosed pleural or pericardial effusion.

Pleural effusion

Up to 10 liters of fluid traverses the pleural space each day. Under normal circumstances, the rate of fluid resorption is equal to the rate of production, so there is no net change in the amount of fluid that is present (only 5–10 ml). Four factors maintain this balance. These include the hydrostatic and colloid pressures of fluid in capillaries, capillary permeability, and fluid absorption by lymphatics. Changes in any of these factors can result in accumulation of pleural fluid. Thus, in patients with malignancy, effusions may arise because of increased production (for example because of changes in capillary permeability due to tumor deposits on the pleural surface) or reduced absorption (for example due to obstruction of mediastinal lymphatics). Malignant effusions are typically exudates (protein content >3 g/100 ml).

The most common causes of pleural effusions differ between men and women (Table 62.1). Overall, combining both sexes, breast cancer, lung cancer, and lymphoma account for 75% of all malignant pleural effusions. The typical presentation of a pleural effusion in a patient with known malignancy is of increasing dyspnea. Other symptoms may include a dry cough or dull chest pain. The major

Table 62.1. Primary tumors in patients with malignant pleural effusions

Male	%	Female	%
Lung	49	Breast	37
Lymphoma	21	Genitourinary	21
Gastrointestinal	7	Lung	15
Genitourinary	6	Lymphoma	8
Melanoma	1	Gastrointestinal	4
Mesothelioma	1	Melanoma	3
Other	4	Other	2
Unknown	11	Unknown	9

signs are of dullness to percussion and diminished breath sounds. These symptoms and signs are not specific to malignant pleural effusions, however, and further investigations are required to confirm the nature of the effusion. For example, in a patient with a past history of malignancy, and no previously identified site of tumor recurrence, other causes of effusion, such as cardiac failure and infection, need to be excluded. There is a major difference in prognosis between these causes of effusion and recurrence of malignancy, and this will be of importance to the patient.

The presence of a pleural effusion is usually confirmed with a chest x-ray. The presence of 200–300 ml of fluid results in blunting of the costophrenic angle, with opacification of the hemithorax indicating an effusion of several liters. Ultrasound is also able to demonstrate the presence of an effusion, and may be useful for identifying an appropriate location for thoracentesis to be performed. Generally, the radiologic appearances are straightforward, but occasionally effusions confined to interlobar fissures or the subpulmonic space may be difficult to identify.

The diagnosis of a malignant pleural effusion requires the demonstration of malignant cells within the pleural fluid. This is most easily achieved by removing a sample of fluid and submitting it for cytological examination. Whilst other features, such as protein content, glucose and LDH may be of value, ultimately it is the demonstration of malignant cells within the effusion that is of importance, and which guides both therapy and prognosis.

In patients known to have neoplasms, cytologic identification of tumor cells occurs in 40–95% of cases. There is a low false positive rate, which ranges from 0–3%. The likelihood of a positive finding can be increased by taking a larger volume of fluid and producing a cell block, or by the use of immunocytochemistry. In addition, the use of pleural biopsy, which can be performed at the same time as thoracentesis, may add to the diagnostic accuracy. On rare occasions, thoracotomy or thoracoscopy may be required in order to make a diagnosis. This is more commonly the case in patients without a pre-existing diagnosis of malignancy, who simply present with an undiagnosed pleural effusion, than in patients with a previously identified tumor.

The approach to the management of pleural effusions depends upon the type and extent of the underlying malignancy. If there is a reasonable prospect that systemic therapy will produce tumor response and control of the disease (for example, in a patient with lymphoma, or previously untreated small cell carcinoma of the lung), then it is likely that the effusion will also be controlled. By contrast, if disease control is not likely to be achieved systemically, then local therapies are usually required. In these cases, the goal of treatment is almost always palliation of symptoms, in particular dyspnea and cough. The method chosen for treatment must take into account the patient's overall condition and estimated prognosis, and should aim to provide relief for the remainder of the expected life span.

Needle aspiration (thoracentesis) is the simplest local treatment for pleural effusions and may be both a diagnostic and therapeutic procedure. The relief gained by patients who undergo thoracentesis is usually immediate, although some patients may develop a transient increase in cough. The procedure is straightforward, although there are associated risks including bleeding, pneumothorax, and re-expansion pulmonary edema. Unfortunately, the improvement produced by thoracentesis alone is only short-lived, with the majority of effusions and symptoms recurring within a month. In addition, in patients undergoing repeated thoracenteses, effusions may become loculated, making adequate drainage increasingly difficult. Hence, in a patient with a prognosis estimated to be more than a few weeks, early definitive management is preferable to repeated thoracenteses.

More lasting control of pleural fluid and symptoms is produced by pleurodesis. The principle underlying this procedure is the obliteration of the pleural space by the introduction of a sclerosing agent into the pleural cavity. In order to be effective, it is necessary that the pleural space be thoroughly drained prior to instillation of the sclerosant. This allows the visceral and parietal pleura to come into contact, so that they may fuse together when an inflammatory reaction is produced by the sclerosant. Drainage to dryness can be achieved with an intercostal catheter or using video-assisted thoracoscopy. When an intercostal catheter is used, drainage should be allowed to fall to less than 100 ml over 24 hours, before the sclerosant is introduced. If there is significant residual fluid when the sclerosant is introduced, dilution and lack of apposition of the pleural surfaces may prevent the development of an adequate reaction. Following insertion of the sclerosant, an intercostal catheter is left in place until drainage again decreases to less than 100 ml per day. There have been no adequately controlled comparisons between the different methods of drainage of effusions prior to pleurodesis. Often, the choice of method will be determined by factors such as the performance status of the patient, availability of thoracic surgical services, and the urgency of the procedure.

A variety of sclerosants have been used to achieve pleurodesis. These include talc (either insufflated or as a slurry), tetracycline (using the intravenous formulation, which is no longer available in most parts of the world), doxycycline (which is now commonly used in place of tetracycline), bleomycin, mitoxantrone, doxorubicin, and nitrogen mustard. In addition, biological agents such as *Corynebacterium parvum* have also been employed. It has generally been felt that talc is the most effective sclerosant, and it is the most widely used agent in patients undergoing surgical drainage with thoracoscopy. However, there are no adequately performed randomized trials that clearly demonstrate talc to be superior to other agents. There are however randomized trials comparing several of the other agents, and although there are shortcomings in their design, these demonstrate that bleomycin and tetracycline have similar efficacy, with fewer side effects than the other agents. Most sclerosants can produce a painful pleuritis when instilled. Consequently it is important that patients receiving these agents be given adequate analgesia.

There are some patients in whom pleurodesis (no matter how it is carried out) is unlikely to be successful. This is the case in patients who have underlying pulmonary collapse due to factors other than pleural fluid. For example, if there is collapse due to bronchial obstruction, there will be inadequate expansion of the lung at the time of attempted pleurodesis to allow apposition of the pleural surfaces.

A newer approach to the management of malignant effusions is the use of a chronic indwelling pleural catheter. The catheter is introduced into the pleural space and then left in situ, with drainage occurring on an intermittent basis (usually every second day). In a randomized trial this approach has been shown to have similar efficacy to doxcycline pleurodesis, but required less time in hospital.

It is uncommon for a malignant pleural effusion itself to be the cause of death in such patients. Hence, the prognosis is variable, and is related to the extent and location of other sites of metastatic disease, and the availability and efficacy of systemic therapy. When all patients are considered, 65% will die within 3 months. However, some patients will have prolonged survival. For example, women with metastatic breast cancer who develop a pleural effusion have a median survival of 10–15 months. Even amongst women with this diagnosis, there is variability, based on whether the effusion is an early or late manifestation of metastatic malignancy.

Pericardial effusions

Pericardial effusions are most commonly caused by breast cancer, lung cancer, or lymphoma. Although common at autopsy (25–35% of patients with breast or lung cancer), symptomatic pericardial effusion is a relatively uncommon problem. The pathophysiology is similar to that of malignant pleural effusions. Thus, pericardial effusions may be caused by parietal or visceral pericardial metastases, or by lymphatic obstruction following infiltration of mediastinal lymphatics. In addition, the usual non-neoplastic causes of pericardial effusion may also be responsible, even in patients with malignancy.

The most common symptoms of pericardial effusion reported in large series are dyspnea (which is experienced by almost all patients), orthopnea, and cough, while chest pain may also occur. Clinical signs include jugular venous distension, distant heart sounds, peripheral edema, and hepatomegaly. The most serious clinical manifestation is of cardiac tamponade, where cardiac output is impaired as a result of pressure from a pericardial effusion. Signs of tamponade include pulsus paradoxus and hypotension.

The diagnosis of pericardial effusion is often suspected when a change in the cardiac contour is observed on serial chest radiographs. This finding is commonly made in the absence of symptoms. However, a normal chest radiograph does not exclude the possibility of a pericardial effusion. The least invasive and most accurate method for demonstrating the presence of pericardial fluid is with echocardiography, which is able to show not only the presence of fluid but also whether or not atrial compression and inspiratory reduction in mitral flow (the echocardiographic correlate of pulsus parodoxus) is present. Although electrocardiographic abnormalities may occur, these are usually nonspecific, and of little assistance in making a diagnosis.

The management of pericardial effusions depends upon the nature and extent of the underlying malignancy, and whether or not tamponade is present. The mere presence of pericardial fluid is not of itself usually a reason to intervene in an asymptomatic patient. This is particularly the case if the patient has a malignancy that is widespread and for which effective systemic therapy is lacking, since their prognosis may be so poor that the pericardial effusion may not become a clinical problem during their remaining life. The major exception is the asymptomatic patient in whom the pericardial effusion is the first manifestation of metastatic malignancy, and in whom aspiration may be performed to make this diagnosis. This is an uncommon situation, however, with most pericardial effusions occurring in patients with other sites of metastatic disease. By contrast, patients presenting with cardiac tamponade require urgent pericardiocentesis, which usually results in rapid and dramatic improvement in their condition.

There are no randomized trials that evaluate different approaches to the management of pericardial effusion, and most reported series are small. This makes determination of the optimal method of control of pericardial effusions difficult. In general however, local therapies, such as pericardiocentesis, with or without the instillation of a sclerosant are used. The exception is in patients with a malignancy for which highly effective systemic therapy exists, such as previously untreated lymphoma.

The use of pericardial drainage alone produces lasting control of effusions in 20–80% of patients, although interpretation of these results is complicated by the differing definitions of "lasting control" as well as the variety of underlying diseases and their prognoses in the reported series. Instillation of sclerosants has been used in a manner analogous to that for malignant pleural effusions. However, as there are no randomized trials comparing this approach with drainage alone, the seemingly improved results reported in many studies may be the result of patient selection, and pericardiocentesis alone remains the most common method of management.

Surgical therapy, with the formation of a pericardial window, is used in patients who have recurrent pericardial effusions despite pericardiocentesis, and who either have no distant disease, or distant disease that can be controlled by appropriate systemic therapies. Formation of a pericardial window is associated with a good outcome in terms of control of pericardial fluid, which is achieved in over 90% of patients. Several different surgical approaches have been used in order to form windows, and more recently, balloon pericardiostomy has been introduced as a noninvasive method of achieving the same result. In rare patients in whom pericardial window fails to control pericardial fluid, or in those in whom pericardial constriction is present, pericardiectomy may be considered.

The prognosis for patients with a malignant pericardial effusion is determined primarily by the nature and extent of the underlying malignancy, rather than by the presence of the pericardial effusion itself. Therefore decisions about the management of the pericardial effusion need to be made after considering the likely outcome for the patient from their systemic disease. Patients with slowly growing or controllable malignancies (for example, lymphoma, or some women with breast cancer) may have a prognosis measured in months or years.

Box 62.1 Summary – pleural and pericardial effusions

Pleural and pericardial effusions are common complications of advanced malignancy and the cause of substantial morbidity.

The most common symptoms are of dyspnea, cough, and chest pain. In addition, pericardial effusion with tamponade can cause hemodynamic collapse.

Treatment needs to be considered in the context of the nature and extent of the underlying malignancy, and the prospects for its therapy.

Pleural effusions are usually managed by pleurodesis using a sclerosing agent instilled after drainage of the effusion.

Pericardial effusions are usually managed by pericardiocentesis.

The prognosis for patients with pleural or pericardial effusions is usually determined by their underlying disease, rather than by the effusion itself.

BIBLIOGRAPHY

Sentinel article

Putnam JB, Light RW, Rodriguez RM et al. A randomized comparison of indwelling pleural catheter and doxycycline pleurodesis in the management of malignant pleural effusions. *Cancer* 1999;86:1992–9.

Review articles

Hausheer FH, Yarbro JW. Diagnosis and treatment of malignant pleural effusion. *Semin Oncol* 1985;12:54–75.

Rodriguez-Panadero F. Current trends in pleurodesis. *Curr Opin Pulm Med* 1997;3:319–25.

Vaitkus PT, Herrmann HC, LeWinter MM. Treatment of malignant pericardial effusion. *J Am Med Assoc* 1994;272:59–64.

Internet sites

www.meds.com/pdq/effusion_pro.html

http://www.cancerweb.ncl.ac.uk/cancernet/

63

Superior vena cava syndrome

Paul W. Read and Maria Kelly

University of Virginia Health Science Center, Charlottesville

Superior vena cava syndrome (SVCS) is the clinical manifestation of obstructed blood flow through the superior vena cava (SVC) secondary to extrinsic compression, tumor invasion, or thrombosis. The SVC is the main venous conduit of blood return from the head, upper extremities, and upper torso. It begins at the confluence of the right and left innominate veins and continues in the middle mediastinum 6–8 cm to drain into the right atrium. During its course the SVC is surrounded by rigid structures including the trachea, right bronchus, sternum, aorta, and pulmonary artery. Due to the physiologic requirements of high volume and low pressure flow it is a large diameter vessel with a thin wall making it susceptible to extrinsic compression by tumor against its rigid surroundings. SVC obstruction results in increased collateral blood flow through the azygos, internal mammary, lateral thoracic, paraspinous, and esophageal veins.

Over 90% of cases of SVCS result from a neoplastic process. Approximately 65–80% of cases are due to lung cancer with small cell cancer being the most common histology, 10–15% of cases are due to lymphoma, and the remainder are caused by thymomas, germ cell tumors, and metastatic disease. Benign causes include mediastinal fibrosis, histoplasmosis, and iatrogenic thrombosis of the SVC secondary to central venous catheters and cardiac pacemakers.

SVCS is a relatively easy clinical diagnosis to make. The presenting symptoms in decreasing order of frequency include dyspnea (63%), facial swelling or head fullness (50%), cough (24%), arm swelling (18%), chest pain (15%), and dysphagia (9%). Physical exam findings in decreasing order of frequency include venous distension of the neck (66%), venous distension of the chest wall (54%), facial edema (46%), cyanosis (20%), plethora of the face (19%), and upper extremity edema (14%). Symptoms and physical exam findings depend on how acutely the SVC is obstructed with slower obstruction times allowing for greater collateral blood flow to develop. Acute thrombosis of the SVC can cause laryngeal edema with associated respiratory distress and increased intracranial pressure with associated headache, confusion, and lethargy, but the vast majority of cases of SVCS are not true medical emergencies with only one out of 1986 patients dying as a direct consequence of SVCS in the review by Ahmann (1984).

Radiographic evaluation of SVCS includes a chest x-ray that shows mediastinal widening in 50–60% of cases, contrast-enhanced chest computed tomography (CT), and venography if stent placement is anticipated. Since the management of the various neoplastic causes of SVCS differ and some of these cancers are potentially curable it is critical to obtain a pathologic diagnosis prior to initiating cytotoxic therapy. The pathologic diagnosis can be obtained in almost all cases by an ordered biopsy approach including sputum cytology, bronchoscopic washings and biopsy, thoracentesis of a pleural effusion, CT-guided fine needle aspiration of a thoracic mass, biopsy of superficial lymph nodes, mediastinoscopy, and finally thoracotomy if necessary. Diagnostic procedures are not reported to carry excessive risk in patients with SVCS in modern reports.

Medical management is aimed at symptomatic relief and treatment of the underlying etiology of the obstruction. Symptomatic management includes elevation of the head, oxygen, salt-restricted diet and diuretics for peripheral edema, and corticosteroids for laryngeal or cerebral edema. Patients who have evidence of thrombus can be managed with anticoagulation and/or catheter-directed thrombolytic therapy with urokinase or tissue plasminogen activator as long as contraindications to such therapy do not exist (i.e., recent hemorrhagic cerebral vascular accident, recent brain surgery, history of a bleeding disorder, pregnancy or recent delivery, active gastrointestinal bleeding, or metastatic cancer to the brain or spinal cord). Patients with severe symptoms at presentation or who have recurrent SVCS following chemotherapy and/or radiotherapy can be managed with angioplasty and intravascular stent placement with complete resolution of SVCS in 69–100% of patients over 2–3 days. Patients with less severe presenting symptoms should have their underlying neoplastic process treated with appropriate chemotherapy and/or radiotherapy; 70–95% of such patients will be symptom-free in 2–3 weeks from initiation of therapy, and only 10–30% of responding patients will have recurrent SVCS prior to death.

REFERENCES

Sentinel articles

Ahmann F. A reassessment of the clinical implications of the superior vena cava syndrome. *J Clin Oncol* 1984;2:961–9.

Armstrong B, Perez C, Simpson J, Hederman M. Role of irradiation in the management of superior vena cava syndrome. *Int J Radiat Oncol Biol Phys* 1987;13:531–9.

Bell D, Woods R, Levi J. Superior vena caval obstruction: A 10-year experience. *Med J Aust* 1986;145:566–8.

Chan R, Dar R, Yu E et al. Superior vena cava obstruction in small-cell lung cancer. *Int J Radiat Oncol Biol Phys* 1997;38:513–20.

Davenport D, Ferree C, Blake D, Raben M. Radiation therapy in the treatment of superior vena caval obstruction. *Cancer* 1978;42:2600–3.

Dombernowsky P, Hansen H. Combination chemotherapy in the management of superior vena caval obstruction in small-cell anaplastic of the lung. *Acta Med Scand* 1978;204:513–16.

Nicholson A, Ettles D, Arnold A, Greenstone M, Dyet J. Treatment of malignant superior vena cava obstruction: metal stents or radiation therapy. *J Vasc Intervent Radiol* 1997;8:781–7.

Parish J, Marschke R, Dines D, Lee R. Etiologic considerations in superior vena cava syndrome. *Mayo Clin Proc* 1981;56:407–13.

Porte H, Metois D, Finzi L et al. Superior vena cava syndrome of malignant origin. Which surgical procedure for diagnosis? *Eur J Cardio-thorac Surg* 2000;17:384–8.

Salsali M, Cliffton E. Superior vena caval obstruction in carcinoma of lung. *N Y State J Med* 1969;69:2875–80.

Review articles

Aurora R, Milite F, Vander Els N. Respiratory emergencies. *Semin Oncol* 2000;27:256–69.

Schindler N, Vogelzang R. Superior vena cava syndrome: experience with endovascular stents and surgical therapy. *Surg Clin N Am* 1999;79:683–94.

Yim C, Sane S, Bjarnason H. Superior vena cava stenting. *Radiol Clin N Am* 2000;38:409–24.

64

Chronic nausea

Ahmed Elsayem and Michael Fisch

U.T. M.D. Anderson Cancer Center, Houston

Chronic nausea is a common, unpleasant symptom in patients with advanced cancer. The distress associated with nausea has enormous impact on the quality of life of this group of patients. More than half of cancer patients report nausea as one of the most distressing symptoms they encounter during the trajectory of their illness. Nausea is particularly prevalent in patients under age 65, females, patients receiving opioid analgesics, and patients with stomach, breast, or gynecologic cancer.

There is no consensus on the definition of chronic nausea, but for the purpose of research it is defined as nausea lasting longer than 4 weeks.

Etiology

Causes of nausea in cancer patients are often multifactorial – they may be related to the cancer itself or the treatment for the cancer. Figure 64.1 summarizes common causes of nausea in cancer patients.

Gastrointestinal causes are common. Amongst the gastrointestinal causes of nausea, constipation is probably the most prevalent etiology. Advanced cancer patients are frequently taking opioid analgesics that cause delayed gastric emptying and slower intestinal transit time. In addition, decreased mobility, poor hydration, and co-exposure to other medications that contribute to constipation are often seen in this population (see Chapter 49).

Nausea and constipation may also be manifestations of chronic malignant bowel obstruction (see Chapter 59). Such obstruction can result from locally advanced disease such as gynecologic and gastrointestinal malignancies or adhesions in patients with prior abdominal surgeries or previous abdominal radiation. Irritation of the upper gastrointestinal mucosa as in postradiation mucositis or infection may stimulate the glossopharyngeal or the vagus nerve and precipitate nausea as well.

Autonomic dysfunction frequently presents as nausea, early satiety, anorexia, and a constellation of cardiovascular symptoms and signs including postural

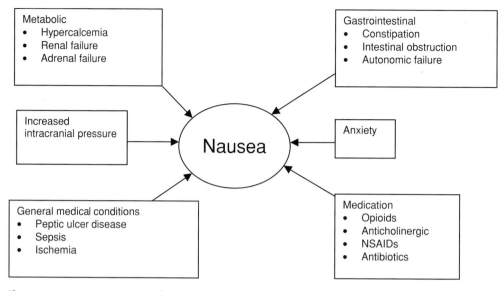

Figure 64.1   Common causes of nausea.

hypotension, syncope, and fixed heart rate. The nausea in this syndrome is believed to be due to gastroparesis manifested as delayed gastric emptying. There is a good body of evidence relating this syndrome to anorexia/cachexia syndrome. Autonomic dysfunction is believed to be prevalent in advanced cancer patients, where in some series it was reported to be present in more than 50% of the cases.

Opioids may induce nausea directly or through their constipating effect. Nausea is observed in about one-third of patients upon initiation of opioid therapy or rapid escalation of the dose. In some cases the onset of nausea may denote the onset of opioid toxicity from accumulation of active metabolites such as morphine-6-glucuronide. Other medications that are known to slow gastric emptying include anticholinergic agents, tricyclic antidepressants, and anti-emetics such as 5-HT$_3$ antagonists or phenothiazines. It is well known that many other medications may cause nausea in some individuals, including antibiotics, digoxin, anticoagulants, and imidazoles.

Metabolic causes of nausea include hypercalcemia, hyponatremia, or uremia. Nausea may be the presenting symptom of renal failure. It is also a known feature of hepatic or adrenal failure. Increased intracranial pressure may present as nausea, headache, and altered mental status. Brain metastasis and metabolic disarray should both be considered in the differential diagnosis of cancer patients presenting with new onset nausea in addition to considering gastrointestinal causes and medication side effects.

Pathophysiology of nausea

Nausea and vomiting are controlled by the vomiting center located in the medulla near the nucleus of the tractus solitarius and the reticular formation. The vomiting center receives afferent fibers from the gastrointestinal tract, thorax, and cerebral cortex. Figure 64.2 illustrates the possible pathophysiologic mechanism of nausea. The vomiting center is under direct effect of the chemoreceptor trigger zone (CTZ) in the area postrema near the fourth ventricle. Chemical mediators in the bloodstream may stimulate CTZ and this in turn relays information to the vomiting center to induce nausea. It has been postulated that the CTZ is under continuous inhibition from an inhibitory center, called the vomiting inhibitory center, the exact nature of which is not clear. The vomiting center receives direct descending impulses from higher centers such as the cerebral cortex, thalamus, vestibular system, and higher brain stem. It also receives ascending impulses from lower centers such as the gastrointestinal tract, pharynx and serosa through the vagus, glossopharyngeal and splanchnic nerves.

The vomiting cascade is complex and poorly understood. The prodromal symptoms may involve respiratory, salivary, vasomotor, and motor components. The presence of the vomiting center near the origin of the vagus nerve may be a factor in these prodromal symptoms. Nausea without vomiting may be due to insufficient stimulation of the vomiting center. On the other hand, persistent nausea after vomiting may denote persistent stimulation.

Important chemoreceptors and mechanoreceptors in the gastrointestinal tract and the central nervous systems have been identified. Pharmacological disruption of these receptors is the major target of anti-emetic medications. The major neurotransmitters interacting with these receptors include dopamine, acetylcholine, serotonin, and histamine.

Assessment

The assessment of chronic nausea plays a major role in proper management of the patient and should be part of a multidimensional approach to assess different symptoms simultaneously. These symptoms include pain, anxiety, appetite, and constipation, all of which are well known to interact with each other. The etiology of nausea should be determined if at all possible. Since nausea is a subjective feeling, the intensity of its expression may vary from patient to patient. Simple tools, such as a numerical 0–10 rating scale, verbal descriptor, or visual analog scale are valid assessment tools. The onset, duration, aggravating and relieving factors, and frequency of nausea are essential components of the patient history. If there is associated vomiting, then the nature and quantity of the vomitus may give a clue as to

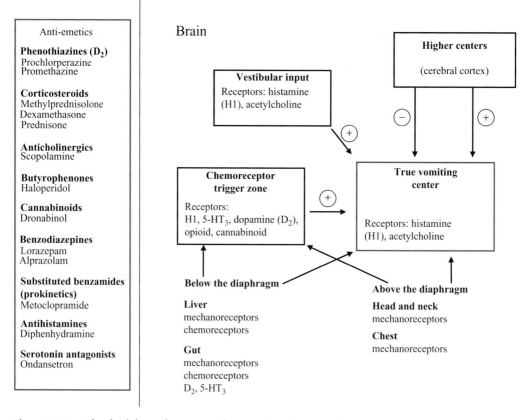

Figure 64.2 Pathophysiology of nausea and categories of anti-emetics.

the etiology of nausea. Large volume emesis may indicate gastric outlet obstruction from gastrointestinal malignancies and place the patient at risk of dehydration. Patients should be asked about the regularity and frequency of bowel movements. The presence of headache (especially early-morning headaches) may denote the onset of cerebral edema in patients known to have cancers that frequently metastasize to the brain. Finally, review of all medications being used is very important and this should include any over-the-counter or alternative medications, their onset, dosage and timing in relation to the time of nausea.

The physical examination may reveal valuable information as to the cause of nausea such as the presence of increased intracranial pressure or intestinal obstruction. Orthostatic hypotension and a fixed heart rate on standing may point towards autonomic dysfunction. Rectal examination may show fecal impaction, and such impaction may not be obvious to the patient or the clinician based on the history alone.

Laboratory examination should include measurement of electrolytes, calcium, and renal and hepatic functions. Abdominal radiographs may reveal the presence of intestinal obstruction or unsuspected significant obstipation. Brain imaging may be required if the history or physical examination suggest the possibility of increased intracranial pressure.

Management

Management of chronic nausea requires detailed assessment as to the etiology of the problem. Symptomatic management should go hand in hand with attempts to reverse the cause of nausea. Fluid and electrolyte imbalances should be corrected. Patients with severe vomiting may require parenteral hydration. If the patient is terminally ill a subcutaneous route may be a suitable alternative to an intravenous one, especially in the home or hospice setting. Subcutaneous hydration is sometimes referred to as hypodermoclysis. The use of an enema may be required to reverse nausea caused by constipation or fecal impaction. Sometimes, the diagnosis of constipation is difficult and an enema may be used as a therapeutic trial. If bowel obstruction is the cause of vomiting, then decompression, rehydration and analgesia are valuable for palliation. Opioid-induced nausea may respond to opioid rotation (also called opioid switching). Raised intracranial pressure symptoms may respond rapidly to use of corticosteroids. Infections may be treated with appropriate antimicrobial agents even when the goal of therapy is comfort care. Hypercalcemia may respond to rehydration and bisphosphonates. Most of these maneuvers are discussed in more detail in other chapters.

Pharmacological measures

Drug therapy should be directed at the probable causes and therefore the mediators of nausea (i.e., dopamine, serotonin, histamine, and acetylcholine). Table 64.1 illustrates the most commonly used anti-emetics.

Dopamine-2 antagonists

Metoclopramide is widely used, especially in chronic nausea and constipation. Although the drug has antidopaminergic activity at the CTZ, its major effect is in the gut, to antagonize peripheral D_2 receptors and stimulate 5-HT_4 receptors. The stimulation of 5-HT_4 results in the release of acetylcholine which stimulates peristalsis, relieves gastroperesis, and improves constipation. At higher doses the drug blocks 5-HT_3 receptors in the CTZ and may improve chemotherapy-induced nausea. The drug is inexpensive and well tolerated by many patients. It has been used successfully in patients with cachexia and anorexia to stimulate the appetite.

Table 64.1. Drugs useful for the treatment of chronic nausea

Drug[a]	Main receptor	Main indication	Starting p.o. dose/route	Equivalent price[b]	Side effects
Metoclopramide	D2	Opioid induced, gastric stasis	10 mg every 4 hours *p.o., s.c., i.v.*	1	EPS (akathisia, dystonia, dyskinesia)
Prochlorperazine	D2	Opioid induced	10 mg every 6 hours *p.o., i.v.*	3	Sedation, hypotension
Cyclizine	H1	Vestibular causes, intestinal obstruction	25–50 mg every 8 hours *p.o., s.c., p.r.*		Sedation, dry mouth, blurred vision
Promethazine	H1	Vestibular, motion sickness, obstruction	12.5 mg every 4 hours *p.o., p.r., i.v.*	2	Sedation
Haloperidol	D2	Opioid, chemical, metabolic	1–2 mg bid *p.o., i.v., s.c.*	1	Rarely EPS
Ondansetron	5-HT$_3$	Chemotherapy	4–8 mg every 8 h *p.o., i.v.*	84	Headache, constipation
Diphenhydramine	H1, Ach	Intestinal obstruction vestibular, ICP	25 mg every 6 hours *p.o., i.v., s.c.*	0.2	Sedation, dry mouth, blurred vision
Hyoscine	Ach	Intestinal obstruction, colic, secretions	0.2–0.4 mg every 4 hours *s.l., s.c., t.d.*	0.4	Dry mouth, blurred vision, urine retention, agitation

[a]Corticosteroids not included because of varied doses and limited indications (see text).

[b]Prices are compared to metoclopramide 10 mg tablets every 4 hours for 10 days based on the formulary prices at M.D. Anderson Cancer Center, November 2001.

p.o., orally; s.c., subcutaneously; i.v., intravenously; p.r., per rectum; t.d., transdermal; s.l., sublingual; D2, dopamine; H1, histamine; Ach, acetylcholine; ICP, intracranial pressure; EPS, extrapyramidal symptoms.

The major side effects are extrapyramidal symptoms (akathisia, torticollis) which are most commonly seen in children and younger adults. This side effect can be managed by using diphenhydramine and by discontinuing the metoclopramide (or other offending agent such as a phenothiazine). Metoclopramide should be avoided in patients with nausea associated with significant intestinal obstruction, as it can contribute to the experience of crampy abdominal pain due to its prokinetic effects on the bowel.

Phenothiazines also target the D2 receptor, but they have a greater effect on the central D2 receptor compared with metoclopramide. The phenothiazines have antagonistic activities on other receptors as well. For example, chlorpromazine blocks the α-1 adrenergic receptor and may cause sedation and hypotension. Haloperidol is more potent as an antagonist of the dopamine receptor at the CTZ than chlorpromazine or prochlorperazine and it is less sedating because it has less effect at the α-1 adrenergic receptor. Phenothiazines are generally safe, but extrapyramidal symptoms can be caused by these drugs, and more rarely, tardive dyskinesia.

Corticosteroids

Corticosteroids are very effective anti-emetic medications either alone or in combination with other anti-emetics. The exact mechanism of action is not clear. They may reduce the permeability of the blood–brain barrier to emetogenic stimuli or antagonize certain mediators or cytokines. The benefit–risk ratio is quite favorable for using these agents in the short term to relieve bothersome nausea, but over the course of several weeks this benefit–risk ratio declines due to the hazards of long-term use of corticosteroids.

5-HT3 receptor antagonists

In the last decade, the introduction of selective antagonists of 5-HT$_3$ receptors has improved chemotherapy-related nausea. These receptors are abundant in the CTZ as well as the vomiting center, and there is a good body of evidence that suggests these receptors are also present in the gastrointestinal tract. Serotonin in the gastrointestinal tract is released as a result of insults to the body such as chemotherapy or radiation therapy. Granisetron, ondansetron, and tropisetron are the three well-studied 5-HT$_3$ receptor antagonists and their role in chemotherapy- and radiation therapy-induced nausea is well documented. This class of drugs is much less appropriate in the setting of chronic nausea because (a) these agents are expensive; (b) they can contribute to constipation; and (c) based on the complete assessment of the patient, the 5-HT$_3$ receptor is not often the most logical target for patients with advanced cancer and chronic nausea.

Other anti-emetics

Benzodiazepines may be useful in anxiety-induced nausea. They may also decrease the severity of anticipatory nausea. The sedation associated with their use can be limiting, especially when other sedating medications are coadministered.

Octreotide is a somatostatin analogue which reduces the gastrointestinal secretions and slows peristalsis. The drug can be useful for reducing the intestinal colic and nausea/vomiting associated with chronic, malignant bowel obstruction. This agent is relatively expensive, and an alternative is to use anticholinergic drugs (such as hyoscine) for the same indication.

There is growing evidence that cannabinoids produce substantial anti-emetic effects in patients receiving chemotherapy. Unlike in young patients, these agents are sometimes associated with dysphoria in elderly cancer patients. The use of cannabinoids is currently limited not only by the the possibility of CNS side effects, but also by legislative regulations and expense in most settings.

Nonpharmacological measures for the treatment of chronic nausea

Psychological techniques such as relaxation therapy and mental imagery are useful in palliation of nausea – especially in chemotherapy-induced nausea. Patients are taught certain techniques to apply at the onset of nausea. The effect of these techniques and cognitive therapy in the palliation of chronic nausea needs further investigation.

Transcutaneous electrical nerve stimulation (TENS) and acupuncture or acupressure have been shown to augment the effect of anti-emetics during chemotherapy. Both maneuvers may exert their effects through endogenous peptides.

Surgical interventions may be useful in intestinal obstruction (when feasible). Laparotomy with or without bypass surgery for gastrointestinal obstruction due to tumor or adhesions can improve symptoms and may improve life expectancy. In more advanced disease percutaneous gastrostomy can greatly alleviate symptoms and may improve quality of life.

Box 64.1 Summary – nausea

Chronic nausea is a highly prevalent and distressing symptom in advanced cancer.

Constipation and opioid-induced gastroparesis are the most frequent causes of nausea in advanced cancer patients.

Proper assessment and identifying the etiology of nausea is crucial for choosing effective management strategies.

Metoclopramide is the drug of first choice in most cases, especially when opioids and constipation are the cause of nausea, because it is effective, less sedating, and inexpensive.

Corticosteroids are effective adjuvant anti-emetics and are generally safe for short-term use.

BIBLIOGRAPHY

Sentinel articles

Gralla RJ, Osoba D, Kris MG et al. Recommendations for the use of antiemetics: evidence-based, clinical practice guidelines. *J Clin Oncol* 1999;17:2971–94.

Lane M, Smith FE, Sullivan RA et al. Dronabinol and prochlorperazine alone and in combination as antiemetic agents for cancer chemotherapy. *Am J Clin Oncol* 1990;13:480–4.

Lundberg JC, Passik S. Controlling opioid-induced nausea with olanzapine. *Primary Care Cancer* 2000;20:35–7.

The Italian Group for Antiemetic Research. Difference in persistence of efficacy of two antiemetic regimens on acute emesis during cisplatin chemotherapy. *J Clin Oncol* 1993;11:2396–404.

Review articles

National Comprehensive Cancer Network: NCCN antiemesis practice guidelines. *Oncology* 1997;11:57–89.

Rhodes VA, McDaniel RW. Nausea, vomiting, and retching: complex problems in palliative care. *Cancer J Clinicians* 2001;51:232–48.

Internet site

National Cancer Institute and National Institute of Health, Supportive Care PDQ section. http://www.cancer.gov/cancerinfo/pdq/supportivecare/nausea

Index